W9-BYZ-079

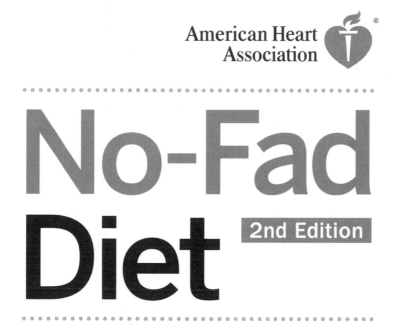

American Heart Association

No-Fad Diet

2nd Edition

Also by the American Heart Association

American Heart Association Healthy Family Meals

*American Heart Association's Complete Guide to
Women's Heart Health*

American Heart Association Quick & Easy Meals

The New American Heart Association Cookbook, 8th Edition

*American Heart Association Low-Fat, Low-Cholesterol Cookbook,
4th Edition*

American Heart Association Low-Salt Cookbook, 3rd Edition

American Heart Association One-Dish Meals

American Heart Association Low-Calorie Cookbook

American Heart Association Low-Fat and Luscious Desserts

WITHDRAWN

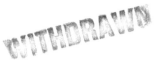

American Heart
Association

No-Fad Diet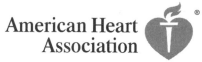

2nd Edition

A Personal Plan for Healthy Weight Loss

Clarkson Potter/Publishers
New York

Dunn Public Library

Copyright © 2005, 2011 by American Heart Association

All rights reserved.

Published in the United States by Clarkson Potter/Publishers, an imprint of the Crown Publishing Group, a division of Random House, Inc., New York.

www.crownpublishing.com

www.clarksonpotter.com

CLARKSON POTTER is a trademark and POTTER with colophon is a registered trademark of Random House, Inc.

A previous edition of this work was published by Clarkson Potter/Publishers, an imprint of the Crown Publishing Group, a division of Random House, Inc., New York, in 2005.

Library of Congress Cataloging-in-Publication Data
American Heart Association no-fad diet : a personal plan for healthy weight loss / American Heart Association.—2nd ed.
   Rev. ed. of: No-fad diet. 1st ed. c2005.
   Includes index.
   1. Reducing diets. 2. Weight loss. I. American Heart Association. II. No-fad diet.
   RM222.2.N6 2011
   613.2'5—dc22   2010013381

ISBN 978-0-307-40759-7

Printed in the United States of America

Design by Amy Sly based on an original design by Jan Derevjanik

10 9 8 7 6 5 4 3 2 1

Second Edition

acknowledgments

American Heart Association Consumer Publications

Director: Linda S. Ball

Managing Editor: Deborah A. Renza

Senior Editor: Janice Roth Moss

Science Editor/Writer: Jacqueline F. Haigney

Assistant Editor: Roberta Westcott Sullivan

American Heart Association Staff Contributors

Chief Science Officer: Rose Marie Robertson, MD

Vice President, Science and Medicine: Gail R. Whitman, PhD, RN

Science and Medicine Advisor: Dorothea K. Vafiadis, MS

Expert Contributors

Stephen R. Daniels, MD, PhD

Robert H. Eckel, MD

Barry A. Franklin, PhD

John M. Jakicic, PhD

Expert Advisors

Claire M. Bassett

Marc-Andre Cornier, MD

Coni Francis, PhD, RD

Barbara V. Howard, PhD

Donna Israel, PhD, RD, LD, LPC

Penny M. Kris-Etherton, PhD, RD

Alice Lichtenstein, DSc

F. Xavier Pi-Sunyer, MD, MPH

Lawrence Rudel, PhD

Frank Sacks, MD

Linda Van Horn, PhD, RD

Judith Wylie-Rosett, EdD, RD

Meg Zeller, PhD

Recipe Developers

Barbara Seelig Brown

Christine Caperton

Linda Drachman

Nancy S. Hughes

Annie King

Nadja Piatka

Carol Ritchie

Julie Shapero, RD, LD

Nutrition Analyst

Tammi Hancock, RD

contents

preface

Are you one of the many people struggling to stop yo-yo dieting and reach a healthy weight? If so, the *American Heart Association No-Fad Diet* is for you. This book will show you step by step how to develop a personalized plan to make better food choices, become more physically active, and create a healthy environment so that you can achieve and maintain your weight-loss goals. The tools provided in the *No-Fad Diet* will help you devise weight-management strategies that work specifically for *you*.

If you are overweight, you are not alone. Current statistics show that about two-thirds of adults and nearly one-third of children and adolescents in the United States are overweight or obese. Many factors, including environmental and biological influences, have contributed to this obesity epidemic, but you don't need to be one of these statistics. If you're looking to successfully take control of your weight, you have turned to the right source. The *No-Fad Diet* was conceived and developed under the guidance of leading experts in the fields of nutrition, physical activity, and behavior change. This second edition has been updated with the latest scientific information on weight loss and weight control and includes revised sample weekly menu plans, along with easy-to-follow instructions on how to create your own menus, an expanded toolkit to help you build an actionable and personalized weight-loss plan, and 50 new recipes to tempt your taste buds while you trim your waistline.

You may wonder why the American Heart Association would write a book on weight loss. The fact is that obesity is the fastest-growing health issue that Americans currently face. As the nation's premier authority on heart health, we know that being overweight contributes to the risk of heart disease by greatly increasing the likelihood of high blood pressure, unhealthy cholesterol and tri-glyceride levels, and type 2 diabetes. Each of these conditions alone raises the risk of cardiovascular disease; together, they are a serious medical problem.

The key to losing weight and keeping off the lost pounds is finding a *proven* and *healthy* approach that meets your individual needs and fits into your lifestyle. With the plethora of diet and weight-loss books on the market, why should you choose this one? Because the strategies and resources of the *No-Fad Diet* come from the American Heart Association, which means you can trust that they are scientifically sound. Start today to build your own comprehensive plan for long-term weight loss. We know you can be successful, so do it for yourself—*and for your heart*.

Rose Marie Robertson, MD
Chief Science Officer,
American Heart Association/American Stroke Association

INTRODUCTION

Our goal at the American Heart Association is to help you be as heart healthy as possible, and it's our business to give you the information and tools to achieve that goal. An important part of the process is learning how to eat well and control your body weight throughout your life. If, like so many other Americans, you're looking for a long-term, livable way to lose weight and keep it off, we're here to help.

Everyday lifestyle habits, including your diet and physical activity routine, have a profound effect on your health and well-being. By choosing well, you can improve many of the factors—your health factors—that delay or prevent heart disease. These factors include having a healthy body weight and being physically active on a regular basis, being a nonsmoker, and having normal blood pressure, cholesterol, and glucose levels. Generally speaking, the lower your weight, the lower your blood pressure and levels of blood cholesterol and glucose, and the lower your risk for heart disease and stroke. Because of the direct correlation between weight and the other health factors, the American Heart Association is committed to helping you find your own personal approach to making smart, healthy lifestyle choices every day.

what is the no-fad diet?

You may have tried several times to lose weight but without much long-term success. As frustrating as that might be, there's no point in feeling bad about yourself. The truth is that losing weight is not easy, and keeping it off is even harder. Unfortunately, no magic bullet exists. Fad diets, gimmicky meal plans, and get-thin-quick schemes don't work over the long haul. For lasting weight loss, you need to choose a no-fad approach that incorporates lifestyle changes that fit into the context of your life and that you can maintain.

The No-Fad Diet is based on the concept of *energy balance*—that is, to keep from gaining weight, you must balance the calories you eat (Calories In) with the calories your body uses up through metabolic function and physical activity (Calories Out). Once you understand the role energy balance plays in whether you lose, gain, or maintain your weight, you can use the three basic principles of the No-Fad Diet to achieve your target weight:

- **Think smart**
- **Eat well**
- **Move more**

Each of these individual components contributes to healthy weight loss, but when you combine them in a way that reflects your personal needs, they can form a strong, cohesive plan for lifelong weight control.

be wary of fad diets

In the midst of so many conflicting and confusing messages and promises about diet, exercise, and health, it's important to rely on reputable sources for information. A weight-loss plan should never endanger your long-term health. Fad diets and quick fixes may work temporarily but do not lead to permanent weight loss. To spot an unhealthy or fad diet, look for these signs:

- Reduces calories drastically without regard for adequate nutrition
- Depends on powders, herbs, or pills
- Relies on certain foods or food combinations
- Eliminates carbohydrates, fat, or any other type of food
- Recommends skipping meals or replaces meals with drinks or food bars

The No-Fad Diet offers a scientifically supported, safe approach to reaching your target weight without jeopardizing your health. The American Heart Association recommendations reflect the opinions of many experts—physicians, nutritionists, and specialists in physical activity and behavior modification. Our panel of scientists has reviewed the most current research and come to a consensus so you can cut through the confusion with confidence. We know that our no-fad approach can bring you lasting success and a lifetime of better health.

circles of success

If you're reading this book, you are already interested in the process of healthy weight loss and how to move from awareness to action. Here we give you specific action steps to help you lose extra weight—and lose it for good. Your weight-loss plan will focus on areas in your life that you can control, represented by the three circles of success—thinking smart, eating well, and moving more. Each circle represents an important influence on your personal choices. You need to include *all three* actions in the circles to achieve successful weight control for life. As the graphic below shows, the three circles interlock, representing the cohesiveness and integration of these three actions.

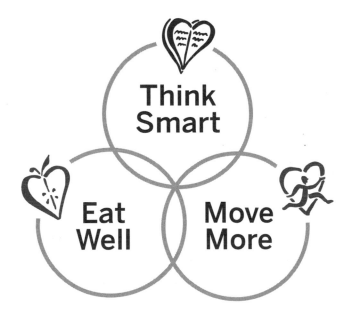

Think
Smart

Eat
Well

Move
More

We know that fads and gimmicks don't work and neither does a one-size-fits-all approach. That's why, for each circle of success, the No-Fad Diet allows you to choose strategies that fit your individual environment, needs, and comfort level. The better your choices suit your usual habits and preferences, the greater the chance these actions will become a permanent part of your lifestyle. Remember that a weight-loss plan should work for *you*.

think smart

Making good lifestyle choices is the cornerstone of sustained weight loss, yet barriers and negative thoughts can get in the way and derail the best intentions. Once you identify your personal and environmental barriers, you can begin to overcome them. Chapter 1, "Think Smart: Make a New Start," offers you different strategies to help analyze the obstacles you face and to reprogram your thinking and rework your environment. As you recognize and change the influences that lead you away from your weight-loss goals, you will also start to think about how to make healthier choices that support what you are working toward. You'll learn to set realistic goals and create a personal action plan designed just for you.

eat well

Eating well is defined not only by the quantity of food but also by the quality. As you reduce calories to lose weight, your goal is to make every calorie count for both energy and nourishment. Chapter 2, "Eat Well: Good Food for Better Health," gives you the tools you need to both decrease your calorie intake and increase your nutrient intake. You'll learn to use a food diary to assess your eating habits so you can see both how they contribute to your current weight and whether you are eating a balanced diet. Understanding how your lifestyle habits influence your eating patterns will help you choose the most effective strategy to lose weight while keeping your body healthy.

move more

Calorie reduction is a key component of weight loss, but to lose weight more quickly and to keep off the pounds for good, you have to get moving and keep moving. Extensive scientific evidence shows that physical activity is an essential part of maintaining weight loss, fitness, and good health. Chapter 3, "Move More: More Fit and Less Fat," outlines three practical strategies to make regular exercise a part of your schedule. From a starting point of just 10 minutes a day of moderate-intensity activity, this chapter also explains how to progress to an ongoing physically active lifestyle. If you're not physically active now, this approach will help you move past the feeling of inertia, become energized, and add more physical activity to your daily routine.

make the most of your knowledge

To get the most benefit from our no-fad approach, you also need the tools to continue living a healthy lifestyle once you've achieved initial weight-loss success. In Chapter 4, "Maintain Momentum: Keep Up the Good Work," you'll learn how to control your environment and behavior to manage your weight for good. You'll also find tips and techniques for integrating the three circles of success into your everyday life.

Chapter 5, "Pass It On: Family, Food, and Fitness," discusses how to share your knowledge of weight management with your entire family. In the face of growing concern about childhood obesity, you can keep your children fit and healthy by teaching them the same basic principles for good health that you use to manage your own weight. We offer six practical strategies so you can work effectively *with* your children to help them avoid becoming overweight now—and in the future.

use the tools for success

In Part II, "Menu Planning and Recipes," we've provided sample menu plans for three calorie levels, nearly 200 recipes, and information on how to build your own menu plans. In Part III, "No-Fad Toolkit," you'll find an assortment of tools to help you put your weight-loss plan into action. Including charts, lists, and templates, these resources will help you record your current eating and physical activity habits; show you how to implement strategies for change, such as making simple food substitutions; help you track calories in common foods, as well as calories used during various physical activities; and much more. All these tools will help you think smart, eat well, and move more as you progress in your journey to a healthy weight.

commit to success

Losing weight and keeping it off is not easy, but with credible science-based information and the right tools in hand—all provided in this book—you *can* achieve your weight-loss goals. Remember that the best diet plan is actually not a diet at all: Successful weight management comes from living a healthy lifestyle that you can maintain for the rest of your life. With that idea in mind, think of the American Heart Association's No-Fad Diet as both a flexible life plan and a greater opportunity for lifelong vitality.

part I
Losing Weight and Keeping It Off

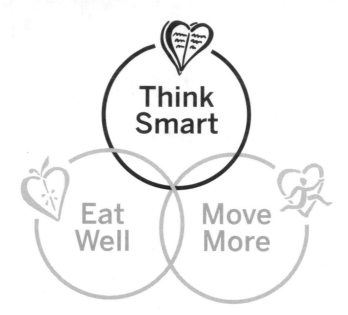

chapter 1

THINK SMART:
make a new start

Think about the running dialogue inside your head. How does it encourage or excuse your behaviors and choices? These thoughts—and the actions they lead to—can either contribute to or hinder your weight-loss success. "Thinking smart" means learning how to change your mind-set so you can change the behaviors that contribute to weight gain. Change is not always welcome, however, because it can involve risk and the unknown. Trying something new takes courage and commitment. If you've been unsuccessful in losing weight before or have lost weight only to regain it, you may be discouraged and reluctant to try again. So how can you make the experience different to improve your chances of success? First, think about why your past experiences were not successful, and decide which aspects of previous diets made them unworkable for you. Whatever your answer, if you tried a diet that was not sustainable for the long run, it's time to think smart and make a new start with the No-Fad Diet approach.

You make hundreds if not thousands of decisions every day. You are constantly reacting to internal messages based on past experience and personal bias, as well as receiving external messages from the people and environment around you. Your overall lifestyle represents the sum of all the choices—big and small—you have made in processing these messages. To change behavior as deeply ingrained as your eating and lifestyle habits, you have to determine whether the messaging in your brain is helping or hurting your well-being. By understanding the influences on your decision making, you can start to strategize and adopt behaviors that will lead you toward a healthy weight that's right for you.

believe in the benefits

Although we live in a society obsessed with being thin and looking good, being overweight or obese is much more than an outward cosmetic issue; it's an internal health issue, too. The more extra pounds you carry, the more you lose in terms of health, fitness, and quality of life because the extra weight requires your heart to work harder to pump blood throughout your body. This heavier workload can damage your heart and arteries. Other potential negatives include high blood pressure, unhealthy levels of cholesterol and triglycerides, and diabetes, which are all major risk factors for heart disease and all common conditions in overweight and obese people.

The advantages of reaching and maintaining a healthy weight and following a healthy lifestyle, on the other hand, include:

- Improved cardiovascular function, including lower blood pressure

- Lower levels of blood cholesterol and glucose

- Reduced risk of heart disease and type 2 diabetes

- Decreased likelihood of developing the metabolic syndrome (a cluster of conditions that increase heart disease risk)

- Better physical functioning, such as easier breathing and more restful sleep

- More energy, with greater physical strength and stamina

- Increased chance for achieving overall fitness

- Increased confidence and self-esteem

- Increased vitality

In this chapter, we'll guide you through the four steps you'll need to learn to think smart about losing weight.

Step 1: Assess your lifestyle choices and behaviors.
Step 2: Analyze your attitude.
Step 3: Set goals.
Step 4: Expect the unexpected.

step 1
assess your lifestyle choices and behaviors

Your mind is a powerful tool that can help you analyze the factors that caused you to gain extra weight. Think about your personal habits, your environment, and the associations that influence your behaviors, especially the things that trigger your eating and physical activity choices. Consider:

- Messages from advertising and marketing

- Daily routines that are developed around food and provide comfort

- Family culture and/or social networks

- Social events that revolve around food

- Work or home environments that are conducive to poor eating habits

Any or all of these and other factors can set in motion a cycle of pleasure, familiarity, and expectation that becomes a habit. For example, one day you pass a coffee shop on your way to work. You skipped breakfast at home, so you stop to buy a latte and a giant banana-nut muffin. You liked the experience, and you do the same the next morning. Each time you repeat this set of choices, you are establishing a stronger association. After just a few repeated experiences, by the time you leave for work, you are programmed to anticipate that latte and muffin. To stop this kind of chain reaction, you must learn which social or environmental cues trigger the behavior you want to change. Then you can work to avoid or eliminate the cue (take a different route to work to bypass the coffee shop) or change the circumstances surrounding the cue (take a banana with you and eat it as you pass the coffee shop). In general, it is the easily accessible foods that you come across in your daily life that become the cues for unplanned eating.

Once you understand how your eating patterns have been programmed, you can replace an unwanted behavior by establishing a new association between a healthier food and a desired habit. The most successful losers are the people who learn to change their thinking and set the right goals as they go about the process of controlling their weight.

step 2
analyze your attitude

While you're trying to manage your weight, it's important to keep your expectations in check. You probably didn't gain weight quickly, so it's unreasonable to expect to lose it quickly. Think of weight loss as a journey, so you can lose weight at a comfortable pace and still like who you are along the way. Instead of beating yourself up for being overweight, examine how and why you gained the extra pounds and look ahead for ways to achieve healthy weight loss.

Armed with solid information and practical tools, you can learn to recognize destructive thinking and turn it off—before it derails you. Stay positive and don't make negative comparisons. Instead of fretting about not looking "skinny," celebrate the fact that people come in all shapes and sizes. Instead of trying to look a certain way, focus on what you can do and make the most of your unique body type. Your long-term goal should be to reach a reasonable, individualized weight that benefits your overall health. Try these techniques:

- **Be aware of your inner voice.** Acknowledge that your inner voice feeds you information or messages that can be destructive more often than you may realize. Differentiate what you tell yourself from more reliable, external sources of information.

- **Watch out for rationalizations and negative self-talk that can get in your way.** If your inner voice says, "I just don't have enough time to exercise" or "I'll have these french fries now but just a salad for dinner," you are talking yourself into making poor choices.

- **Turn negative messages into positive ones.** If you are sending yourself a negative message, such as "I had a bad day at work. I'm not in the mood to take a walk," try to rephrase it into a positive statement, such as, "I had a bad day at work. Walking will help me clear my head."

step 3
set goals

Good planning, not willpower, is the key to successful sustained weight loss. When you establish concrete goals and plan your day-to-day activities to support your weight-loss efforts, you will find it much easier to reach and maintain your target weight. Here are some strategies to help you create effective goals.

- **Be reasonable, specific, and realistic.** It is natural to be enthusiastic about a new weight-loss plan, but also be sensible about how to make the changes that will best fit your lifestyle. You need a reasonable goal so you will be pleased with realistic results. Instead of setting your bar too high, start with small, specific goals that will give quick results. If you face obstacles that just can't be changed, figure out how to adjust your planning so you can best work around those barriers. For example, if you prefer to exercise in the morning but you drive your children to school, try to arrange a morning carpool that will allow you more time to exercise. If your work often requires you to eat in restaurants, try to determine a specific change in how you order to decrease your calorie intake. Can you order smaller portions or choose more healthy offerings?

- **Set short-term goals.** A short-term goal is something that is tied to a specific action that happens every day, every few days, or once a week. Try to set short-term goals that help pave the way to your long-term goals. When you set your short-term goals, choose a time frame that will allow you to see progress. For example, you might decide that your goals are to replace your usual dessert with fruit every day, have a low-calorie lunch twice a week, and cook a healthy dinner once a week. Other examples include planning to walk after dinner or going to the park to play with your dog twice a week instead of turning on the television.

- **Set checkpoints to assess your progress.** By evaluating your progress at regular intervals (perhaps after the first six weeks and every six weeks after that), you'll be able to see the payback from your efforts along the way. When you reach a goal, celebrate your achievement, but don't stop there. Continue to set new goals that keep you moving in the right direction.

- **Set long-term goals.** When you set long-term goals, choose a manageable amount of time that will accommodate the inevitable ups and downs of life. You're more likely to reach your long-term goals if you continue to reevaluate your progress. To make all your goals measurable, clearly define them in terms of what, when, and how.

- **Keep a diary.** Writing down your goals and keeping track of what you eat and when you exercise lead to a much better awareness of your habits. They focus your attention and provide a record of the triggers that lead to your behavior at specific moments. Analyzing the entries in your diary will tell you how your thoughts work for or against your weight-loss goals.

The chapters "Eat Well" and "Move More" provide more information on the specifics of keeping diaries and goal setting for weight loss and weight control. We also have included blank work sheets for setting goals for weight loss (page 414) and physical activity (page 432), a food diary page (page 415), and an activity tracker (page 433) to help you define your goals and record the milestones and achievements along the way.

step 4
expect the unexpected

Food comes into play in many different business and social settings, as well as in emotional contexts. You will be more likely to make good choices if you plan for potential pitfalls and decide how to react to them.

- **Rehearse saying, "Thanks but no thanks."** If your boss brings in homemade cookies, you might say something such as, "They look delicious and I would love to have one, but I'm trying to cut back on sweets. Thanks anyway." Most people will understand, but if they press you to accept food, just remain firm. Your first responsibility is to your own well-being.

- **Keep your options open.** When your colleagues ask you to join them for a movie but you've made plans to go to the gym the same night, consider other times when you can work out. You don't have to give up a fun night with co-workers, but don't let a change in plans override your commitment to exercise. Be flexible—the more options you have, the more likely you'll be to follow through when you do change your plans.

- **Ask for what you need.** Don't hesitate to speak up and politely request something different from what's offered, such as a diet drink or sparkling water instead of a sugary beverage. Most people are more than happy to help you if you ask.

- **Don't procrastinate.** When you know you are behaving in counterproductive ways, figure out how to make changes right away. If you ate too much dinner and missed a workout on Saturday, you can decide you have totally blown it and just give up, you can tell yourself you will start dieting next month or get on the treadmill next week, or you can decide to skip dessert right now and spend a little extra time walking tonight. The better choice always is to change your behavior at the first opportunity, not to wait until later.

- **Learn to cope with stress.** If you have learned to reach for food whenever you feel stressed, it's important to think through a healthier alternate plan that will work with your own needs. Try to imagine different scenarios that would calm you after a stressful day or divert your attention from comfort foods.

  - To restore your inner resolve, try isolating yourself for a few of minutes of peace and quiet so you can reflect on your successes and the many benefits of continuing to work toward your goals.

  - Sit down and plan your meals for the next few days. A formal meal plan can be a big help in preventing "unconscious eating" during a period of stress.

  - Bump up your exercise routine—a good workout will help relieve stress and boost your confidence.

Techniques like these are all skills that need practice to become habit. It's not about giving up everything you love—it's a matter of choosing what makes sense for you and your health. The more you apply these "think smart" strategies, the easier it will be to make better choices about how to eat well and move more, and the sooner weight control will become a natural, permanent part of your life.

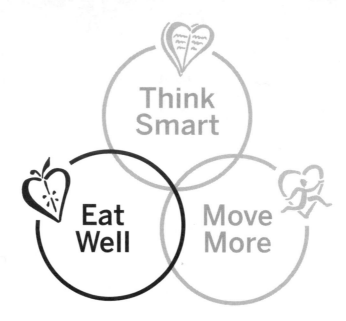

chapter 2

EAT WELL:
good food for better health

Most diets, even the fads, work in the beginning. When you are highly motivated to follow a new program, you probably will lose weight because most plans lead you to eat fewer calories than before. However, the diets that focus on eliminating certain foods or eating foods in certain combinations don't magically burn away calories. Whatever approach you take, unless you can sustain the behaviors that allow you to lose weight for a lifetime, it's unreasonable to expect the weight loss to last. Just as important, you may be depriving your body of important nutrients. If you've spent your energy "dieting" instead of looking honestly at your normal eating habits, don't be discouraged. By using proven and effective eating strategies, you can develop a no-fad weight-loss plan that is tailored to your lifestyle, and you can avoid the yo-yo effect so many dieters experience.

The term "yo-yo dieting," or weight cycling, refers to the destructive pattern of quickly losing weight only to quickly regain it. When a dieter severely limits calories without including regular exercise, the body adapts after a short time by lowering its metabolic rate so it uses fewer calories. Because these dieters are burning fewer calories, they are now more prone to weight gain than before. As well, most extreme diets are too difficult to maintain for a very long period of time, so dieters who follow them usually return to their original eating habits—or eat even more—after the initial period of weight loss, regaining the lost weight and a few extra pounds.

In this chapter, we'll guide you through the four simple steps you'll need to take to successfully—and healthfully—eat well to lose weight.

Step 1: Assess your eating habits.

Step 2: Set your personal weight-loss goal. First lose 10 percent of your body weight, then aim for a healthy target weight.

Step 3: Choose an eating strategy to lose 1 to 2 pounds each week:

- The Switch and Swap Approach
- The 75% Solution
- The American Heart Association Menu Plans

Step 4: Monitor and assess your progress.

understanding energy balance

Weight management is based on the concept of energy balance. Imagine a scale with your daily Calories In (the food you eat) on one side and your daily Calories Out (the average of calories you burn through both basic metabolic function and physical activity) on the other. Regardless of how much you weigh, if your weight stays relatively stable, that scale will stay balanced, like this:

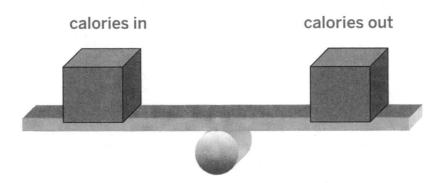

To create weight loss, you must change the balance in favor of Calories Out.

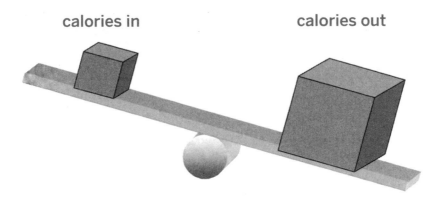

In other words, to lose weight, you must eat fewer daily calories than the number of calories your body uses each day. You can subtract calories from your daily total by eating less, moving more, or doing both. In fact, for most people, it doesn't take a lot to affect—negatively or positively—the balance of

Calories In and Calories Out. Eating just 100 extra calories per day can add up to about 10 pounds of weight gain in one year! On the other hand, walking an extra mile or cutting out one 8-ounce can of regular soda each day may seem like a small change, but that 100-calorie subtraction can make a meaningful difference over time with respect to weight and health.

To safely lose weight, follow these guidelines:

- Subtract about 500 calories per day to lose about 1 pound per week.

- Subtract about 1,000 calories per day to lose about 2 pounds per week.

As a general rule, we don't recommend that you try to lose more than 2 pounds per week without the guidance of a healthcare professional.

a calorie is a calorie

For several decades, reducing the amount of total fat in the average American diet was believed to be the best approach to losing weight. The unintended consequence of this message in the marketplace was a glut of low-fat but high-calorie products. People who ate these products believed they were getting "diet foods," but in many cases these foods actually contained more calories than their full-fat versions.

The next approach encouraged people to limit carbohydrates, which in turn started another diet fad that was taken to extremes. In a recent study from the National Institutes of Health, experts compared four different diets representing a range of percentages of fat, protein, and carbohydrates, and they found that all subjects lost about the same amount of weight. This landmark study reinforces the idea that, regardless of the hype for each new fad diet, a calorie is a calorie no matter what the source is. That's good news because it gives you the flexibility to cut calories in the way that best suits your individual needs.

step 1
assess your eating habits

To develop an effective, personalized approach to weight loss, you need to know exactly what you are eating—and why. Studies continue to show that the best way to find out is to keep a food diary. On page 415, you'll find a sample food diary page that you can use to create a daily log. Write down everything you eat and drink for one week, even if you think the amount is too small to matter. You'll need to be prepared to record:

- What you ate for each meal and snack and how much

- The calorie values for each food

- What prompted you to eat

- Why you chose that food

As you track your eating habits, don't forget to record the "hidden" calories. These calories come from the foods you eat either without thinking or in such small amounts that you forget to count them. For example, when you are cooking, do you often taste for seasoning or automatically add margarine to vegetables? Do you eat the last few mouthfuls of mashed potatoes or clean your children's plates because you think you shouldn't waste food? One bite may not seem to make much difference, but every calorie counts. If you eat or drink it, write it down. Keeping track takes only a few minutes each day, but the payback in self-discovery can be huge.

Once you've collected about a week's worth of information, read it over and look for patterns. Analyzing this information is crucial to understanding why you eat the way you do. You may be surprised by how many times you grabbed a candy bar for a quick pick-me-up, downed a high-calorie soda, or went back for extra helpings.

As part of your self-assessment, it's especially useful if you can identify the different reasons you eat besides satisfying hunger, as well as why you choose a particular food. In addition to the physical cues, such as hunger pangs, pay attention to the emotional triggers that make you think you're hungry or cause you to gravitate toward certain foods. Often what you really need is reassurance or distraction from boredom. Almost everyone experiences cravings, but there are healthy ways to deal with them. The Sample Daily Food Diary of Original Eating Habits on page 15 shows how one person's entries might look at the initial assessment, with comparison entries on pages 25 and 27 using different weight-loss strategies.

sample daily food diary of original eating habits

Time/Place	Food or Beverage (type and amount)	Calories*	What Prompted You to Eat? Why This Food Choice?
BREAKFAST 8:00 A.M. Home	1 large plain bagel with 1 Tb tub cream cheese	410	Hunger; needed fuel for the day
	8 oz orange juice	110	
	8 oz coffee with 2 Tb half-and-half	40	
	Subtotal	560	
SNACK 10:30 A.M. Work	8 oz low-fat strawberry yogurt	240	Stress
LUNCH 12:00 P.M. Fast-food restaurant	1 6-inch meatball sub	580	Hunger; fast and cheap
	1 oz potato chips	150	
	16 oz cola	205	
	Subtotal	935	
SNACK 3:00 P.M. Work	1¼ oz Cheddar cheese	145	Needed energy
DINNER 6:30 P.M. Home	6 oz T-bone steak	420	Dinner time with my family; comfort foods
	1 large baked potato with 2 Tb sour cream and 2 Tb margarine	540	
	1 cup green beans with 1 Tb margarine	140	
	1 cup mixed salad greens with 2 Tb creamy Italian dressing	190	
	1 serving bakery pineapple upside-down cake	365	
	8 oz whole milk	135	
	Subtotal	1,790	
SNACK 9:00 P.M. Home	1 cup chocolate ice cream	260	Habit while watching TV; I love ice cream
	Total	3,930	

*Calorie numbers are rounded to the nearest multiple of 5.

Most human behaviors and responses are learned, and they become habits over time. Use your food diary to identify eating habits and cravings that are working against your weight-loss efforts. Then you can unlearn those habits, replace them, or find healthier ways to work *with* them. For example, if you discover you are a grazer who needs small amounts of food all day long, use that information to develop a plan that incorporates lots of low-calorie, high-nutrient snacking. Be honest with yourself, and it will be easier to find a workable strategy to satisfy cravings without caving. Learn to listen to your body.

counting calories

Another important part of your self-assessment is to determine how many calories you are eating on a regular basis. Unless you're actively losing or gaining weight over a period of time, you can assume that you are consuming the calories it takes to maintain your energy balance, or current weight. To change that energy-balance equation in favor of weight loss, you know you need to cut back on Calories In and increase Calories Out. Before you can decide how many calories to subtract, you need to know your average daily intake of calories and then compare that number with the ideal number of calories your body needs to maintain energy balance.

Using the following formula to quickly calculate about how many calories you need on an average day to maintain your weight, multiply your current weight by the values shown. (Most people experience a decrease in metabolism at middle age, which is why you should subtract 10 percent of your total calories if you are over 50 years old.) The final adjusted total is your baseline, or the number of calories you'll subtract *from* in order to reach a daily calorie intake that will allow you to lose weight.

Multiply current weight in pounds _____   X 10 = Base Calories _____

Multiply current weight in pounds _____

If not active: X 3 =   _____

If moderately active: X 5 =   _____

If very active: X 8 = Activity Calories _____

Add Base + Activity Calories = Total Calories to Maintain Weight _____

If you are older than 50 years, subtract 10% of that total.   (−10%) _____

Total Adjusted Calories _____

For example, here's what this calculation would look like for a woman who weighs 180 pounds, is not active, and is 55 years old. To lose weight, this woman must reduce her calorie intake to an average of fewer than 2,106 calories each day. The more calories she subtracts, the faster she will lose.

Multiply current weight in pounds __180__ X 10 = Base Calories __1,800__

Multiply current weight in pounds __180__

If not active:	X 3 =	__540__
If moderately active:	X 5 =	_____
If very active:	X 8 = Activity Calories	_____

Add Base + Activity Calories = Total Calories to Maintain Weight __2,340__

If you are older than 50 years, subtract 10% of that total.   (−10%) __234__

Total Adjusted Calories __2,106__

To determine a healthy target weight and set a reasonable personal weight-loss goal, start with your baseline calorie intake and your current weight level. Then decide how fast you want to lose and which weight-loss strategy is the best for you. Let's use our 180-pound, 55-year-old woman as an example. She is currently eating an average of about 2,100 calories each day. As explained, if she cuts back by only 500 calories each day, she will lose about 1 pound a week; in this case, that means 18 pounds in about 18 weeks, which is 10 percent of the woman's original body weight. If she increases her activity level, she also will burn additional calories and increase the likelihood of maintaining that weight loss for good. As she chooses how to eliminate those 500 calories, she can also gradually start making more healthy choices to reap better nutritional benefits from the foods she does eat. Again, small changes can lead to big rewards.

step 2
set your personal
weight-loss goal

Are you trying to have a picture-perfect body like the ones we often see in the entertainment and advertising industries? When setting your goals, remember that movie stars and models benefit from lots of professional help, both behind the scenes and in front of the camera. The work of personal chefs and trainers, make-up artists, and lighting experts—as well as careful editing, cropping, and airbrushing—all help create the ideals that we have come to see as "normal." It just isn't fair to yourself, however, to think your mirror will show the same images.

- **Start with reasonable expectations.** Most likely you gained those extra pounds in small increments over a long time, and, realistically, it will take time to lose them. To avoid setting yourself up for failure, allow yourself enough time to be successful in the long run. Armed with a good (and honest) understanding of what you are eating now, you can make an educated decision about how much weight you can lose in a healthy way.

- **Decide on a reasonable goal. We recommend that you begin by aiming to lose about 10 percent of your body weight.** A good rule of thumb is to lose no more than 2 pounds each week. That's a sensible amount of weight loss that you will be able to maintain over time. Interestingly, according to behavior experts, starting with a greater daily calorie reduction to lose faster, as opposed to cutting just a few calories, may help "train" you and make it easier to stick to the program—even if you cut back that much for only the first two weeks.

Making lifestyle changes is very individual, however; do what works for you. If smaller changes fit more easily into your lifestyle, start there. You can always cut back more sharply if you find that you want to lose weight faster, but do not aim for more than 2 pounds a week without checking with your healthcare provider. Be aware, too, that if you eat fewer than 1,200 calories per day, you run the risk of not getting all the nutrients you need.

The good news is that you don't have to lose every pound before your health will benefit. For most people, losing even 10 pounds may help reduce your risk of heart disease, stroke, and diabetes.

If after several weeks of following your chosen plan, you find that the target calorie intake level does not produce the weight loss you would expect, you may need to reevaluate. You will probably have to increase your level of physical activity and possibly further restrict your daily calories to the point where you can achieve the right energy balance for weight loss, but if you are in this situation, it's best to work with a healthcare professional who advises patients on individualized approaches to weight loss.

defining a healthy weight

Healthcare professionals often use body mass index (BMI), which assesses body weight relative to height, to classify levels of overweight and obesity. A BMI of less than 25 indicates that you are at a weight that is healthy for you (less than 18.5 is considered underweight, however). If your BMI is between 25 and 29.9, you are considered overweight. A BMI of 30 or more indicates obesity.

The chart below shows you how to determine your BMI. Find your height in the left-hand column and see whether your weight falls into either range listed. If you prefer to calculate your exact BMI, multiply your weight in pounds by 705. Divide by your height in inches; divide again by your height in inches.

body mass index (BMI)

Height	Overweight (BMI 25.0–29.9)	Obese (BMI 30.0 and above)
4'10"	119–142 lbs	143 lbs or more
4'11"	124–147	148
5'0"	128–152	153
5'1"	132–157	158
5'2"	136–163	164
5'3"	141–168	169
5'4"	145–173	174
5'5"	150–179	180
5'6"	155–185	186
5'7"	159–190	191
5'8"	164–196	197
5'9"	169–202	203
5'10"	174–208	209
5'11"	179–214	215
6'0"	184–220	221
6'1"	189–226	227
6'2"	194–232	233
6'3"	200–239	240
6'4"	205–245	246

If your weight puts you in the overweight or obese range, work to bring your BMI down to a healthy level. Although there are exceptions, for most people a high BMI means you're carrying too much body fat for your build. Try calculating your BMI at different weights to find a weight-loss goal that will eventually bring you into the normal range.

recording your target goals

As simple as it seems, having to write down your goals helps you clarify what you want to do and commit to doing it. Start by planning checkpoints, or times you will assess your progress, at two-week intervals. You can use the personal weight-loss plan (page 414) and the personal physical activity plan (page 432) in the No-Fad Toolkit to record your long- and short-term goals, as well as the rewards you intend to enjoy as you reach your two-week, four-week, and six-week targets. The more specific your objectives, the better. Persistence is the key: If you don't reach your target on occasion, realize that every step you make toward your goal is a sign of success.

step 3
choose an eating strategy

Good food and good health go together, and you can enjoy both as part of a sensible approach to managing your weight. For lasting weight control, however, you also need to feel satisfied by your choices so you can stick with a healthy eating plan for life. That's why it's so important to personalize your approach and calorie goals.

We offer three eating strategies to help you reach your weight-loss goals:

- **The Switch and Swap Approach:** Substitute lower-calorie foods for high-calorie foods.

- **The 75% Solution:** Eat three-quarters of the amount of food that you eat now.

- **The American Heart Association Menu Plans:** Follow easy-to-use two-week menus for three calorie levels and learn how to build your own.

You can use one, two, or all three strategies in whatever combination leads to personal results. If you're not sure which strategy to choose, answer the questions on pages 22 and 23 to help identify the plan that will work best for you.

The Switch and Swap Strategy is best for people who usually follow a routine. Once they see how their eating habits lead to weight gain, they can see what changes they need to make for effective weight loss.

The 75% Solution is best for people on the go. Their schedules may not allow them to control *what* foods they eat, but they can learn to control *how much.*

The American Heart Association Menu Plans are best for people who prefer a defined and nutritious approach that takes the guesswork out of making food choices.

which eating strategy is best for you?

1. How often do you eat out? (Count breakfasts, brunches, lunches, and dinners.)
   A. A few times a week
   B. Every day
   C. Seldom or never _____

2. How aware are you of the number of calories you are consuming?
   A. Haven't a clue
   B. Sort of aware
   C. Very aware _____

3. Do you like to go with the flow or plan ahead?
   A. Go with the flow
   B. Plan when I can
   C. Planning is my strong suit _____

4. Do you feel you have already cut high-calorie, nutrient-poor foods from your diet?
   A. Haven't really paid attention
   B. Somewhat
   C. Absolutely _____

5. Do you enjoy cooking at home?
   A. When I have time
   B. Not really
   C. Love it _____

6. Do you look up nutrition facts (in brochures, books, or on the Web) about the food you're eating and/or read food ingredient labels?
   A. Can't be bothered
   B. Sometimes
   C. Most of the time/always _____

7. Do you like to try new foods and new cooking methods?
   A. Somewhat
   B. Not really
   C. Absolutely _____

8. How balanced are your meals?
   A. Somewhat
   B. Very
   C. Haven't a clue   _____

9. Do you like to follow routines?
   A. Somewhat
   B. Not really
   C. Absolutely   _____

10. Are you comfortable with change?
   A. If it's not too drastic
   B. New things make me uneasy
   C. Yes, very comfortable   _____

                              Total Number of As   _____
                              Total Number of Bs   _____
                              Total Number of Cs   _____

WHAT YOUR SCORE MEANS

6 to 10 As   See page 24 for the Switch and Swap Approach.
6 to 10 Bs   See page 26 for the 75% Solution.
6 to 10 Cs   See page 28 for the American Heart Association Menu Plans.

What if your scores are fairly evenly split? Try combining the two methods that have the highest number. For example, if you have mostly As and Bs, try both the Switch and Swap Approach and the 75% Solution.

These three simple strategies will help you cut back on extra calories and follow a nutritionally balanced diet while still enjoying what you eat. No one diet plan is best for everyone. It's up to *you* to decide which approach or approaches best fit your preferences and your individual weight-loss needs.

the switch and swap approach
substitute lower-calorie foods for high-calorie foods

This strategy is based on the concept of subtracting calories by making small but effective changes in your daily eating patterns. Where are your daily calories coming from? What can you replace with a lower- or no-calorie substitute? Find about 500 calories of substitutions each day for the high-calorie foods you eat frequently, and you're already on your way to losing about 1 pound each week.

Keeping a food diary is an essential part of the substitution approach. Base your switches on the information and patterns you find there. Just swapping the margarine on your toast for a teaspoon of all-fruit spread and using fat-free milk instead of whole milk, for example, can save you a substantial number of calories. Keep in mind that you still need to eat a variety from all the food groups as you make substitutions. Using the entries from your food diary and the information on balanced nutrition on pages 30–36, you will be able to see where you can cut calories without cutting nutritional quality. For example, if you pick up a cinnamon roll on the way to work every morning, just switching to a cinnamon-raisin English muffin will save you about 300 calories! For more ideas on how to make some simple switches, refer to "Switch and Swap Food Substitutions" (page 416) in the No-Fad Toolkit. You can also refer to the list of common foods by calorie count found there (page 428).

To see how to apply the principles of the Switch and Swap Approach, review the following Sample Switch and Swap Daily Food Diary and compare it with the Sample Daily Food Diary of Original Eating Habits on page 15. You'll see how many calories you can eliminate just by making substitutions for high-calorie foods or beverages that have become part of a routine. (Calories have been rounded to the nearest multiple of 5 for easier adding.) It's really just a matter of swapping one habit for another.

The Switch and Swap Approach is especially good for people who usually follow a routine and can see how their eating habits may be contributing to weight gain. You can change the way you think about eating and food as you opt to make healthier choices. If you look at the entries in your daily food diary and can find several foods to replace with lower-calorie, higher-nutrition choices, the substitution plan may be your best bet to find a leaner, trimmer you.

sample switch and swap daily food diary

Time/Place	Food or Beverage (type and amount)	Calories	Switch and Swap Choices	Calories	Calories Saved
BREAKFAST 8:00 A.M. Home	1 large plain bagel with 1 Tb tub cream cheese	410	2 mini bagels with 1 Tb light tub cream cheese	170	240
	8 oz orange juice	110	1 medium orange	80	30
	8 oz coffee with 2 Tb half-and-half	40	8 oz coffee with 2 Tb fat-free half-and-half	20	20
	Subtotals	560		270	290
SNACK 10:30 A.M. Work	8 oz low-fat strawberry yogurt	240	8 oz fat-free, sugar-free yogurt with ¼ cup strawberries	140	100
LUNCH 12:00 P.M. Fast-food restaurant	1 6-inch meatball sub	580	1 6-inch turkey sub	220	360
	1 oz potato chips	150	1 oz baked potato chips	110	40
	16 oz cola	205	16 oz diet cola	0	205
	Subtotals	935		330	605
SNACK 3:00 P.M. Work	1¼ oz Cheddar cheese	145	1¼ oz low-fat Cheddar cheese	60	85
DINNER 6:30 P.M. Home	6 oz T-bone steak	420	1 serving Beef Tenderloin with Horseradish Cream (page 274)	175	245
	1 large baked potato with 2 Tb sour cream and 2 Tb margarine	540	1 large baked potato with 1 Tb light sour cream	300	240
	1 cup green beans with 1 Tb margarine	140	1 cup green beans with salt-free lemon pepper	40	100
	1 cup mixed salad greens with 2 Tb creamy Italian dressing	190	1 cup mixed salad greens with 2 Tb light Italian dressing	50	140
	1 serving bakery pineapple upside-down cake	365	1 serving Peach and Pineapple Upside-Down Cake (page 392)	100	265
	8 oz whole milk	135	8 oz fat-free milk	85	50
	Subtotals	1,790		750	1,040
SNACK 9 P.M. Home	1 cup chocolate ice cream	260	1 sugar-free frozen fudge bar	50	210
	Totals	3,930		1,600	2,330

the 75% solution
eat three-quarters of the amount of food that you eat now

Portion control is a major issue for most people. If you are one of the many who have gotten into the habit of eating too much too often, the 75% Solution may be the simplest way to work toward a healthy weight. Although we don't recommend that you continue indefinitely to eat many foods that have little nutritional value, the simplicity of just cutting back across the board can be a great help in starting to change lifetime habits.

You might be pleasantly surprised at how easy it can be to cut out 500 to 1,000 calories each day if you cut back on the amount of food you eat overall. You don't need to think too hard: Concentrate at first on reducing your daily calorie intake by about 25 percent. You can continue to eat most of the things you like—just eat less of each one.

As you serve yourself each meal, mentally draw a line on your plate to portion out 75 percent of what you normally eat. Compare the size of your average portions with the recommendations on page 33 or with the following visual estimates of reasonable servings. If your 75 percent portions are larger than these suggestions, gradually reduce your serving sizes to bring your overall intake in line with your target goals.

> 3 ounces cooked meat = a computer mouse
> 3 ounces cooked fish = a checkbook
> 1½ ounces cheese = six stacked dice
> 1 teaspoon mayonnaise = tip of a thumb
> 1 medium fruit = a baseball
> ½ cup cooked pasta = a baseball

To see how the 75% Solution can help you, review the following Sample Daily Food Diary. (Calories have been rounded to the nearest multiple of 5 for easier adding.) The changes from the sample original eating habits illustrate how the 75% Solution can save you calories. This approach to cutting back seems especially appropriate for people on the go. If you find yourself eating three slices of deep-dish pizza at your kid's football game every Friday night, cut back to two pieces of pizza with a lightly dressed salad if it's available. You can't always control where or what you are going to eat, but in most circumstances, you are the only one who decides how much you will eat.

sample 75% solution daily food diary

Time/Place	Food or Beverage (type and amount)	Calories	75% Solution Choices	Calories	Calories Saved
BREAKFAST 8:00 A.M. Home	1 large plain bagel with 1 Tb tub cream cheese	410	¾ large plain bagel with ¾ Tb tub cream cheese	305	105
	8 oz orange juice	110	6 oz orange juice	80	30
	8 oz coffee with 2 Tb half-and-half	40	6 oz coffee with 1½ Tb half-and-half	30	10
	Subtotals	560		415	145
SNACK 10:30 A.M. Work	8 oz low-fat strawberry yogurt	240	6 oz low-fat strawberry yogurt	180	
LUNCH 12:00 P.M. Fast-food restaurant	1 6-inch meatball sub	580	1 4½-inch meatball sub	435	145
	1 oz potato chips	150	¾ oz potato chips	110	40
	16 oz cola	205	12 oz cola	155	50
	Subtotals	935		700	235
SNACK 3:00 P.M. Work	1¼ oz Cheddar cheese	145	1 oz Cheddar cheese	110	35
DINNER 6:30 P.M. Home	6 oz T-bone steak	420	4 oz T-bone steak	315	105
	1 large baked potato with 2 Tb sour cream and 2 Tb margarine	540	1 medium baked potato with 1½ Tb sour cream and 1½ Tb margarine	405	135
	1 cup green beans with 1 Tb margarine	140	¾ cup green beans with 2¼ tsp margarine	105	35
	1 cup mixed salad greens with 2 Tb creamy Italian dressing	190	¾ cup mixed salad greens with 1½ Tb creamy Italian dressing	140	50
	1 serving bakery pineapple upside-down cake	365	¾ serving bakery pineapple upside-down cake	275	90
	8 oz whole milk	135	6 oz whole milk	100	35
	Subtotals	1,790		1,340	450
SNACK 9 P.M. Home	1 cup chocolate ice cream	260	¾ cup chocolate ice cream	195	65
	Totals	3,930		2,940	990

Need to grab a meal on the run? You can still enjoy your favorites if you commit to eating less. Order what you would usually choose and remove one-quarter of the food. Then enjoy the remaining three-quarters free of guilt. In most cases, you'll feel satisfied but will have eliminated those crucial extra calories. Hate the waste? Take the leftovers home for a snack or to add to another meal. If that's not feasible, recognize that the cost of a little wasted food is a small price to pay for better health, especially if you consider what you would be willing to pay to lose 10 pounds.

As you continue to make better meal choices, gradually transition to include enough servings from each important food group. It takes about six weeks to form new habits, so make it part of your six-week strategy to replace the foods that aren't contributing nutrients to your diet. Your food diary will help you see which foods to replace. If you usually have a doughnut for breakfast, start cutting calories by eating only three-quarters of it. Once you've adjusted to eating less, find an alternative food, such as a small whole-grain muffin, that will give you more nutritional benefit. These types of small changes really do add up to long-lasting weight loss.

the american heart association menu plans
follow our easy-to-use two-week menu plans

For the many people who prefer a defined and well-planned program, we offer two weeks' worth of delicious menus for three calorie levels that take the guesswork out of shopping and calorie counting. These menus, developed using some of the more than 190 recipes found on pages 126 to 412, are based on the American Heart Association dietary recommendations. To promote heart health, the menus and recipes are low in sodium, added sugars, saturated fat, trans fat, and cholesterol, as well as being low in calories for better weight management.

To decide which menu plan to follow, use the formula on page 16 to establish your current calorie intake. Depending on your calorie needs, choose from the 1,200-, 1,600-, or 2,000-calorie menus to safely lose between 1 and 2 pounds each week. Let's return to our 180-pound woman as an example. Since she is now eating about 2,100 calories each day, she could choose the 1,600-calorie menus to subtract 500 calories each day to lose 1 pound a week. If she wants to lose faster, she could follow the 1,200-calorie plan, reducing her intake by about 900 calories for a loss of just under 2 pounds per week.

You can also use the recipes and resources in this book to make your own menu plans. Planning your meals allows you to be creative and to control your calorie intake at the same time. Organizing in advance also reduces the stress of wondering what to have for dinner and making last-minute shopping trips. By keeping a grocery list and stocking your pantry with the core items used in these plans, you'll be sure to have what you need on hand. These foods fit right into a low-calorie, healthy eating plan and are quite versatile, too. With a wide selection of items in your kitchen, on the spur of the moment you can put together many simple combinations with a variety of seasonings.

The following section, "Eating Well for Good Health," provides a brief overview of what foods constitute a balanced and nutritious diet. For more information on how to create your own healthy menu plans, turn to "Part II: Menu Planning and Recipes," starting on page 77. The No-Fad Toolkit also includes handy reference tools, such as a blank menu planner (page 419), a list of common foods by calorie count (page 428), and smart low-calorie snacking ideas (pages 426 and 427).

eating well for good health

Reducing calories, no matter how you do it, will result in weight loss. In most cases, the loss will make you healthier. But when cutting calories, you also want to choose foods that nourish your body, especially as you make choices over time. Start with small changes to find workable ways to cut calories, but as soon as you've adjusted to eating less, it's time to incorporate nutritional balance into your dietary habits. Eating too many foods from certain groups and cutting back on others leads to nutritional imbalance. In fact, it's best not to think in terms of "good" or "bad" foods. Rather, think about finding the right balance to best fuel your body. When you focus on eating well instead of eating less, you will discover many options that are both low in calories *and* high in nutrition.

Every day, you have options on how to put together the meals you consume; with each choice, your aim should be to get the most return from each calorie. For optimal health, base your personal eating strategy on sound nutritional guidelines and include foods in the amounts you need from all the major food types. (See the table on page 33 for specific information on healthy food choices and recommended numbers of servings.) A basic knowledge of good nutrition will be a big help no matter which eating strategy you choose.

Choosing a wide variety of foods in the right amounts gives you the best chance of getting all the nutrients your body needs. For all phases of weight loss and maintenance, the American Heart Association recommends a balanced diet that is rich in nutrient-dense foods. In following any eating strategy, focus most on including these major food groups.

- **Vegetables and fruits** provide essential vitamins, minerals, and fiber, and because they're also low in calories, they can help you manage your weight and your blood pressure.

- **Fiber-rich whole grains** contain both soluble and insoluble fiber that can help you feel full as well as help lower your blood cholesterol. At least half your daily grain servings should be whole grain.

- **Fat-free and low-fat (1%) dairy products** provide calcium and protein without the saturated fat found in whole milk and whole-milk products.

- **Fish** is an important part of a heart-healthy diet. The omega-3 fatty acids in fish such as salmon, tuna, and trout have been shown to reduce the risk of heart disease.

- **Lean and extra-lean meats and skinless poultry** are excellent sources of protein, but you probably don't need as much as you think. Visualize your plate divided into fourths, with two sections for vegetables and fruits, one for grains or starches, and one for a protein source.

- **Legumes, nuts, and seeds** provide meatless protein and fiber and are great additions to a balanced diet. Rich in heart-healthy unsaturated oils, most nuts and seeds provide energy without empty calories when eaten in moderation and without added salt.

- **Unsaturated oils and fats** provide a combination of monounsaturated and polyunsaturated fats, both of which have heart-health benefits. All fats are high in calories, though, so use them in moderation to replace the unhealthy saturated and trans fats found in products such as butter and stick margarine.

To maximize the benefit you get from each calorie, aim to include fewer nutrient-poor foods, such as regular soda and french fries. To protect your heart health, it's also important to limit the amount of sodium, added sugars, saturated fat, trans fat, and cholesterol in your diet. When shopping, read package labels carefully—the nutrition facts panel will help you understand how much of those nutrients each food or beverage contains.

To achieve the right balance of nutrient-rich and nutrient-poor foods, follow these general recommendations.

- Choose the leanest cuts of meat and skinless poultry, and prepare them without added saturated and trans fats.

- Replace whole-fat dairy products with fat-free and low-fat alternatives to reduce your intake of saturated fat and cholesterol.

- Cut back on foods containing partially hydrogenated oils to reduce your intake of trans fats.

- Cut back on foods high in dietary cholesterol, which comes primarily from foods made from animal products. Try to eat less than 300 mg of cholesterol each day.

- Read labels and choose foods with little or no added salt (sodium), and use less salt in cooking and at the table. Limit prepared and packaged foods because most of them contain high levels of sodium. Ideally, most people should limit their intake of sodium to less than

1,500 mg each day for significant health benefits. To transition to lower levels of sodium in your diet, begin by aiming to eat less than 2,300 mg of sodium per day. As your taste buds adjust, look for ways to continue to cut back on sodium. A reduced sodium intake can lower blood pressure, prevent and control high blood pressure, and help prevent cardiovascular disease.

- Limit your intake of added sugars to half of your discretionary calories. For most women, that means 100 calories a day, or roughly 6 teaspoons or 25 grams of added sugars. For most men, it means no more than 150 calorie, or about 9 teaspoons or 38 grams per day.

- If you drink alcohol, limit your daily intake to one drink for a woman, two for a man. One drink is 12 ounces of beer, 4 ounces of wine, or 1½ ounces of 80-proof hard liquor.

The following chart lists the major food groups with the recommended number of servings daily for three calorie levels, as well as examples of serving sizes. Before you decide it's too complicated to do the math, remember that in many cases the servings add up easily. For example, if you eat a sandwich with two slices of whole-wheat bread, you are getting two servings' worth of the nutrients from fiber-rich whole grains. If you eat 1 cup of cooked broccoli instead of the standard serving size of ½ cup, you've eaten two vegetable servings for that day.

suggested servings of food groups

Food Group	Calorie Range			Sample Serving Sizes
	1,200	1,600	2,000	
Vegetables Eat a variety of colors and types.	3 to 4 servings per day	3 to 4 servings per day	4 to 5 servings per day	1 cup raw leafy vegetable ½ cup cut-up raw or cooked vegetable ½ cup vegetable juice
Fruits Eat a variety of colors and types.	3 to 4 servings per day	4 servings per day	4 to 5 servings per day	1 medium fruit ¼ cup dried fruit ½ cup fresh, frozen, or canned fruit ½ cup fruit juice
Fiber-rich whole grains Choose whole grains for at least half of your grain servings.	3 to 4 servings per day	6 servings per day	6 to 8 servings per day	1 slice bread 1 oz dry cereal (check nutrition label for cup measurements) ½ cup cooked rice, pasta, or cereal
Fat-free or low-fat (1%) dairy products Choose fat-free when possible.	1 to 2 servings per day	2 to 3 servings per day	2 to 3 servings per day	1 cup fat-free or low-fat milk 1 cup fat-free or low-fat yogurt 1½ oz fat-free or low-fat cheese
Fish Choose fish high in omega-3 fats.	6 to 7 oz (cooked) per week	6 to 7 oz (cooked) per week	6 to 7 oz (cooked) per week	3 to 3½ oz cooked fish
Lean meats and poultry Choose lean and extra-lean.	Less than 6 oz (cooked) per day	Less than 6 oz (cooked) per day	Less than 6 oz (cooked) per day	3 oz cooked meat or poultry
Nuts, seeds, and legumes Choose unsalted products.	2 to 3 servings per week	3 to 4 servings per week	4 to 5 servings per week	⅓ cup or 1½ oz nuts 2 Tb peanut butter 2 Tb or ½ oz seeds ½ cup dry beans or peas
Fats and oils Use liquid vegetable oil and spray or light tub margarines most often.	1 to 2 servings per day	2 servings per day	2 to 3 servings per day	1 tsp light tub margarine 1 Tb light mayonnaise 1 tsp vegetable oil 1 Tb regular or 2 Tb light salad dressing (Fat-free dressing does not count as a serving.)

eating out

For most of us, it's easier to stick to a healthy eating plan when we prepare our own food than when we eat away from home. Given today's busy schedules, however, it isn't realistic to expect to cook all your own meals at home. But if you regularly apply the same techniques of substitution or portion control in a restaurant as you would at home, you *can* enjoy the experience of eating out without derailing your weight-loss efforts.

When in a restaurant, take some time to study the menu and find options that will fit with your eating plan. Once you decide what to order, stick to your decision regardless of what your companions select. Remember too that most restaurants are happy to provide lower-calorie alternatives—if you ask for what you want. Try these questions the next time you are eating away from home.

- *Can you broil, grill, or poach my selection?*

- *Would you explain how this dish is prepared?* (See the box on page 35 for calorie-conscious food-preparation terminology.)

- *May I have a lunch-size portion?* Even at dinnertime this option may still be available.

- *May I substitute salad for french fries? Fat-free milk for cream?*

- *May I have soft corn tortillas?* Eat these instead of the fried tortilla chips served in Mexican restaurants.

- *May I have a to-go box with my meal?* Restaurant portions are so large these days that it's easy to eat almost twice what you need without thinking. Place half your order in the to-go box *before* you start eating so you'll know when to stop.

- *Would you take the bread/chips away?* Have your server remove temptation after your companions have helped themselves and given their okay.

- *May I have the sauce/salad dressing/gravy on the side?* These food toppings often drown food and add lots of expendable calories. Instead of pouring a sauce, dressing, or gravy over your food, dip the tines of your fork into it before spearing each bite—you'll eat a great deal less and still enjoy the flavor.

These tricks can help you get used to smaller portions and still enjoy eating out.

- Drink a glass or two of water while you wait for your food to be served. It will help you feel full and take the edge off your hunger.

- Eat slowly and savor your food. It takes about 20 minutes for your brain to register the signal from your stomach that it is full. Putting your utensils down between bites will help you slow down.

- Consider eating something low in calories—and preferably high in fiber (it's filling)—before leaving for the restaurant if you are very hungry. A small apple is one of many great choices.

- Try having two lower-calorie appetizers instead of a full entrée. The greater taste variety will help you feel more satisfied and full even with smaller portions.

common menu terms

Low Calorie	High Calorie
au jus	au gratin
baked	battered
braised	béarnaise
broiled	béchamel
fresh	breaded
grilled	buttered/buttery
poached	creamed/creamy
lean	fried
roasted	hollandaise
steamed	scalloped
stewed	tempura

We know that eating fast food is a reality for many Americans. Most fast-food restaurants are quick, inexpensive, and conveniently located. As society moves toward a more health-conscious age, however, many of these restaurants are offering healthier options. Review the nutrition guides on menus or the Web sites of restaurants you visit often so you'll know the best choices in advance. If you don't have that option, you can always ask for nutrition information at individual restaurants. When you do eat fast food, try the following techniques.

- Use the 75% Solution and eat only three-quarters of your order, or split an entrée with a companion.

- Ask for special preparation, such as no sauce or cheese.

- Order the kid's meal; the portion is smaller than the adult's meal.

- Choose from à la carte selections to get exactly what you want rather than buying the meal option, even if it seems like a "good deal." The extra calories in the added foods such as french fries are not worth the savings.

- When you opt for a salad, use the dressing sparingly if at all, and watch for hidden calories and sodium in items such as croutons and cheese.

- Choose vegetable or fruit options, if available, for the side item.

step 4
monitor and assess your progress

Once you've chosen an eating strategy and put it into action, stay focused on your progress. Ask yourself what's working—and what isn't. If you aren't meeting your goals, spend some time and energy to analyze why. You can also reassess and change your short- and long-term goals if needed, as well as choose a new strategy.

If you find you're not reaching your weight-loss goals, you probably aren't reducing your calorie intake as much as you think. Try to figure out where you may be underestimating how much you're eating, and adjust your plan accordingly. For example, if you've chosen to use the Switch and Swap Approach to cut 500 calories a day by switching five foods, try switching eight foods and see whether cutting back more helps you meet your goals.

Another approach is to try a combination of strategies. For example, find substitutes for your favorite high-calorie foods *and* cut back on your portion sizes. Perhaps you'd rather prepare some of the suggested menu plans (starting on page 78) on certain days of the week and then follow the 75% Solution on days when you have less time to cook or when you know you will eating out. Also be sure that your current level of physical activity is adequate for your expectations; you may need to add more physical activity to your routine to meet your goals. The bottom line is that you should use whatever tools you need to get the job done.

overcoming barriers

When you do hit a barrier, the important thing is that you don't give up. Instead of letting obstacles stop you, try these barrier-busting suggestions.

- **Eat snacks that don't add significant amounts of calories.** You can snack or round out a meal so you feel full without sabotaging your diet efforts. See the list of low-calorie snack foods in the No-Fad Toolkit.

- **Begin your meals with a zero-calorie drink or low-calorie starter.** A glass or two of water or a cup of hot tea can help you feel less hungry before you actually eat. Also, try eating a tossed green salad or light soup before your entrée to help curb your appetite.

- **Give in to a craving—within reason.** When you can't think of anything but a certain food, it might be best to go ahead and satisfy your craving by eating just a small amount of it. When you feel too denied and frustrated, you may actually overeat as a consequence. Don't forget to record what you ate in your food diary, including the amount, the calories, and the reason you ate that particular food.

- **Be mindful of whether you are actually hungry.** Make a habit of asking yourself before you put something in your mouth, "Am I really hungry enough to eat this? If this were something I didn't like very much, am I hungry enough to eat it anyway? Am I truly hungry, or do I just crave the sensation of eating?" More often that not, your honest answer will help you make a healthier choice.

- **Be conscious of what you're eating as well as with whom.** Your social circle really does influence how much you eat. In a recent study, researchers found that when in the company of friends or family members, adults tend to eat more than when eating with strangers. Especially among other overweight people, it's easier to relax and encourage each other to overeat. Stay aware of this potential pitfall so you can keep your meals as healthy and lean as possible, regardless of what others around you are eating. On the other hand, family members and friends can be a huge help in keeping you on track.

- **Bookmark some No-Fad Diet favorites.** Flag a few easy go-to meals and snacks in this book that you can rely on when your schedule is particularly hectic. No time to sit down and have breakfast at home? Instead of skipping the meal, whip up Banana-Blueberry Smoothies (page 139) and pour one serving into a travel cup. Instead of visiting the vending machine at work during mid-afternoon, have a serving of the Lemon-Ginger Trail Mix (page 136) that you prepared over the weekend.

staying focused

Family, work, and social obligations all claim large portions of the hours in a day. Although it's tempting to let time constraints threaten your resolve, you'll need to stay focused to keep on course. In a comparison of the most popular weight-loss plans, researchers found that long-term success had much less to do with the type of diet than with the perseverance of the participants. The people who focus on making changes to their lifestyles, not just to their diets, are the ones who are able to maintain their weight loss for life. Keeping on track won't always be easy, but the reward is that you will gain the control to make lasting changes. To stay focused on eating well to lose weight, you'll need to:

✓ Get used to eating less by making small changes that you can live with.

✓ Set reasonable goals and write them down. Track your progress with regular assessments and self-monitoring so you know what works for you.

✓ Transition to healthful eating habits that promote good nutrition.

✓ Get support from your family and friends.

✓ Focus on developing a long-term healthy eating plan and lifestyle that you can stick with for the rest of your life.

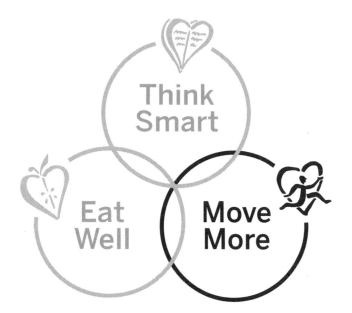

chapter 3

MOVE MORE:
more fit and less fat

Although cutting calories and eating healthier food will have a large impact on your weight and your health, it's important to remember that there is another key part of the weight-loss equation. Changing your diet alone is not enough to keep you fit and trim, especially for the long term. To reach and maintain the right energy balance over time, you need to incorporate regular physical activity into your lifestyle.

Calorie control is much more effective when integrated with a consistent exercise routine that incorporates aerobic and muscle-strengthening activities. Regular exercise burns unused calories to increase the Calories Out component of the energy-balance equation. Staying physically active is also essential to keep lost weight from creeping back. In fact, the best predictor of whether people will regain lost weight is whether they make physical activity a regular part of their life. If you are committed to breaking the yo-yo cycle—gaining weight, losing weight, and regaining weight—it's important to get moving and keep moving.

The benefits of being physically active go much further than just burning calories. Studies have established that physical activity improves overall health and fitness and can help prevent or help manage chronic diseases, including coronary heart disease, stroke, type 2 diabetes, osteoporosis, and depression. Being active also helps manage many cardiovascular risk factors, such as high blood pressure, high blood cholesterol, metabolic syndrome, and especially excess body weight. A recent study found that, in terms of heart health risk, being physically *inactive* is roughly equivalent to smoking a pack of cigarettes a day! In addition to all these health advantages, regular physical activity can help boost your mood, increase your confidence, and manage stress.

In this chapter, we guide you through the four simple steps you'll need to take to successfully—and healthfully—move more to lose more.

✓ Step 1: Assess your physical activity habits and levels.

✓ Step 2: Set your personal fitness goal. Start with at least 10 minutes of activity each day.

✓ Step 3: Choose a physical activity strategy:
  ○ The Lifestyle Approach
  ○ The Walking Program
  ○ The Organized Activity Option

✓ Step 4: Monitor and assess your progress.

move it to lose it

The American Heart Association recommends that all healthy adults engage in at least 150 minutes (2 hours and 30 minutes) of moderate-intensity, or 75 minutes (1 hour 15 minutes) of vigorous-intensity, aerobic activity each week. However, when working to lose weight, you should aim for 150 to 300 minutes each week of moderate-intensity activity or the equivalent 75 to 150 minutes of vigorous activity. If that seems overwhelming, bear in mind that in meeting your physical activity needs, regular moderately intense activities such as brisk walking can be just as effective as higher-intensity jogs and bike rides. Additionally, you can divide the total time into shorter sessions (a minimum of 10 minutes) spread out through the week. Just remember that any exercise is better than none, and making time to be active is a crucial part of a successful weight-loss plan and an overall healthy lifestyle.

If you are relatively active now, look for ways to add to your routine so you will burn more calories. If you need a jump-start off the couch, start today with a 10-minute walk, then read on to find some practical, workable solutions to increase the level of physical activity in your busy life. The sample progression chart on the next page shows how you can add a few minutes each week to go from just 10 minutes a day to 60 minutes of daily activity, or 300 minutes a week. You don't need to join a gym or buy expensive equipment, because the No-Fad approach offers you options to tailor your exercise routine to your personal needs. Just find something you enjoy and can fit into your life—and get moving!

should you consult your healthcare provider before starting an exercise program?

Many authorities feel that you don't need a medical examination or stress test before starting an activity program such as brisk walking. However, if you have a chronic medical condition or experience any symptoms that might affect your activity level—such as chest pain or pressure, dizziness, or heart palpitations—be sure to talk with your healthcare professional.

sample progression to 60 minutes of daily activity*

Weeks	Physical Activity** for 5 Days		Average Number of Steps Taken***	
	Total Daily Minutes	Total Weekly Minutes	Daily	Weekly
1 and 2	10	50	1,670	8,350
3 and 4	15	75	2,500	12,500
5 and 6	20	100	3,330	16,650
7 and 8	25	125	4,170	20,850
9 and 10	30	150	5,000	25,000
11 and 12	35	175	5,830	29,150
13 and 14	40	200	6,670	33,350
15 and 16	45	225	7,500	37,500
17 and 18	50	250	8,330	41,650
19 and 20	55	275	9,170	45,850
21 on	60	300	10,000	50,000

*Numbers are rounded to the nearest multiple of 5.

**Activity does not need to be continuous, but sessions lasting at least 10 minutes do more to increase fitness, maintain weight loss, and reduce risk factors for heart disease.

***These figures represent the average between walking at a pace of 4,000 to 6,000 steps in 30 minutes.

step 1
assess your physical activity habits and levels

In the same way you kept a daily food diary to help you understand your eating habits, you'll need to do an honest (but not harsh) self-assessment of how active you are—or aren't—at this point in your life. To help complete your assessment, use My Activity Tracker (page 433) in the No-Fad Toolkit. Check out the Sample Activity Tracker for reference. As you record your daily activities for one week, you'll need to include:

- The physical activities you do and when you do them
- The duration, level of effort/intensity, and level of enjoyment of the activities.

After you've completed this initial assessment, determine your current baseline activity level so you can decide how to set goals for improvement.

sample activity tracker

Date: *January 11* ❑ Mon ❑ Tues ☒ Wed ❑ Thurs ❑ Fri ❑ Sat ❑ Sun				
Time of Day	Activity	Duration	Level of Perceived Effort	Level of Enjoyment
6:00 A.M.	*Walked around the neighborhood with the dog*	*15 minutes*	*4*	*3*
8:25 A.M. *5:30 P.M.*	*Walked up and down the stairs in the parking garage*	*3 minutes*	*4*	*2*
3:00 P.M.	*Walked around the building at work*	*10 minutes*	*3*	*3*
6:00 P.M.	*Walked from the back of the parking lot to and from the grocery store*	*2 minutes*	*4*	*2*
7:00 P.M.	*Took an aerobics class at the local recreation center*	*30 minutes*	*5*	*3*

TOTAL DAILY ACTIVITY IN MINUTES: *60*

TOTAL DAILY NUMBER OF STEPS: *10,672*

Notes

Had a stressful day at work and didn't feel like going to aerobics class. Went anyway and am glad I did—it relieved a lot of my stress!

If You Did Not Exercise Today, Why?

❑ Not enough time

❑ Didn't want to

❑ Other:

Level of Perceived Effort	Level of Enjoyment
0 = Nothing at all	1 = Did not enjoy
1 = Very, very light	2 = Neutral
2 = Very light	3 = Did enjoy
3 = Light	
4 = Moderate/brisk	
5 = Somewhat hard	
6 = Hard	
7 = Very hard	
8 = Very, very hard	
9 = Extremely hard	
10 = Absolute maximal effort	

To help define your baseline activity level, try using a reliable pedometer. It will record every step you take, giving you a good idea of how everything you do during the day adds up. Wear the pedometer for one week. Add the daily totals and divide by 7 to find your average number of daily steps. That average is your current baseline, the starting point you'll use to set your fitness goals. (Record your average in My Personal Physical Activity Plan on page 432.) For comparison, the average American takes 2,500 to 3,500 steps in one day. On average, your activity level can be classified according to the number of daily steps taken:

- 2,000 to 4,000 steps is considered not active.

- 5,000 to 7,000 steps is considered moderately active.

- 10,000 or more steps is considered very active.

learn to gauge intensity

In addition to identifying your physical activity level, you need to determine its intensity. To gauge the relative intensity of an exercise session, pay attention to your breathing and heart rate while you are exercising. If you can talk but not sing, the activity is considered moderate intensity; if you cannot say more than a few words without pausing for a breath, the activity is classified as vigorous. The table below shows the typical intensity level of several common activities; of course, the actual intensity for you depends on your personal level of fitness.

selected common activities by intensity level

Moderate Intensity	Vigorous Intensity
Walking briskly (3 miles per hour)	Jogging/running
Bicycling (slower than 10 miles per hour)	Bicycling (faster than 10 miles per hour)
Ballroom dancing	Aerobic dancing
Water aerobics	Swimming laps
Doubles tennis	Singles tennis
General gardening	Heavy gardening that increases heart rate

Source: U.S. Department of Health and Human Services, *2008 Physical Activity Guidelines for Americans.*

To help you gauge the intensity of your daily activities, think about rating them on a scale of 1 to 10. The scale is based on the idea that you are the best judge of how hard you are working. Your body provides that information in the ways it reacts during physical activity: increased heart rate, increased breathing rate, increased perspiration, and fatigue. Use your perception of these reactions and the Level of Perceived Effort scale in the Activity Tracker to guide your ratings.

step 2
set your personal fitness goal

Your individual level of fitness will affect how you set your goals. What result is most important to you? In addition to losing and maintaining a healthy weight, are you especially interested in increasing your strength and stamina? Maybe you are concerned about your blood pressure or another health factor that exercise can improve. Once you know your priorities, you can establish your short- and long-term goals.

A *long-term* activity goal is something you want to achieve in six months to a year. It can be specific, such as being able to exercise for 60 minutes each day without feeling exhausted or sore the next day, but it should also be flexible enough to accommodate both unforeseen difficulties and opportunities. Long-term goals keep you focused on the end result. *Short-term* goals are the smaller steps that lead you to your desired result and help you feel successful. For example, you can decide to buy a new pair of walking shoes if you have walked for 150 minutes by the end of the week. Your short-term goals must be specific to be useful, so decide exactly what you want and how you will go about making your goal happen. Use My Personal Physical Activity Plan in the No-Fad Toolkit to organize how you are going to make physical activity a priority. Be sure to record:

- Short- and long-term goals

- Checkpoints at regular intervals

- Specific actions to make regular physical activity a part of your lifestyle

- Rewards for reaching your goals

After you've set your goals and begun to act on them, be sure to continue to record your ongoing efforts in My Activity Tracker (page 433) so you can monitor your progress.

If you are not used to much activity now, get moving. You may feel a sense of inertia, or think there are barriers, such as lack of time or procrastination, that keep you from being more active. Just 10 minutes a day of some form of light activity will get you past the inertia. Perhaps that activity will be a walk around your office building before you go home from work or adding five 2-minute walks to your usual workday. The first step is the hardest, but every step counts.

If, on the other hand, you already are an active weekend athlete or a daily neighborhood stroller, *keep adding activity.* You can always find ways to bump up your existing activity level to aid your weight-loss efforts and work up to the recommended number of minutes of activity each day. All activities, those that are part of everyday life as well as targeted exercise, count. Current research has not identified a limit to the level of health benefit achieved by adding physical activity. That means that the more active you are, the better for your health. The good news is that regular physical activity continues to provide major health benefits, no matter how your weight changes over time.

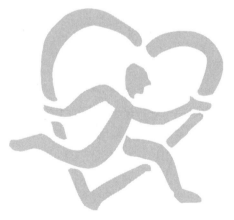

step 3
choose a physical activity strategy

Physical activity should be an enjoyable part of your life, not something you see as a chore or punishment for eating. Finding one or more physical activities that you can incorporate into your lifestyle and that you enjoy is key to sticking with an exercise plan for good. That's why it's so important to personalize your approach and physical activity goals.

We offer three physical activity strategies to help you reach your weight-loss goals and maintain long-term weight control:

- **The Lifestyle Approach:** Find ways to integrate more fitness into your daily routine.

- **The Walking Program:** Add walking to your routine in 10-minute increments.

- **The Organized Activity Option:** Participate in classes, group activities, or scheduled workouts.

You can select one strategy or try a combination of two or all three. The important thing is to choose activities that you will stick with and that are in addition to what you are currently doing. Any type of physical activity is beneficial if it makes your muscles work more than usual. Aerobic exercise that involves moving the legs and arms is especially good for the heart. Common aerobic activities include walking, running, swimming, and dancing, but you certainly don't have to limit yourself to these choices. Any activity that requires steady, rhythmic movement of the legs and arms will help condition your heart, get blood pumping through your body, and burn calories.

As you develop your workout routine, include stretching and strengthening activities to keep your muscles in good working order. Strengthening exercises (also called resistance training) pit your muscles against a force of resistance, such as gravity or a weight of some type. In addition to increasing your stamina, toning your muscles, and maintaining bone density, strength training can help boost your metabolism so you can maximize the effects of your aerobic activities and lose weight faster.

Keep in mind that it is the regularity, not the intensity, of activity that gives you the most benefit over time. No fitness routine can deliver the results you want if you don't follow through on a regular basis. Take the questionnaire on the following pages to help you determine which of the No-Fad Diet physical activity strategies will work best for your lifestyle.

which physical activity strategy is best for you?

1. Do you enjoy regular physical activity?
   A. Not really
   B. Somewhat
   C. Absolutely   _____

2. Do you enjoy participating in organized activities and sports?
   A. Hate it
   B. It's okay
   C. Love it   _____

3. Can you make time to be involved in a specific activity for a
   total of 150 minutes spread throughout each week?
   A. Not a chance
   B. Maybe
   C. Definitely   _____

4. Do you like to learn new activities?
   A. No way
   B. If they aren't too hard
   C. Absolutely   _____

5. Do you like to be around others when you participate in
   physical activity?
   A. Not really
   B. When they help motivate me
   C. Absolutely   _____

6. How do you feel about perspiring?
   A. Hate it
   B. It's okay
   C. Like it because it means I'm getting the most out of my workout   _____

7. Do you have a place to participate in physical activity?
   A. Not really
   B. Safe walking trail or quiet streets
   C. Home (with exercise equipment or DVDs), gym, or sports center   _____

8. Did you enjoy playing sports when you were younger?
   A. Never
   B. Loved it as a kid
   C. Still enjoy it   _____

9. How ready are you to get moving?
   A. Not really
   B. Somewhat ready
   C. Can't wait to get started   _____

10. How much variety do you want in your physical activity?
    A. Some variety
    B. Stick to one thing
    C. Lots of variety   _____

                          Total Number of As   _____
                          Total Number of Bs   _____
                          Total Number of Cs   _____

WHAT YOUR SCORE MEANS

6 to 10 As   See page 50 for the Lifestyle Approach.
6 to 10 Bs   See page 52 for the Walking Program.
6 to 10 Cs   See page 56 for the Organized Activity Option.

What if your scores are fairly evenly split? Choose the strategy that appeals to you most or try combining the two that have the highest number. For example, if you have mostly As and Bs, try the Lifestyle Approach on some days and the Walking Program on others. For real variety, try some of each activity.

the lifestyle approach

One of the simplest ways to live a more active lifestyle is through the Lifestyle Approach. Success using this strategy doesn't depend on which activity you choose but rather on how well and vigorously you add activity to your lifestyle. In the past decade, studies have shown that for adults who are not physically active to start, the Lifestyle Approach and a typical structured exercise program resulted in similar benefits regarding heart and lung fitness, overall body fat, and risk factors for coronary heart disease.

Taking the Lifestyle Approach means that you commit to performing enough small activities throughout your day—on top of what you normally do—to add up to an increased amount of overall total activity.

Identify ways you can fit more physical activity into your everyday life; the more you do, the better for your health. Also look for the obstacles that keep you from being more active, and plan to work against those barriers. To build on your baseline exercise level, climb the stairs instead of taking the elevator. Park your car as far as possible from your workplace so you will walk farther than you do now. Everyday tasks such as housework and raking leaves also count as physical activity if you act with vigor and speed. Instead of finding ways to lessen the physical activity of tasks—using a leaf blower rather than raking, for example—embrace the idea of doing more to burn calories and improve fitness. Remember, all activities—both baseline and physical activity—count in your energy-balance equation.

Step Up Your Activity Level. If you used a pedometer to determine your current level of activity, your baseline number of daily steps will be a big help in setting your goals when using the Lifestyle Approach. If you're like the average sedentary American, your baseline is about 2,500 to 3,500 daily steps. You should aim to add an average of between 4,000 and 6,000 steps to your baseline, which reflects about 30 minutes of additional walking. Ideally, your eventual target for weight loss should be about 60 minutes or more of daily activity. (If you are already active, be sure to set your personal goal well *above* your baseline number of steps.) To gradually reach your goal, each week add just 250 steps per day, averaged out over the week. That means that if your baseline daily average is about 2,500 steps, your daily average in Week 2 should be about 2,750 steps. In Week 3, it should be about 3,000 steps, and so on.

Try adding steps while walking through the places you go as part of your everyday life. For example, walk around your grocery store twice before you grab a cart. Use your pedometer to track how many steps that adds. Or when you go shopping, walk around the perimeter of the mall or shopping center. Walk through your workplace or across campus. If possible, walk your children to and from school. Look for ways to add steps as you progress toward more and more activity.

Fit in Fitness. One of the great benefits of the Lifestyle Approach is that you can choose what works best in your daily routine. The chart below will help you incorporate many of the things you already do into a personalized activity routine that fits into your life. People of different weights burn calories at different rates when doing the same physical activity at the same intensity for the same amount of time, so remember to check your approximate weight level. In general, the heavier you are, the more calories you burn for any given activity. The activities you choose—and how long and energetically you do them—will make a big difference in the long-term effect on your energy balance.

selected activities for the lifestyle approach

ACTIVITY**	Calories Burned in 30 Minutes of Continuous Activity by Approximate Weight*			
	150 lb	175 lb	200 lb	225 lb
Washing a car	100	120	140	150
Vacuuming	120	140	160	180
Cleaning windows	135	160	180	200
Raking leaves	150	170	195	220
Shoveling snow	205	240	270	310

*Calorie numbers are rounded to the nearest multiple of 5.

**For a more comprehensive list of activities, go to page 434 in the No-Fad Toolkit.

How can you check your progress as you implement the Lifestyle Approach? Because the effectiveness of this strategy is based on the intensity of your daily activities, the interim targets are up to you. Each week, check

Dunn Public Library

your activity tracker to see how your daily activity level compares to your initial goals. You can use simple tests to check your progress: How long does it take you to walk 200 steps? How far can you walk in 10 minutes? How winded are you after walking around the block? You'll know you're reaching your goal when you can walk farther (more steps), bike faster (more distance), or garden more easily (lower heart rate and better breath control).

the walking program

Walking is one of the most popular forms of physical activity in America today. It's inexpensive, easy, convenient, and the simplest way to start and continue a fitness program. That's probably why people who walk for exercise tend to stick with it; in fact, it has the lowest dropout rate of any physical activity. In addition to promoting weight loss, walking briskly for as little as 30 minutes a day will improve your circulation; build muscle tone and strength; help lower blood pressure, cholesterol, and triglycerides; increase energy and stamina; and reduce stress and anxiety. For such a small investment, walking provides a huge payoff.

What You Need to Get Going. It doesn't take much to start a walking program. Of course, you need a safe and convenient place to walk. Try walking around your neighborhood, the track at the local school, a trail at a community center, a park trail, a hiking trail, in your local shopping mall, or on a treadmill. Be sure to use a pedometer so you can track your efforts.

- **Choose the right clothing.** Loose clothing will make walking more comfortable and enjoyable. Dress in layers so you can easily remove the outer ones as you warm up. Loose-fitting clothing made of lightweight breathable fabric is ideal.

- **Wear good supportive shoes.** For each mile you walk, your feet will hit the ground between 1,500 and 2,000 times. Any athletic-type shoe will do, but your best bet is a walking shoe. Walking shoes have a curved sole that helps transfer weight from the back to the front of the foot with each step forward.

- **Try on new shoes to be sure they fit well.** Check fit in the toe box, arch, and heel. Walk briskly around the store so you'll know whether the shoe is comfortable. If it isn't, try another style or a different brand.

- **Check the condition of your shoes periodically,** especially the inside cushioning and tread. Replace shoes when they become worn or no longer support your feet.

Before You Walk. It's good to stretch and warm up before walking—or doing any other exercise. Warm up by walking slowly for about 5 minutes, then limber up your body and prepare it for more strenuous activity with stretching exercises. The basic stretches include:

- **Hamstring stretch.** Prop up one foot on a low, secure bench or stair step. Stand tall. Keeping your chest high, hips square, and tailbone lifted, bend forward from your hips. Feel a stretch in the back of your thigh or knee of the straight leg. Hold for 20 to 30 seconds on each leg.

- **Calf stretch.** Stand facing a wall and place both hands on it. Position one foot forward (knee bent) and the other foot back with the leg straight, toes pointing at the wall. With your stomach tight, lean in toward the wall until you feel a stretch in the lower part of the back leg. Hold for 20 to 30 seconds on each leg.

- **Hip flexor stretch.** With your back leg straight or slightly bent, lunge forward with the other leg, knee bent. Push your hips forward until you feel a stretch in front of your back thigh near the groin. Keep your torso upright and your front knee behind your toes. Hold for 20 to 30 second on each leg.

- **Abductor (inner thigh) stretch.** Keeping your torso upright, lunge to one side with a bent knee over the toe. Keep your other leg straight. Push your weight to the "bent knee" side until you feel a stretch in the inner thigh of your straight leg. Hold for 20 to 30 seconds on each leg.

Remember to drink some water before, during, and after you walk so you stay hydrated. On the other hand, eating too much right before walking (or any other exercise) can cause you to feel sluggish or even have an upset stomach; that's because your muscles and your digestive system are competing with each other for energy resources. Conversely, eating too little can lead to low blood sugar levels, leaving you weak, faint, or tired.

Walk with Purpose. While walking, keep your head up, shoulders relaxed, and stomach pulled in. Let your arms swing naturally and stick with a natural stride length. Warm up by starting out slowly, then pick up the pace. There are different ways to tell what walking pace is right for you. One is the perceived-effort scale included in the Activity Tracker (see page 43). As a general guideline, moderately intense exercise should be rated between 3 and 5—that is, between light and somewhat hard. Another way is to pretend you are walking to a meeting and that you'll be late if you don't pick up the pace. Simply stated, if you think you are just strolling along, you are walking too slowly. Try to find a pace at which you can say a few words but cannot sing. The following chart shows how many calories you will burn at different speeds. At the end of your walk, remember to stretch your muscles again, especially the ones you used the most.

selected activities for the walking program

| | Calories Burned in 30 Minutes of Continuous Activity by Approximate Weight* | | | |
ACTIVITY**	150 lb	175 lb	200 lb	225 lb
Walking (strolling at 1 mph)	70	80	90	100
Walking (at 3½ mph)	130	150	170	190
Hiking and backpacking	205	240	270	310
Jogging (at 5 mph)	270	320	360	410
Running (at 6 mph)	340	400	455	510

*Calorie numbers are rounded to the nearest multiple of 5.

**For a more comprehensive list of activities, go to page 434 in the No-Fad Toolkit.

Step It Up. The secret to long-term success with the walking program is to keep stepping up the activity level. When you are actively trying to lose weight, it's important to walk *in addition to* your current activities. If you now take an evening walk a few times a week, you must decide how to add to that schedule. If you don't already walk regularly, walk for at least 10 minutes every day for two weeks. As you begin Week 3, increase your walking time. On three or four days in the week, walk for 20 minutes—either all at one time or in two sessions of 10 minutes each. Continue to walk 10 minutes on the other days of that week. The chart on the next page shows one example of how to add increments of walking time each week. By the sixth week, you should be comfortable walking 30 minutes on most days.

sample walking times for a 6-week jump start to fitness

Week 1	Week 2	Week 3	Week 4	Week 5	Week 6
10 minutes on most days	10 minutes on 7 days	20 minutes on 3 days; 10 minutes on 4 days	20 minutes on 7 days	30 minutes on 3 days; 20 minutes on 4 days	30 minutes on 7 days

Note: The total walk times shown here can be broken into 10- or 15-minute segments to better fit into your lifestyle.

Each week, review your activity tracker. Evaluate whether you've accomplished what you set out to do—for example, walking for 30 minutes on five days each week. Are you walking farther in that 30 minutes after several weeks? Are you continuing to lose weight? If not, you may want to step up your program. On the other hand, if you find that you have achieved a walking goal that once seemed out of reach, congratulations!

Walk with Buddies. An American Heart Association survey revealed that adult Americans are 76 percent more likely to walk when someone else is counting on them. The more you can integrate your walking program into everyday life, the better, and walking with a partner is one of the most effective ways to stay committed to physical fitness. Need a walking buddy? Go on evening walks with your family, walk your dog or your neighbor's, or start a neighborhood walking club or "talk and walk" group.

Walk at Work. The American Heart Association's Start! program encourages walking as a way to improve Americans' general fitness and cardiovascular health. Visit MyStart! online at StartWalkingNow.org to connect with a network of people who share your interest and walking goals. The site offers tips on how to start a walking program at your workplace; how to find safe, convenient walking paths in your area; and how to stay motivated. You can also go to StartWalkingNow.org to find a buddy in your neighborhood or find a virtual buddy to help encourage you from a distance.

the organized activity option

The Organized Activity Option involves participating in scheduled classes or sports to add physical activity to your weekly routine. Besides getting more fit, you'll benefit from the social support and expectations of your classmates and teammates. It's more difficult to justify skipping out of your planned activity if you know that ten people are counting on you. "Organized" doesn't have to mean a team sport, however. You may want to take a few introductory classes to learn about activities that interest you. Taking lessons is a good way to hone your skills and increase your activity level at the same time.

Check your local newspaper or community newsletter for classes or group activities offered in your area. Try something new. Thousands of people have found dozens of ways to enjoy being physically active—don't hesitate to join them. The activity chart below lists a few sports and activities that lend themselves to group participation. It's important to find a good match—something you can enjoy and do regularly—so experiment until you find the right combination for your lifestyle and personality.

selected activities for the organized activity option

	Calories Burned in 30 Minutes of Continuous Activity by Approximate Weight*			
ACTIVITY**	150 lb	175 lb	200 lb	225 lb
Golfing (carrying the clubs)	190	220	250	280
Bicycling (10 to 12 mph)	205	240	270	310
Racquetball	240	280	320	360
Swimming	240	280	320	360
Tennis (singles)	270	320	360	410

*Calorie numbers are rounded to the nearest multiple of 5.

**For a more comprehensive list of activities, go to page 434 in the No-Fad Toolkit.

You also can work out at home using exercise equipment, video fitness games, or recorded activity sessions. This works well for lots of people, but it means that you need to be disciplined about your routine. Be sure to establish a clear schedule for your regimen. Plan your activities as you would appointments and add them to your calendar or PDA. When you're exercising at home, turn off the phone, shut the door, and don't let distractions disrupt your workout. Once you get into the habit, you'll enjoy the time you spend doing something good for yourself.

combining activities and strategies

Even if you enjoy the activity you have chosen, you can still find additional ways to participate and other groups to join. If you are going to the gym for racquetball two evenings during the week, you may want to join a swimming program on Saturday mornings. If all your activities take place indoors but you would love to be outside in good weather, look for an outdoor organized activity.

Combine two or all three "move more" strategies for maximum benefit, flexibility, and variety. You could use a pedometer to track lifestyle steps on busy days, go for a fitness walk on some days, and play sports on the weekend or in the summer months. Try incorporating other types of exercise. If you are primarily following the Walking Program, try a 20-minute session that consists of cycling for 10 minutes and then walking for 10 minutes. Be creative: if you love the water, try a water aerobics class and then try a rowing club. The key is to find the combination that works for you. For a combined listing of the calories burned in various activities, as shown in the charts on pages 51, 54, and 56, see page 434 in the No-Fad Toolkit.

step 4
monitor and assess your progress

Making regular entries in My Activity Tracker (page 433) will give you a written record of your exercise habits, as well as documentation of when you didn't exercise and the reasons why. Attitude is a big contributor to your success: the positive feelings that come with being more active help you move forward, while negativity makes achieving your goals harder. When you do reach a target checkpoint, be sure to reward yourself with a nonfood treat and keep working toward improving your fitness and health.

If over time your fitness level seems to be improving without a corresponding effect on weight loss, you may be building muscle tissue, which is heavier than fat. You are also developing better cardiovascular health and increased stamina. Remember too that an ongoing program of exercise will help you maintain weight loss in the long run. If your chosen activity doesn't seem to be getting easier, however, try to find out why by reviewing the entries in My Activity Tracker.

overcoming barriers

Depending on the obstacles you face, you may need to reassess and change your short- and long-term goals and perhaps choose a different strategy. The important thing is that you don't give up and give in. Try these barrier-busting suggestions instead:

- **Embrace the buddy system.** Recruit a spouse, other family member, neighbor, friend, or co-worker who will help motivate you and join you in activities such as walking around the neighborhood before or after work, joining a dance class, or shooting hoops in a local park. You're more likely to keep your exercise commitment if you have someone else counting on you.

- **Be prepared for inclement weather.** Identify indoor alternatives for bad weather days so you won't be derailed by rain, snow, cold, or heat.

- **Dedicate a particular time in the day for exercise.** Lack of time is an enemy for most of us, so it's important to carve out and schedule dedicated time or chunks of time for exercising. Add notices to your work calendar as reminders to walk around your workplace for 10 minutes every few hours or block your lunch hour so you can go to a nearby gym or mall for a walk.

- **Work in your workouts even while traveling.** Find yourself with lots of downtime in airports? Instead of sitting while you wait for your flight, take a walk in the airport. Also, pack your workout gear and walking shoes and use the hotel's exercise facilities or explore the city on foot.

debunking common myths

Many commonly held beliefs about how physical activity affects weight loss are based on misconceptions; some of those beliefs are just not true. Advertisements for miracle products and gadgets promise quick and easy weight loss, but the rule of thumb is that if something sounds too good to be true, it probably is. Here are the facts on just a few of the weight-loss myths that continue to pop up.

Myth: All I have to do to lose weight is exercise; then I can eat what I like.
Reality: Exercise alone cannot burn away an unlimited number of extra calories. When you are physically active, you benefit in both body and mind, but that doesn't mean you can then eat anything you want. The truth is that 20 minutes of moderate-intensity activity burns about 100 calories, which won't have much effect on your energy balance if you're overeating at the same time. Good eating habits and regular physical activity go hand in hand to keep you fit and trim.

Myth: Exercise can be targeted to burn fat in certain parts of my body.
Reality: Plain and simple, this is not true. Those heavily advertised exercise devices do more to slim down your wallet than your hips or thighs. A classic study from the 1970s was reinforced by more recent evidence that localized exercise does not "burn off" fat from that target area. Rather, whenever you exercise, fat is taken from stores throughout your body to supply the energy you need. You can build up specific muscles with specific exercises, but you won't lose more fat where you build muscle than in other areas of your body.

Myth: I can lose weight with "effortless" exercise.
Reality: The desire to melt away fat effortlessly is not new. The rubberized "sweat suits" and heated belts on the market are modern versions of the vapor baths of yesteryear. These products create only temporary loss of body water (dehydration), which can be dangerous. Although your body measurements may be less after you wear these garments, the body weight you thought you lost will come right back once your body is rehydrated. Likewise, mechanical vibrating machines and electrical stimulating devices that promise the health benefits of exercise without the effort may make the fat tissue move around, but they do not remove it.

Myth: Exercise increases the appetite.
Reality: Some people believe that exercise will make them feel hungrier and they will eat even more. However, most research suggests that moderate exercise doesn't increase appetite at all, especially for people who were previously inactive. In fact, exercise usually helps regulate appetite and makes people feel less hungry overall.

staying focused

Being physically active is vital to overall good health and is essential if you want to lose weight and keep it off. Enjoying your exercise plan is also important. Having fun in the process makes it much easier to plan with enthusiasm, counteract negative thinking, overcome obstacles, meet your goals, and reap the multitude of benefits of an active life. To stay focused on achieving fitness success and controlling your weight:

✓ Think of yourself as a healthy, fit person.

✓ Write down your short- and long-term goals and keep track of your progress with regular self-monitoring assessments.

✓ Choose an activity that is fun for you.

✓ Start out slowly to avoid injury.

✓ Establish a routine.

✓ Get support from your family or friends.

✓ Seek enthusiastic, capable leaders for group activities.

✓ Vary your activities and enjoy yourself.

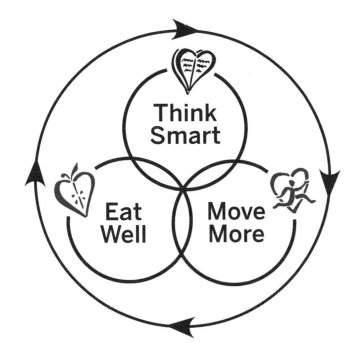

chapter 4

MAINTAIN MOMENTUM:
keep up the good work

For most people, losing weight is hard work. When you do approach your target weight, be proud of your achievement. Keeping weight off can be just as difficult as losing it, if not more so. That's why it's so important to continue to integrate all three key components of the No-Fad Diet—think smart, eat well, and move more—into your everyday life.

The complex interplay of biology, psychology, environment, and commitment is unique for every individual. To successfully reach and *maintain* your target weight, you'll need to determine for yourself what will motivate you and keep your focus on fulfilling your goals instead of returning to old habits.

Given sound information, smart strategies, and appropriate tools, you can manage your weight just as many other Americans have done. For the past 15 years, the U.S. National Weight Control Registry has documented how more than 5,000 people have lost weight and kept it off—and how the lifestyle elements and behaviors they had in common contributed to their success.

✓ Most members continue to eat a low-calorie diet and maintain high levels of physical activity.

✓ 90 percent of them exercise, on average, about 1 hour per day.

✓ 78 percent eat breakfast every day.

✓ 75 percent weigh themselves at least once a week.

✓ 62 percent watch less than 10 hours of TV per week.

When most people go "on a diet," they think of it as a temporary change in eating behavior to achieve their goal weight. Once their goal is achieved, however, many go "off the diet" and ultimately regain the weight they lost—and sometimes even more. Keep in mind that the No-Fad Diet is not actually a diet at all but rather a sustainable way of life. As you work to maintain your own momentum, learn from others' successes. It's a good bet that the same things that have worked for them will work for you, too.

In this chapter, we'll guide you through the steps you'll need to take to successfully—and healthfully—keep off the weight you lose.

✓ Step 1: Monitor your weight and behavior.

✓ Step 2: Maintain your healthy eating habits.

✓ Step 3: Keep up your physical activity routine.

✓ Step 4: Continue to make healthy lifestyle choices.

step 1
monitor your weight and behavior

Staying aware of the triggers and avoiding associations that negatively affect your behavior choices are just as important now as when you first started to work toward energy balance. Well-established habits are hard to break completely, so it's important to stay focused on how your ongoing behaviors affect your weight. Use these strategies to keep your weight control on track.

- **Listen to your body.** You shouldn't obsess about the numbers on the scale, but do check your weight on a regular basis; about once a week works well for most people. Pay attention to how you feel and be ready to respond to the cues your body is giving you. Those extra pounds creep back in small increments and can add up before you know it. A regular weigh-in keeps you aware of changes in your energy balance *before* you experience a major slowdown or setback.

- **Write down and review your goals and achievements.** Maintaining an ongoing record of your progress is a proven way to keep your weight loss a reality. The act of writing makes you focus on your goals and helps you monitor and identify what works and what doesn't. Take a look at your original food diary and your written goals. If you're not making the progress you hoped for, perhaps your goals are less realistic than you thought or you encountered unexpected barriers. In either case, adjust your goals and decide what action you can take right away to solve the problem.

- **Enlist social support.** Although losing weight is often considered a personal or private endeavor, studies show that people who seek social support as they work to maintain their weight loss are most likely to succeed. Spouses in particular can make or break a weight-loss plan. A supportive partner will encourage you and help you maintain the lifestyle changes you need. Sometimes, however, spouses and other people who are overweight themselves will feel threatened by your success. Being aware of this possibility makes it easier for you to ignore people who might subconsciously (or even consciously) sabotage your efforts. Attending meetings of weight-control groups and accessing interactive Web sites can also provide you with helpful input from other people going through the same things as you are.

step 2
maintain your healthy eating habits

It's essential to stay focused and to be vigilant about continuing your healthy eating habits. After the initial thrill of losing a few pounds, it's easy to be tempted to slide back into unhealthy ways of using food, such as easing stress with ice cream. Instead of reverting to your old behaviors, remind yourself of the weight-loss results you achieved by using smart eating strategies. To help you maintain your healthy eating habits, try these suggestions:

- **Learn "flexible restraint."** Manage and maintain good eating habits without becoming obsessive or overly controlled. Eat to live rather than live to eat.

- **Practice "conscious" eating.** Continue to be aware of *why* you are eating. Is it to fill a physical need (hunger) or some type of emotional need (such as stress or loneliness)?

- **Recognize when you have eaten enough.** It takes about 20 minutes for the brain to register when the stomach is full, so it's a good idea to stop eating when you feel you still have some room left. Don't eat more than you need, just to finish what you or the kids didn't finish.

- **Stay clear of your trigger foods.** Replace the candy dish in your office with healthy low-calorie snacks, and don't keep unhealthy foods at home. High-calorie, low-nutrient eating habits can quickly find their way back into your life if you are not careful about monitoring and controlling the food in your environment.

- **Celebrate without food.** Try celebrating some of life's successes and special times in ways other than eating out or indulging in bakery goods. For example, instead of treating your newly promoted girlfriend to lunch at a restaurant, treat her to a manicure or a movie instead.

keep up your physical activity routine

Researchers are confirming what clinicians who work with weight-loss patients have known for years: staying physically active is essential to keep lost weight from creeping back. The exact mechanisms at work aren't understood yet, but in addition to burning calories, regular physical activity seems to affect the body's metabolic systems in ways that discourage weight gain.

Once you've achieved your goal weight, you can focus less on cutting calories and more on exercising and staying in energy balance. To transition from the dieting phase to a permanently active lifestyle, implement these ideas to stay motivated:

- **Exercise with friends.** Hanging out with friends makes working out more fun; you're doing something good for your mental well-being and physical fitness at the same time. You're also less likely to skip a workout if other people are depending on you to join them.

- **Integrate physical activity into your leisure time.** Brainstorm with friends to find physical activities that all of you are interested in trying. For example, go hiking one weekend to enjoy the outdoors or take dance lessons together. Organize a weekend basketball game in the neighborhood park or start a dog-walking club on Saturday mornings. Get creative, think of as many active and entertaining activities as you can, and then try them all.

- **Wear a pedometer to keep track of your activity level.** Keeping track of the steps you take each day is a great reality check and will keep you from becoming complacent about moving more. Add 250 more steps each week until you've hit 10,000 steps a day; that is the benchmark for a very active lifestyle.

- **Lobby for a work culture that supports a more physically active environment.** Many Americans spend the majority of their time at sedentary workplaces. If you are one of them, encourage your co-workers to join you to add more physical activity to your day. Visit the American Heart Association's Start! program at StartWalkingNow.org for more information on workplace walking programs.

continue to make healthy lifestyle choices

Intellectually understanding how to effectively and safely lose weight is not the same as turning that awareness into action. Changing your lifestyle takes effort and resolve, and it doesn't happen overnight. It is reasonable to expect some slips along the way, so it's especially important to *keep* working toward the behaviors that support your efforts.

Hitting a dry spell when you just can't seem to make progress is part of the weight-loss process, so it's best to prepare yourself for those occasional pitfalls and plateaus. Changing your diet may even alter the biochemistry that regulates your appetite and fat storage. When you do hit a plateau, don't give up and don't waste your energy on guilt. Stick to your plan and refocus. Hitting a plateau does not mean you've failed, and it does not mean you've lost control of your weight forever. Try these "think smart" techniques to help you get back on track and continue making healthy lifestyle choices.

- **Change your mind-set and environment to support your success.** None of us is perfect, and the environment in which we live isn't always conducive to eating well. Once you've reached your goal weight, keep watching for the food triggers and destructive thought patterns that can creep back into your life. Likewise, establish routines at home and at your workplace that will help you avoid unwanted eating and encourage more physical activity.

- **Develop effective coping skills to reduce stress and end emotional eating.** Food can temporarily satisfy emotional needs, which is why so many people turn to eating for comfort. Eating, however, doesn't provide lasting solutions, so as soon as you feel yourself leaning toward food when you are not actually hungry, focus on finding a behavior that will replace the emotional gratification you get from eating.

- **Learn from experience.** Use previous weight-loss attempts to learn about your personal behavior and gain better self-awareness. Every failure and every success can teach you how your mind and body react to food, stress, and environmental factors so you can make better lifestyle choices.

- **Strive for good health and fitness, not physical perfection.** Better health is achievable for almost everyone, and living a more vital life is a more worthwhile goal than dreaming of perfect looks.

According to the findings from the U.S. National Weight Control Registry, the first two years after losing weight are the most difficult. If you can stick it out as you learn to adapt to new principles and adopt them as lasting behavior choices, you—like the other successful losers on record—will be most likely to maintain a healthier weight for good. As healthcare professionals, we at the American Heart Association want to help you succeed in attaining that goal. From years of experience in working with real people like you who are trying to reach and maintain a healthy weight, we can offer our observations on how to turn your hopes into reality. We can give you sound advice on how to think about food, as well as how to eat well and keep your body fit. We can provide the information and tools in this book to help you take a healthy approach to permanent weight loss, but it is up to you to put these tools to use. Ultimately, you are the only one who can make the lifestyle changes needed to think smart, eat well, move more, and maintain your momentum for a lifetime of successful weight management.

chapter 5

PASS IT ON:
family, food, and fitness

Adults are not the only ones who can benefit from a No-Fad Diet approach. Because of today's busy schedules, easy access to unhealthy foods, and limited physical activity, it is increasingly more difficult for children to learn the lifetime habits that promote good health. Kids today are taking in record numbers of empty calories, and the fast-rising number of overweight children in the United States is evidence of that trend.

Being obese during childhood increases the risk of being obese as an adult. Like overweight adults, overweight children are at risk for serious health consequences, and more and more kids are developing the conditions and diseases typically associated with adult obesity. If the rise in childhood obesity continues unchecked, it is predicted that the current generation of young people will become the first in American history to live shorter lives than their parents.

You can reverse this frightening trend by using the same basic principles of think smart, eat well, and move more. These same strategies will help you create an alternative to the current fat-friendly atmosphere so kids can learn how to make good choices. Even in today's "toxic" environment, *you can do a lot* to help your kids eat better, be more active, and enjoy the benefits of being healthy. Using the strategies outlined in this book, as well as advice from your healthcare providers and other reliable resources, you can take the steps needed to raise more active, healthier children.

be proactive about your child's good health

More than any other individuals, parents influence their children's food and lifestyle choices. Kids are overweight for the same reasons adults are—too much food, too little activity. When you embrace good eating habits and enjoy physical activity, you establish a home environment that teaches your children to do the same. Family members create their culture of lifestyle habits together, and they can find a healthy approach to weight control together as well.

talk with your kids

Weight gain is a sensitive subject for people of any age, and it can be difficult to know how to approach the issue without hurting a child's self-image and confidence. At the same time, it's important to explain to your child why you might want to make changes in his or her routine. Discuss the physical benefits of eating well and being active, and emphasize the importance of being healthy, not being thin. An overweight child is much more likely to be overweight or obese as an adult, but most kids don't think much about health issues in the future. Help your child see how he or she will be better off *right now* by having more energy, better concentration at school, and stronger performances in sports and social activities. A child who understands these immediate benefits will be more likely to realize that being healthy is a positive experience, not a punishment.

talk with your healthcare provider

Because of how a child's body changes during growth, calculating his or her body mass index (BMI) can be complicated, so work with your healthcare provider to keep track of your child's weight. At each visit, ask how your child's weight compares with the entries in an age-appropriate growth chart. Ideally, your child's weight should be less than the 85th percentile. You should also expect to see occasional shifts up or down; they are a normal part of the growth process. If, however, your doctor thinks your child is gaining weight too quickly or shows a tendency to become overweight, make the necessary changes in your family's diet and physical activity levels right away—for the sake of your child's health.

choose a pass-it-on strategy

Eating habits are set in childhood and tend to stick with us for life, so it's best to help your children develop healthy ones. Help them learn to enjoy physical activity rather than view it as a chore.

We offer six pass-it-on strategies to help you improve your children's eating and physical activity habits:

- Be a good role model.

- Give kids choices.

- Make being healthy practical and fun.

- Work with your schools.

- Pack healthy lunches.

- Limit screen time and encourage sleep.

be a good role model

Every day you have the opportunity to do things—big and little—that affect your children's health in a big way. The lifestyle habits you help them develop early on stay with them as they grow into adults. For example, model good self-esteem; avoid talking negatively about your body. Focus both on eating nutritious foods to keep your body nourished and on working out to keep your body healthy. By demonstrating your commitment to live in a healthy way, you positively influence the family culture that you create and share with your kids.

healthy eating

- Serve meals at home as much as possible. Eating together provides the best chance you have to reinforce good eating habits, and studies show that families who eat together tend to be healthier both physically and mentally. You can see what your kids are eating; and in relaxed conversation, you may gain insight into situations in your children's lives that trigger overeating.

- Practice portion control when you are serving meals. A preschooler and a teenage athlete need different amounts of food, of course, so encourage what is appropriate for each stage of childhood development.

- Enjoy your vegetables, and your kids are more likely to enjoy theirs, too.

healthy physical activity

- Promote and share as much physical activity as you can. Children should get 60 minutes of moderate to vigorous play or physical activity each day. Limit the time the whole family spends in front of the television and computer, and make a point of enjoying many different physical activities together with your children, from tag to T-ball.

- Schedule a special time each week for your whole family to participate in a favorite physical activity. Go bowling, take a hike, or play softball. Enjoying a fun family event makes it clear to your kids that you value them *and* a healthy, active lifestyle.

give kids choices

Instead of thinking in terms of putting your kids on a diet, give them opportunities to make the same healthy choices you intend to make for yourself. Overweight children need to learn how to overhaul their eating patterns, and you can show them how to take small, manageable steps so they will feel good about their progress. You want them to have a good understanding of healthy eating habits so they don't take the battle with weight gain into adulthood. One of the best ways to teach your kids to make healthy choices is to get them involved.

healthy eating

- Make kids part of the whole process of choosing recipes, shopping for ingredients, preparing food, setting the table, and enjoying mealtime. The more they participate, the more they will feel a sense of accomplishment and learn to appreciate different foods.

- Have your kids choose a healthy food that's new to them from the grocery store. Even if they don't like the new food at first, it's important to encourage them to keep trying different things. Kids' taste buds change and develop as they grow, and it may take ten to fifteen tries before a child decides he or she likes a new food. (Adults' tastes evolve with time also, so just because you didn't like spinach as a child, don't let that stop you from trying it now!)

- Encourage your kids to ask for what's good for them. When you eat out, explain that restaurants usually offer better alternatives to the french fries, fried chicken nuggets, and soft drinks that are typical children's fare. Ask for veggies, grilled chicken, and whole-grain rolls when possible. Even most fast-food places now offer salads instead of fries, applesauce or fruit for dessert, and fat-free or low-fat milk instead of soda. Let your kids know it's okay to take a to-go box home or split an entrée.

healthy physical activity

- Let your children have some say in the action. Get their opinions as you discuss different sports, classes, or other options for exercise. Remember that physical activity does not have to be competitive, and not all children are destined to be jocks. Many children who choose not to participate in organized or team sports still like being physically active. Help them find physical activities they can enjoy alone or with a friend; the benefits are the same, but the stress will be gone.

make being healthy practical and fun

Stay positive and be realistic in your expectations for your children. Negative statements and nagging will not help you—or your children—in the long run. Instead of dwelling on the foods your kids *can't* have, make gradual changes that involve the whole family, and let your children adapt to changes at their own pace. Don't aim for a quick fix; help establish good lifetime habits instead.

healthy eating

- Offer nutritious foods regularly; serve them with enthusiasm and positive comments. Reiterate that healthy food is not a chore to be endured. Don't use fast food as a reward or withhold treats as punishment.

- Forget the idea of cleaning one's plate. Teach your children to stop eating when they are no longer hungry and let them know that it's not necessary to feel "full" to be satisfied. The average adult's stomach is about the size of a medium fist; children's stomachs are, of course, even smaller.

- Keep healthy snacks on hand at all times so it's just as easy to grab an apple on the way out the door as to stop for fast food on the way home.

healthy physical activity

- Set concrete and achievable activity goals that will give your child a sense of accomplishment, such as shooting hoops for 20 minutes on Monday, Wednesday, and Friday. Try to avoid the idea of exercise as "work."

- Don't punish your kids by restricting their opportunities for physical activity. (Encourage your children's school to use other ways to keep control in the classroom as well.)

- Use play as a wonderful way for children to use their imaginations and their bodies. From the time your infant begins to move around, create a safe environment for baby to explore, then provide age-appropriate opportunities for active play.

- For young children, set up play dates that involve physical activities; as kids get older, encourage them to get outside with friends to walk, ride bikes, and enjoy other unstructured play activities. Kids are more likely to be active and stay active if their friends are, too. Keep equipment such as bikes and basketball hoops in good working order.

sweet treats

Sugary treats abound from Halloween to Valentine's Day and are offered at birthday parties throughout the year, so it can be hard to feel in control. Instead of fretting about how to limit candy consumption, just keep providing healthy meals and once in a while let your child choose one or two treats at snack time or on the weekends. It's the overall pattern of your child's food choices that counts most, not an occasional splurge. Encourage reasonable restraint, then turn to other ways to enjoy the holiday or celebration. Read a favorite book, do a craft project, play a game, or engage in some active play based on the theme of the special occasion. Your attention and fun times spent together will mean more to your child than any amount of candy.

work with your schools

Once you send kids off to school, it can be hard to get the details about their daily environment and food choices. Visit your school's cafeteria. Ask what meals are available and check out the options in vending machines. Visit the gymnasium and ask about the physical education program. Today's schools have a lot of influence over the types of food and activity levels available to their students. As a parent, you can get involved in your community to be sure your children are given the nourishing meals and physical activity they need. Healthy kids are better able to concentrate on their work, are more likely to attend school on a regular basis, and typically perform better in class. To learn how to make your school a healthier place, visit healthiergeneration.org for free resources and tools. Developed in partnership by the American Heart Association and the Alliance for a Healthier Generation, the Healthy Schools Program helps parents and schools work together to promote physical activity and healthy eating before, during, and after school.

pack healthy lunches

When you send your child to school with a lunch box from home, make sure to pack it with both nutrition and taste in mind. Because so many of the packaged convenience options are high in calories, fat, and sodium, your child is usually much better off with a homemade lunch. A balanced meal includes one serving of vegetables or salad, one serving of fruit (fresh, canned, or dried), one whole-grain food, one serving of a fat-free or low-fat dairy food, one serving of a protein source, and a healthy sugar-free drink, such as water, fat-free or low-fat (1%) milk, or no-sugar-added 100 percent juice. Try these ideas when making healthy lunches for your kids:

- Replace white bread with whole-grain, and try pitas or corn tortillas for variety.

- Spread peanut butter or all-fruit spread on a toasted whole-wheat waffle. Top it off with a second toasted waffle to make a sandwich.

- Cut fat-free, low-sodium turkey or ham into bite-size pieces. Pack them with a plastic fork and a packet of mustard or hot sauce for dipping.

- Pack a salad as an entrée and include a protein, such as beans or a hard-boiled egg. When you serve salad for dinner, make a little extra to set aside for the next day's lunch.

- Kids love finger foods: send grilled asparagus spears cut into 1-inch pieces, or steam broccoli florets and slice them into smaller "trees." Send along a packet or separate container of light dressing.

- Try whole-grain pasta and tomato sauce in a resealable container.

- Pack a fruit for dessert. Bananas, apples, and oranges come "wrapped" and ready to go.

- Mix a handful of unsalted nuts with some dried fruit or high-fiber/low-sugar cereal for a healthy snack.

limit screen time and encourage sleep

"Screen time" includes watching television shows and movies, playing video games, and surfing the Web. With kids spending so much time on passive entertainment, there isn't much left for the daily 60 minutes or more of physical activity that experts recommend. Sitting instead of doing can also encourage unhealthy snacking. Until you do a reality check at home, you may not realize just how much screen time your children are getting in each day. Try these strategies to help everyone cut down:

- Set firm limits for the entire family. You'll be amazed how much extra time you "find" when you turn off the TV or computer.

- Don't use screen time to reward a child or take it away as punishment. Recognize and praise your child for being physically active and let passive activities be a "nonevent."

- Help your kids come up with alternatives to watching TV after school. Write out a list of activities such as riding bikes, shooting hoops, skating, dancing, or even folding laundry or mowing the lawn. Post the list where your kids can check it when they get home.

- Turn off the TV during meals. Use the time at the table to share events of the day.

- Take the TVs and computers out of your kids' bedrooms. Children who have TVs in their rooms spend almost 1½ hours more each day watching them than kids who don't have their own TVs. In addition, if your kids are in their rooms watching TV, they're not interacting with the family.

Although sleep is important for everyone's health, that's especially true for kids. In general, children need a lot of sleep each night to recharge and energize (see the chart below). Over time, lack of restful sleep can lead to serious health problems. Chronically tired kids are low on energy and tend to perform less well in school and other activities. They also tend to rely on unhealthy, high-calorie drinks and snacks to boost their flagging energy levels. To help your child both sleep and eat better, set a defined bedtime and keep the preceding hour calm and soothing. Turn off the TV and computer games for that hour, don't offer anything more to eat or drink, and keep bedrooms quiet, cool, and dark for better sleep.

amount of sleep recommended for children by the national sleep foundation

Age Group	Number of Hours
Infants (3 to 11 months)	9 to 12 at night; 30-minute to 2-hour naps, one to four times a day
Toddlers (1 to 3 years)	12 to 14
Preschoolers (3 to 5 years)	11 to 13
School Age (5 to 12 years)	10 to 11
Adolescents and Teens (13 to 17 years)	8½ to 9¼

Kids who make small, progressive changes in their behavior are likely to stick with new habits for good. Even more important, they will be better equipped to make the right choices when they are on their own. Just like adults, kids who feel valued and good about themselves flourish. Encourage your children to explore activities that develop their unique strengths. If kids are busy with exciting and active interests and hobbies, they won't need to rely on passive entertainment to fill their time. Finally, the best way to avoid weight gain is to prevent it in the first place. By teaching your children good eating habits and the joy of an active lifestyle now, you are setting them up for success that will last a lifetime.

part II
Menu Planning and Recipes

MENU PLANNING

RECIPES

MENU PLANNING

The core approach of the No-Fad Diet is to help you move from high-calorie, nutrient-poor foods to low-calorie, nutritious choices. Following an established eating strategy (see page 28) can set you on a healthy course to make that move. Because your environment and existing habits influence many of your food selections, having such an eating plan in place—one that helps you know what and how much to eat—can teach you how to make lower-calorie, healthier food choices.

about the menu plans

Using the American Heart Association's dietary recommendations as our foundation for creating a healthy diet, we developed two weeks' worth of menu plans for each of three calorie levels—1,200, 1,600, and 2,000. In addition to counting calories, each week's menus offer all the important components of a heart-healthy eating plan, including:

- The suggested number of servings of the different types of foods you need to achieve a proper balance of vegetables, fruit, grains (especially whole grains), dairy products, and foods that provide protein

- Two servings of fish and two or three vegetarian meals, as well as legumes, nuts, and healthy oils

The menus are designed so that most foods are used for the same meal at all calorie levels. This makes it easy for you to stay within your calorie count and still enjoy eating with the rest of the household. For example, if you are on the 1,200-calorie plan and your spouse or roommate is on a higher-calorie plan or is not following the No-Fad Diet, you and the other person can basically eat the same things at the same time, making only minor changes, such as serving size, to suit each person's individual needs.

using and personalizing the menu plans

To get started, you need to know what calorie level is right for you. If you aren't sure, check the calorie worksheet on page 16 for help with determining how many calories you should be consuming to lose weight. Next, review the set of menus for your particular calorie level. (If your calorie level is different from the three calorie levels provided in our sample menu plans, you can identify the menus that come closest to your calorie needs and make adjustments by eating more or less of the suggested foods.)

Now, identify which foods you like and which you don't; then feel free to make comparable substitutions to replace the "don't likes." For example, if the broccoli in a given menu plan doesn't appeal to you, substitute another green vegetable. Eat the afternoon snack in the morning if you'd rather or choose a different snack option, such as one suggested in the Snack Ideas charts on pages 426 and 427. You also might want to create your own list of favorite "flex" foods—vegetables and fruit you already keep on hand and can easily swap for a similar suggested dish in our menu plans.

Let's say you want to try a different entrée instead of the one listed in the sample menu. If dinner calls for grilled salmon but you prefer broiled tuna, go ahead and switch to the tuna. You will, of course, need to note the calorie difference in your eating plan. You can do that in several ways: check the nutrition label on the food package, look in a calorie-counter book, or go online to myfoodapedia.gov. You also can easily make swaps by referring to the list of entrées (page 421) in the No-Fad Toolkit, which provides calories and servings of various food groups in one portion for each recipe. Looking at dinner on the first Tuesday, for example, you'll see that Honey-Lime Flank Steak is the main dish and that it contains 188 calories and counts as one protein. If you don't like beef, just check the chart for entrées that offer roughly the same calorie count and food group profile. Then it's a simple matter of choosing from those recipes the one that's most appealing to you.

The American Heart Association Menu Plans are designed to be suggestions, not prescriptions; at first, it may be easier to follow these sample menu plans as they are, but we encourage you to experiment and customize the food choices to best suit *your* lifestyle and *your* preferences. These menus are geared to be flexible, so go ahead and make substitutions and changes. As you shop, just be sure that your food combinations stay within the parameters of your calorie range, the basic food groups, recommended portion sizes, and limits for sodium, saturated fat, trans fat, and cholesterol. (See Chapter 2, "Eat Well," for more detailed information.)

We recognize that the idea of counting calories and following menu plans may seem daunting at first. However, we've developed our menu plans with a busy and realistic lifestyle in mind, and we've incorporated a number of things to simplify using the plans. You'll find that the menus:

- Offer snack suggestions that are portable so you can easily take the snacks to work, to school, or on errand runs.

- Suggest servings for many of the perishable foods, particularly fruit, on several days of the same week so you can shop in quantity and avoid wasting food.

- Note where leftovers from one meal can be used for another meal.

- Limit cooking from recipes during the week, since most people have more time to cook on the weekends.

- Round the calorie counts for individual portions to the nearest multiple of 5 to make it easier to track total calories. The idea is to stay aware of what you are eating, not to obsess about exact calculations.

> **As you look over the menu plans, you'll see that each day's suggestions are designed to provide a good balance of the basic food groups, which are abbreviated throughout this book as follows:**
>
> GR = Grain
> VG = Vegetable/Legume
> FR = Fruit
> DA = Dairy
> PRO = Protein from seafood, lean meat or poultry, or vegetarian source
> FAT = Healthy fats and oils

creating your own menu plans

To help make healthy eating a habit, you will want to develop a few menu plans that best suit your personal tastes and lifestyle. Once you create some menus that incorporate favorite foods and favorite recipes in a healthy balance, the work is done; you can rotate your menu plans every few weeks for variety yet simplicity.

Before you actually begin menu planning, get an overview of all the helpful resources in the No-Fad Toolkit. Start by reviewing the Menu Planner Chart by Food Group (page 420). This at-a-glance summary makes it a no-brainer to see the numbers of servings you need of the core food groups. Once you get used to thinking in terms of building a plan from servings of the basic food groups, you will find it easier to choose each day's meals and satisfy your preferences. For example, breakfast for the 1,200-calorie plan includes one serving each of grain, fruit, and dairy products. If you keep that in mind, you will easily be able to include those food groups every morning, regardless of which foods you actually choose from each category. (The information on page 33 gives you ideas of different food choices and how much of each equals one portion.)

Next, take a look at My Menu Planner (page 419), a blank template intended to help you build your menus. The Entrée Recipes by Calorie Count and Food Group (page 421), Snack Idea charts (pages 426 and 427), and Common Foods by Calorie Count (page 428) also will help you plan menus. Another important resource is the recipe section (pages 124–412), where you'll find nearly 200 recipes to choose from in creating delicious and healthy meals. Each recipe includes a graphic that shows you at a glance how many calories that recipe contains.

Now you're ready to really get started. There's no right or wrong way to build a menu plan, so it's best to begin wherever makes the most sense for you. For instance, you might want to start with the foods that you know you will eat during the week. Think about what you enjoy having on a regular basis—perhaps bread or a glass of wine with dinner or Friday pizza with your co-workers. You don't need to give up your favorites; you just need to build them into your eating plan. Once you've accounted for these foods, you can fill in the remaining snacks and meals to customize your meal plan according to your calorie level and nutritional needs.

Providing nutritional balance and variety and eating foods that are enjoyable and healthy are the cornerstones to sustaining you through your weight-loss journey and to maintaining your weight-loss success.

1,200 calories
day 1: monday

	Calories	Food Group
breakfast		
¾ cup high-fiber cereal with	115	1 GR
1 cup fat-free milk	85	1 DA
½ cup sliced strawberries	25	1 FR
1 tablespoon chopped walnuts	50	
	275	
snack		
1 medium apple	**95**	1 FR
lunch		
Sandwich of 2 slices whole-grain bread with	140	2 GR
2 ounces grilled chicken breast	95	1 PRO
1 tablespoon light mayonnaise	35	1 FAT
½ cup dark green lettuce and 4 tomato slices	20	1 VG
	290	
snack		
8 ounces fat-free yogurt, plain or sugar-free, with	125	1 DA
½ medium banana	55	1 FR
	180	
dinner		
3 ounces grilled or baked salmon	125	1 PRO
½ cup *Italian Barley and Mushrooms* (page 358)	110	1 GR
1 cup steamed broccoli with salt-free lemon pepper	45	2 VG
2 cups leafy greens and ½ cup chopped cucumber with	30	3 VG
2 tablespoons *Sun-Dried Tomato Vinaigrette* (page 163)	45	1 FAT
	355	
daily totals	**1,195**	**6 VG, 3 FR, 4 GR, 2 DA, 2 PRO, 2 FAT**

1,200 calories
day 2: tuesday

breakfast

	Calories	Food Group
1 cup *Banana-Blueberry Smoothies* (page 139)	185	1 DA, 1 FR
½ whole-wheat English muffin, toasted, with	65	1 GR
1 teaspoon all-fruit spread	15	
	265	

snack

	Calories	Food Group
¾ cup *Smoky Roasted Tomato Soup* without optional ingredients (page 148) or 8 ounces low-sodium mixed vegetable juice	**80**	1 VG

lunch

	Calories	Food Group
2 ounces grilled chicken breast on	95	1 PRO
2 cups leafy greens and ½ cup chopped vegetables with	45	3 VG
2 tablespoons *Sun-Dried Tomato Vinaigrette* (page 163)	45	1 FAT
1 cup green grapes	110	2 FR
	295	

snack

	Calories	Food Group
2 crispbreads, choice of flavor	75	1 GR
1 ounce fat-free Cheddar or Swiss cheese	45	1 DA
	120	

dinner

	Calories	Food Group
1 serving *Honey-Lime Flank Steak** (page 278; extra steak reserved for *Flank Steak Salad with Sesame-Lime Dressing*—Day 4)	190	1 PRO
½ cup brown rice	110	1 GR
½ cup zucchini cooked in 1 teaspoon olive oil	50	1 VG, 1 FAT
1 cup sliced strawberries and blueberries	55	2 FR
	405	

	Calories	Food Group
daily totals	**1,165**	**5 VG, 5 FR, 3 GR, 2 DA, 2 PRO, 2 FAT**

*Prepare the steak in the morning to allow time to marinate.

1,200 calories
day 3: wednesday

	Calories	Food Group
breakfast		
1 serving *Fruit-and-Yogurt Breakfast Parfaits* (page 389)	230	½ DA, 1 FR
½ whole-wheat English muffin, toasted, with	65	1 GR
1 teaspoon all-fruit spread	15	
	310	
snack		
1 medium orange	**80**	1 FR
lunch		
Sandwich of 2 slices whole-grain bread with	140	2 GR
3 ounces very low sodium albacore tuna	90	1 PRO
1 tablespoon light mayonnaise	35	1 FAT
½ cup dark green lettuce	5	½ VG
½ cup raw baby carrots	25	1 VG
	295	
snack		
1 medium apple	95	1 FR
1 ounce fat-free Cheddar or Swiss cheese	45	1 DA
	140	
dinner		
1 serving *Fresh Veggie Marinara with Feta* (page 318)	**375**	1 PRO, 1 GR 3 VG
Time-Saver: Make extra pasta for tomorrow's dinner.		
daily totals	**1,200**	**4½ VG, 3 FR, 4 GR, 1½ DA, 2 PRO, 1 FAT**

1,200 calories
day 4: thursday

	Calories	Food Group
breakfast		
¾ cup high-fiber cereal with	115	1 GR
1 cup fat-free milk	85	1 DA
1 cup sliced strawberries	55	2 FR
	255	
snack		
1 medium apple	**95**	1 FR
lunch		
1 serving *Flank Steak Salad with Sesame-Lime Dressing* (page 184) using steak from *Honey-Lime Flank Steak* (Day 2)	230	1 PRO, 2 VG
4 whole-wheat crackers	80	1 GR
¾ cup *Smoky Roasted Tomato Soup* without optional ingredients (page 148) or 8 ounces low-sodium mixed vegetable juice	80	1 VG
	390	
snack		
2 crispbreads, choice of flavor	75	1 GR
1 ounce fat-free Cheddar or Swiss cheese	45	1 DA
	120	
dinner		
1 serving *Black-Pepper Chicken* (page 239)	155	1 PRO
½ cup whole-wheat penne with dried basil and	85	1 GR
2 teaspoons Parmesan cheese	15	
1 teaspoon olive oil	40	1 FAT
1 cup steamed broccoli with salt-free lemon pepper	45	2 VG
	340	
daily totals	**1,200**	**5 VG, 3 FR, 4 GR, 2 DA, 2 PRO, 1 FAT**

1,200 calories
day 5: friday

	Calories	Food Group
breakfast		
8 ounces fat-free yogurt, plain or sugar-free, with	125	1 DA
½ cup blueberries	40	1 FR
1 slice whole-grain bread, toasted, with	70	1 GR
1 teaspoon all-fruit spread	15	
	250	
snack		
4 whole-wheat crackers	80	1 GR
1 ounce fat-free Cheddar or Swiss cheese	45	1 DA
	125	
lunch		
Restaurant option or choice of meal less than 400 calories, less than 7 g saturated fat, and less than 600 mg sodium	**400**	1 PRO*
snack		
½ cup raw baby carrots with	25	1 VG
1 tablespoon light Ranch dressing	25	½ FAT
	50	
dinner		
1 serving *Cannellini and Black Bean Salad* (page 185)	210	1 PRO, 3 VG, 1 FR
1 medium whole-grain roll	95	1 GR
½ cup green grapes	55	1 FR
	360	
daily totals	**1,185**	**4 VG, 3 FR, 3 GR, 2 DA, 2 PRO, ½ FAT***

*Plus foods from lunch choices.

1,200 calories
day 6: saturday

	Calories	Food Group
breakfast		
1 *Cheesy Florentine Egg Cup* (page 386)	75	1 PRO
1 cup mixed fruit, such as sliced pineapple, strawberries, and bananas	70	2 FR
½ whole-wheat English muffin, toasted, with	65	1 GR
1 teaspoon all-fruit spread	15	
1 cup fat-free milk	85	1 DA
	310	
snack		
1 cup *Cran-Raspberry Smoothies* (page 138)	**125**	1 DA
lunch		
1 *Miami Pita Sandwich* (page 336)	**325**	1 PRO, 2 GR, 1 VG
snack		
2 medium ribs of celery with	20	1 VG
¼ cup *Cucumber and Avocado Dip* (page 127)	55	
	75	
dinner		
1 serving *Grilled Sirloin Kebabs with Creamy Herb Dipping Sauce* (page 282)	220	1 PRO, 1 VG
½ cup *Orzo with Tomato and Capers* (page 367)	105	1 GR
	325	
daily totals	**1,160**	**3 VG, 2 FR, 4 GR, 2 DA, 3 PRO**

1,200 calories
day 7: sunday

	Calories	Food Group

breakfast

	Calories	Food Group
1 *Peach Cornmeal Waffle* (page 384) topped with	190	1 GR, ½ FR
½ cup sliced peaches	40	1 FR
2 tablespoons sugar-free maple syrup	10	
	240	

snack

8 whole-wheat crackers	160	2 GR
1 cup fat-free milk	85	1 DA
	245	

lunch

1 serving *Taco Salad with Avocado Dressing* (page 186)	**330**	1 PRO, 1 GR, 1 VG

snack

1 medium orange	**80**	1 FR

dinner

1 serving *Slow-Roasted Sage Turkey Breast** (page 238)	125	1 PRO
½ cup *Smashed Potatoes with Aromatic Herbs* (page 369)	105	1 VG
½ cup *Stewed Zucchini and Cherry Tomatoes* (page 375)	50	1 VG
2 cups leafy greens with	20	2 VG
2 tablespoons *Sun-Dried Tomato Vinaigrette* (page 163)	45	1 FAT
	345	

	Calories	Food Group
daily totals	**1,240**	**5 VG, 2½ FR, 4 GR, 1 DA, 2 PRO, 1 FAT**

*Use leftovers in meals for Days 9 and 10.**

1,200 calories
day 8: monday

	Calories	Food Group
breakfast		
¾ cup cooked oatmeal with	125	1 GR
2 tablespoons raisins or other dried fruit	60	½ FR
2 tablespoons chopped pecans	95	
1 cup fat-free milk	85	1 DA
	365	
snack		
1 serving *Lemon-Ginger Trail Mix* (page 136)	**120**	½ GR
lunch		
Sandwich of 2 slices whole-grain bread with	140	2 GR
1 ounce (2 slices) fat-free American cheese	40	1 DA
2 teaspoons mustard, if desired	5	
½ cup dark green lettuce and 4 tomato slices	20	1 VG
½ cup raw baby carrots	25	1 VG
	230	
snack		
½ cup cooked edamame	**100**	1 PRO
dinner		
1 95% lean broiled beef patty (3 ounces cooked) with	130	1 PRO
1 tablespoon ketchup (lowest sodium available)	15	
½ cup *Lemon-Herb Brown Rice* (page 371)	90	1 GR
8 spears steamed asparagus with lemon and	30	2 VG
1 teaspoon light tub margarine	15	1 FAT
1 cup sliced strawberries	55	2 FR
	335	
daily totals	**1,150**	**4 VG, 2½ FR, 4½ GR, 2 DA, 2 PRO, 1 FAT**

1,200 calories
day 9: tuesday

	Calories	Food Group
breakfast		
1 cup *Banana-Blueberry Smoothies* (page 139)	185	1 DA, 1 FR
½ whole-wheat English muffin, toasted, with	65	1 GR
1 teaspoon all-fruit spread	15	
	265	
snack		
1 medium apple	**95**	1 FR
lunch		
1 serving *Fruit and Spinach Salad with Fresh Mint* (page 165)	135	2 VG, 1 FR
Roll-up of 2 ounces sliced turkey breast* with	75	1 PRO
1 ounce (2 slices) fat-free Swiss cheese	40	1 DA
	250	
snack		
2 servings *Lemon-Ginger Trail Mix* (page 136)	**245**	1 GR
dinner		
1 serving *Tuna and Broccoli with Lemon-Caper Brown Rice* (page 219)	265	1 PRO, 1 GR, 1 VG
½ cup steamed baby carrots with cinnamon and	20	1 VG
1 teaspoon light tub margarine	15	1 FAT
	300	
daily totals	**1,155**	**4 VG, 3 FR, 3 GR, 2 DA, 2 PRO, 1 FAT**

*Use leftover *Slow-Roasted Sage Turkey Breast* from Day 7.

1,200 calories
day 10: wednesday

	Calories	Food Group
breakfast		
¾ cup cooked oatmeal with	125	1 GR
½ cup blueberries	40	1 FR
1 cup fat-free milk	85	1 DA
	250	
snack		
8 ounces fat-free, sugar-free vanilla yogurt or choice of flavor	**125**	1 DA
lunch		
Sandwich of 2 slices whole-grain bread with	140	2 GR
2 ounces sliced turkey breast* or chicken breast	75	1 PRO
1 tablespoon light mayonnaise	35	1 FAT
½ cup dark green lettuce	5	½ VG
½ medium green bell pepper	10	1 VG
	265	
snack		
1 medium banana with	105	2 FR
1 tablespoon low-sodium peanut butter	100	
	205	
dinner		
1 serving *Slow-Cooker Black Bean Chili* (page 332) topped with	325	1 PRO, 2 GR, 1 VG
1 medium tomato, chopped	20	1 VG
	345	
daily totals	**1,190**	**3½ VG, 3 FR, 5 GR, 2 DA, 2 PRO, 1 FAT**

*Use leftover *Slow-Roasted Sage Turkey Breast* from Day 7.

1,200 calories
day 11: thursday

	Calories	Food Group
breakfast		
1 slice whole-grain bread, toasted, with	70	1 GR
2 tablespoons low-sodium peanut butter	200	
½ cup cubed cantaloupe	25	1 FR
1 cup fat-free milk	85	1 DA
	380	
snack		
1 medium Bartlett pear	**105**	1 FR
lunch		
1 serving *Spinach and Salmon Salad with Spicy Orange Dressing* (page 179)	210	1 PRO, 1 GR, 2 VG
2 crispbreads, choice of flavor	75	1 GR
	285	
snack		
3 medium ribs of celery with	30	2 VG
3 tablespoons whipped low-fat cream cheese	60	1 DA
	90	
dinner		
1 serving *Pork Tenderloin with Cranberry Salsa* (page 306)	205	1 PRO, 1 FR
½ medium sweet potato, baked, with	50	1 VG
2 tablespoons sugar-free maple syrup and cinnamon	10	
½ cup steamed green beans with lemon and	20	1 VG
1 teaspoon light tub margarine	15	1 FAT
	300	
daily totals	**1,160**	**6 VG, 3 FR, 3 GR, 2 DA, 2 PRO, 1 FAT**

1,200 calories
day 12: friday

	Calories	Food Group
breakfast		
1 cup *Banana-Blueberry Smoothies* (page 139)	185	1 DA, 1 FR
½ whole-wheat English muffin, toasted, with	65	1 GR
1 teaspoon all-fruit spread	15	
	265	
snack		
4 whole-wheat crackers with	80	1 GR
2 tablespoons whipped low-fat cream cheese	40	½ DA
	120	
lunch		
Restaurant option or choice of meal less than 400 calories, less than 7 g saturated fat, and less than 600 mg sodium	**400**	1 PRO*
snack		
½ cup raw baby carrots	**25**	1 VG
dinner		
1 serving *Tilapia en Papillote* (page 204)	130	1 PRO
1 cup *Mixed Vegetable Grill* (page 376) on	75	2 VG
½ cup brown rice	110	1 GR
1 medium orange	80	1 FR
	395	
daily totals	**1,205**	**3 VG, 2 FR, 3 GR, 1½ DA, 2 PRO***

*Plus foods from lunch choices.

1,200 calories
day 13: saturday

	Calories	Food Group
breakfast		
1 cup cubed cantaloupe	55	2 FR
1 *Cheesy Florentine Egg Cup* (page 386)	75	1 PRO
1 slice whole-grain bread, toasted, with	70	1 GR
1 teaspoon all-fruit spread	15	
	215	
snack		
½ cup sliced strawberries	**25**	1 FR
lunch		
1 serving *Chicken Minestrone* (page 156)	**230**	1 PRO, 1 GR, 1 VG
snack		
8 ounces fat-free yogurt, plain or sugar-free, with	125	1 DA
½ cup sliced peaches	30	1 FR
	155	
dinner		
1 serving *Stuffed Shells with Arugula and Four Cheeses* (page 324)	280	1 PRO, 1 GR, 1 DA
2 cups leafy greens and ½ cup chopped vegetables with	45	3 VG
2 tablespoons *Sun-Dried Tomato Vinaigrette* (page 163)	45	1 FAT
2 *Pumpkin Oatmeal Cookies* (page 400)	165	1 GR
	535	
daily totals	**1,160**	**4 VG, 4 FR, 4 GR, 2 DA, 3 PRO, 1 FAT**

1,200 calories
day 14: sunday

	Calories	Food Group
breakfast		
1 serving *Crisp French Toast* (page 385) with	170	1½ GR
3 tablespoons sugar-free maple syrup	20	
1 cup fat-free milk	85	1 DA
½ cup sliced strawberries	25	1 FR
	300	
snack		
1 medium apple	95	1 FR
1 ounce fat-free Cheddar or Swiss cheese	45	1 DA
	140	
lunch		
1 serving *Egg Drop Soup with Crabmeat and Vegetables* (page 152)	120	1 PRO, 1 VG
2 crispbreads, choice of flavor	75	1 GR
	195	
snack		
3 cups light (94% fat-free) microwaved popcorn	**60**	2 GR
dinner		
1 serving *Beef Stroganoff with Baby Bella Mushrooms* (page 288)	340	1 PRO, 1 GR, 1 VG
1 cup steamed broccoli with salt-free lemon pepper with	45	2 VG
1 teaspoon light tub margarine	15	1 FAT
½ cup pineapple chunks in their own juice	70	1 FR
	470	
daily totals	**1,165**	**4 VG, 3 FR, 5½ GR, 2 DA, 2 PRO, 1 FAT**

1,600 calories
day 1: monday

	Calories	Food Group
breakfast		
1½ cups high-fiber cereal with	225	2 GR
1 cup fat-free milk	85	1 DA
1 cup sliced strawberries	55	2 FR
1 tablespoon chopped walnuts	50	
	415	
snack		
1 medium apple	95	1 FR
1 ounce fat-free Cheddar or Swiss cheese	45	1 DA
	140	
lunch		
Sandwich of 2 slices whole-grain bread with	140	2 GR
2 ounces grilled chicken breast	95	1 PRO
1 tablespoon light mayonnaise	35	1 FAT
½ cup dark green lettuce and 4 tomato slices	20	1 VG
	290	
snack		
8 ounces fat-free yogurt, plain or sugar-free, with	125	1 DA
½ medium banana	55	1 FR
	180	
dinner		
3 ounces grilled or baked salmon	125	1 PRO
1 cup *Italian Barley and Mushrooms* (page 358)	215	2 GR, 1 VG
1 cup steamed broccoli with salt-free lemon pepper	45	2 VG
2 cups leafy greens and ½ cup chopped cucumber with	30	3 VG
2 tablespoons *Sun-Dried Tomato Vinaigrette* (page 163)	45	1 FAT
10 animal crackers	110	
	570	
daily totals	**1,595**	**7 VG, 4 FR, 6 GR, 3 DA, 2 PRO, 2 FAT**

1,600 calories
day 2: tuesday

	Calories	Food Group
breakfast		
1 cup *Banana-Blueberry Smoothies* (page 139)	185	1 DA, 1 FR
1 whole-wheat English muffin, toasted, with	135	2 GR
1 tablespoon all-fruit spread	40	
	360	
snack		
¾ cup *Smoky Roasted Tomato Soup* without optional ingredients (page 148) or 8 ounces low-sodium mixed vegetable juice	80	1 VG
6 whole-wheat crackers	120	1 GR
	200	
lunch		
3 ounces grilled chicken breast on	140	1 PRO
2 cups leafy greens and ½ cup chopped vegetables with	45	3 VG
2 tablespoons *Sun-Dried Tomato Vinaigrette* (page 163)	45	1 FAT
1 cup green grapes	110	2 FR
	340	
snack		
4 crispbreads, choice of flavor	145	2 GR
1 ounce fat-free Cheddar or Swiss cheese	45	1 DA
	190	
dinner		
1 serving *Honey-Lime Flank Steak** (page 278; extra steak reserved for *Flank Steak Salad with Sesame-Lime Dressing*—Day 4)	190	1 PRO
½ cup brown rice	110	1 GR
1 cup zucchini cooked in 1 teaspoon olive oil	60	2 VG, 1 FAT
½ cup fat-free frozen yogurt, choice of flavor, with	80	½ DA
1 cup sliced strawberries and blueberries	55	2 FR
	495	
daily totals	**1,585**	**6 VG, 5 FR, 6 GR, 2½ DA, 2 PRO, 2 FAT**

*Prepare the steak in the morning to allow time to marinate.

1,600 calories
day 3: wednesday

	Calories	Food Group
breakfast		
1 serving *Fruit-and-Yogurt Breakfast Parfaits* (page 389)	230	½ DA, 1 FR
1 whole-wheat English muffin, toasted, with	135	2 GR
1 tablespoon all-fruit spread	40	
	405	
snack		
1 medium apple	95	1 FR
2 ounces fat-free Cheddar or Swiss cheese	90	2 DA
	185	
lunch		
Sandwich of 2 slices whole-grain bread with	140	2 GR
3 ounces very low sodium albacore tuna	90	1 PRO
1 tablespoon light mayonnaise	35	1 FAT
½ cup dark green lettuce	5	½ VG
½ cup raw baby carrots	25	1 VG
1 medium orange	80	1 FR
	375	
snack		
2 medium ribs of celery	20	1 VG
2 tablespoons low-sodium peanut butter	200	
	220	
dinner		
1 serving *Fresh Veggie Marinara with Feta* (page 318)	**375**	1 PRO, 1 GR, 3 VG
Time-Saver: Make extra pasta for tomorrow's dinner.		
daily totals	**1,560**	**5½ VG, 3 FR, 5 GR, 2½ DA, 2 PRO, 1 FAT**

1,600 calories
day 4: thursday

	Calories	Food Group
breakfast		
1½ cups high-fiber cereal with	225	2 GR
1 cup fat-free milk	85	1 DA
1 cup sliced strawberries	55	2 FR
	365	
snack		
8 ounces fat-free yogurt, plain or sugar-free, with	125	1 DA
½ medium banana	55	1 FR
	180	
lunch		
1 serving *Flank Steak Salad with Sesame-Lime Dressing* (page 184) using steak from *Honey-Lime Flank Steak* (Day 2)	230	1 PRO, 2 VG
¾ cup *Smoky Roasted Tomato Soup* without optional ingredients (page 148) or 8 ounces low-sodium mixed vegetable juice	80	1 VG
1 medium orange	80	1 FR
	390	
snack		
2 cups light (94% fat-free) microwaved popcorn	**40**	2 GR
dinner		
1 serving *Black-Pepper Chicken* (page 239)	155	1 PRO
½ cup whole-wheat penne with dried basil and	85	1 GR
2 teaspoons Parmesan cheese	15	
1 teaspoon olive oil	40	1 FAT
1 cup steamed broccoli with salt-free lemon pepper	45	2 VG
2 *Pumpkin-Oatmeal Cookies* (page 400)	165	1 GR
1 cup fat-free milk	85	1 DA
	590	
daily totals	**1,565**	**5 VG, 4 FR, 6 GR, 3 DA, 2 PRO, 1 FAT**

1,600 calories
day 5: friday

	Calories	Food Group
breakfast		
8 ounces fat-free yogurt, plain or sugar-free, with	125	1 DA
½ cup blueberries	40	1 FR
2 slices whole-grain bread, toasted, with	140	2 GR
1 tablespoon all-fruit spread	40	
	345	
snack		
1 cup green grapes	**110**	2 FR
lunch		
Restaurant option or choice of meal less than 500 calories, less than 7 g saturated fat, and less than 600 mg sodium	**500**	1 PRO*
snack		
½ cup chopped raw vegetables of choice	25	1 VG
¼ cup *Cucumber and Avocado Dip* (page 127)	55	
2 crispbreads, choice of flavor	75	1 GR
	155	
dinner		
1 serving *Cannellini and Black Bean Salad* (page 185)	210	1 PRO, 3 VG, 1 FR
1 medium whole-grain roll	95	1 GR
1 cup fat-free frozen yogurt, choice of flavor	190	1 DA
	495	
daily totals	**1,605**	**4 VG, 4 FR, 4 GR, 2 DA, 2 PRO***

*Plus foods from lunch choices.

1,600 calories
day 6: saturday

	Calories	Food Group
breakfast		
1 *Cheesy Florentine Egg Cup* (page 386)	75	1 PRO
1 cup mixed fruit, such as sliced pineapple, strawberries, and bananas	70	2 FR
1 whole-wheat English muffin, toasted, with	135	2 GR
1 tablespoon all-fruit spread	40	
1 cup fat-free milk	85	1 DA
	405	
snack		
1 cup *Cran-Raspberry Smoothies* (page 138)	**125**	1 DA
lunch		
1 *Miami Pita Sandwich* (page 336)	325	1 PRO, 2 GR, 1 VG
1 medium apple	95	1 FR
	420	
snack		
2 medium ribs of celery with	20	1 VG
¼ cup *Cucumber and Avocado Dip* (page 127)	55	
	75	
dinner		
1 serving *Grilled Sirloin Kebabs with Creamy Herb Dipping Sauce* (page 282)	220	1 PRO, 1 VG
¾ cup *Orzo with Tomato and Capers* (page 367)	160	1½ GR
½ cup green beans with	20	1 VG
1 teaspoon light tub margarine	15	1 FAT
½ cup sliced peaches	40	1 FR
1 cup fat-free milk	85	1 DA
	565	
daily totals	**1,565**	**4 VG, 4 FR, 5½ GR, 3 DA, 3 PRO, 1 FAT**

1,600 calories
day 7: sunday

	Calories	Food Group
breakfast		
2 *Peach Cornmeal Waffles* (page 384) topped with	385	2 GR, 1 FR
1 cup sliced peaches	80	2 FR
¼ cup sugar-free maple syrup	25	
	490	
snack		
8 ounces fat-free yogurt, plain or sugar-free, with	125	1 DA
½ medium banana	55	1 FR
	180	
lunch		
1 serving *Taco Salad with Avocado Dressing* (page 186)	**330**	1 PRO, 1 GR, 1 VG
snack		
1 1-ounce 2% milk mozzarella cheese stick	80	1 DA
1 Roma tomato and fresh basil	10	1 VG
2 crispbreads, choice of flavor	75	1 GR
	165	
dinner		
1 serving *Slow-Roasted Sage Turkey Breast** (page 238)	125	1 PRO
½ cup *Smashed Potatoes with Aromatic Herbs* (page 369)	105	1 VG
½ cup *Stewed Zucchini and Cherry Tomatoes* (page 375)	50	1 VG
1 medium whole-grain roll	95	1 GR
2 cups leafy greens with	20	2 VG
2 tablespoons *Sun-Dried Tomato Vinaigrette* (page 163)	45	1 FAT
	440	
daily totals	**1,605**	**6 VG, 4 FR, 5 GR, 2 DA, 2 PRO, 1 FAT**

*Use leftovers in meals for Days 9 and 10.

1,600 calories
day 8: monday

	Calories	Food Group

breakfast

¾ cup cooked oatmeal with	125	1 GR
2 tablespoons raisins or other dried fruit	60	½ FR
2 tablespoons chopped pecans	95	
1 cup fat-free milk	85	1 DA
	365	

snack

2 servings *Lemon-Ginger Trail Mix* (page 136)	**245**	1 GR, ½ FR

lunch

Sandwich of 2 slices whole-grain bread with	140	2 GR
1½ ounces (3 slices) fat-free American cheese	65	1 DA
2 teaspoons mustard, if desired	5	
½ cup dark green lettuce and 4 tomato slices	20	1 VG
½ cup raw baby carrots	25	1 VG
1 medium Bartlett pear	105	1 FR
	360	

snack

½ cup cooked edamame	**100**	1 PRO

dinner

1 95% lean broiled beef patty (3 ounces cooked) with	130	1 PRO
1 tablespoon ketchup (lowest sodium available)	15	
1 cup *Lemon-Herb Brown Rice* (page 371)	180	2 GR
8 spears steamed asparagus with lemon and	30	2 VG
1 teaspoon light tub margarine	15	1 FAT
1 cup sliced strawberries with	55	2 FR
½ cup fat-free frozen yogurt, choice of flavor	80	½ DA
	505	

	Calories	Food Group
daily totals	**1,575**	**4 VG, 4 FR, 6 GR, 2½ DA, 2 PRO, 1 FAT**

1,600 calories
day 9: tuesday

	Calories	Food Group
breakfast		
1 cup *Banana-Blueberry Smoothies* (page 139)	185	1 DA, 1 FR
1 whole-wheat English muffin, toasted, with	135	2 GR
1 tablespoon all-fruit spread	40	
	360	
snack		
1 medium apple	95	1 FR
1 cup fat-free milk	85	1 DA
	180	
lunch		
1 serving *Fruit and Spinach Salad with Fresh Mint* (page 165)	135	2 VG, 1 FR
Sandwich of 1 whole-wheat 6-inch pita with	160	2 GR
2 ounces sliced turkey breast*	75	1 PRO
1 ounce (2 slices) fat-free Swiss cheese	40	1 DA
	410	
snack		
2 servings *Lemon-Ginger Trail Mix* (page 136)	**245**	1 GR
dinner		
1 serving *Tuna and Broccoli with Lemon-Caper Brown Rice* (page 219)	265	1 PRO, 1 GR, 1 VG
1 cup steamed baby carrots with cinnamon and	40	2 VG
1 teaspoon light tub margarine	15	1 FAT
½ cup fat-free frozen yogurt, choice of flavor	80	½ DA
	400	
daily totals	**1,595**	**5 VG, 3 FR, 6 GR, 3½ DA, 2 PRO, 1 FAT**

*Use leftover *Slow-Roasted Sage Turkey Breast* from Day 7.

1,600 calories
day 10: wednesday

	Calories	Food Group
breakfast		
¾ cup cooked oatmeal with	125	1 GR
½ cup blueberries	40	1 FR
1 cup fat-free milk	85	1 DA
	250	
snack		
8 ounces fat-free yogurt, plain or sugar-free, with	125	1 DA
½ cup sliced strawberries	25	1 FR
1 whole-wheat mini bagel	100	1 GR
	250	
lunch		
Sandwich of 2 slices whole-grain bread with	140	2 GR
3 ounces sliced turkey breast* or chicken breast	115	1 PRO
1 tablespoon light mayonnaise	35	1 FAT
½ cup dark green lettuce	5	½ VG
1 serving *Multicolored Marinated Slaw* (page 171)	80	1 VG
	375	
snack		
1 medium banana with	105	2 FR
2 tablespoons low-sodium peanut butter	200	
	305	
dinner		
1 serving *Slow-Cooker Black Bean Chili* (page 332) topped with	325	1 PRO, 2 GR, 1 VG
1 medium tomato, chopped	20	1 VG
½ medium green bell pepper, chopped	10	1 VG
1 6-inch corn tortilla	60	1 GR
	415	
daily totals	**1,595**	4½ VG, 4 FR, 7 GR, 2 DA, 2 PRO, 1 FAT

*Use leftover *Slow-Roasted Sage Turkey Breast* from Day 7.

1,600 calories
day 11: thursday

breakfast

	Calories	Food Group
1 slice whole-grain bread, toasted, with	70	1 GR
2 tablespoons low-sodium peanut butter	200	
½ cup cubed cantaloupe	25	1 FR
1 cup fat-free milk	85	1 DA
	380	

snack

1 medium Bartlett pear	105	1 FR
4 whole-wheat crackers	80	1 GR
	185	

lunch

1 serving *Spinach and Salmon Salad with Spicy Orange Dressing* (page 179)	210	1 PRO, 1 GR, 2 VG
1 6-inch whole-wheat pita	160	2 GR
1 medium apple	95	1 FR
	465	

snack

4 medium ribs of celery with	40	2 VG
¼ cup whipped low-fat cream cheese	80	1 DA
	120	

dinner

1 serving *Pork Tenderloin with Cranberry Salsa* (page 306)	205	1 PRO, 1 FR
½ medium sweet potato, baked, with	50	1 VG
2 tablespoons sugar-free maple syrup and cinnamon	10	
½ cup steamed green beans with lemon	20	1 VG
1 medium whole-grain roll with	95	1 GR
1 teaspoon light tub margarine	15	1 FAT
	395	

daily totals	**1,545**	**6 VG, 4 FR, 6 GR, 2 DA, 2 PRO, 1 FAT**

1,600 calories
day 12: friday

	Calories	Food Group
breakfast		
1 cup *Banana-Blueberry Smoothies* (page 139)	185	1 DA, 1 FR
1 whole-wheat English muffin, toasted, with	135	2 GR
1 tablespoon all-fruit spread	40	
	360	
snack		
4 whole-wheat crackers with	80	1 GR
2 tablespoons whipped low-fat cream cheese	40	½ DA
	120	
lunch		
Restaurant option or choice of meal less than 500 calories, less than 7 g saturated fat, and less than 600 mg sodium	**500**	1 PRO*
snack		
½ cup raw baby carrots with	25	1 VG
2 tablespoons light Ranch dressing	45	1 FAT
	70	
dinner		
1 serving *Tilapia en Papillote* (page 204)	130	1 PRO
1 cup *Mixed Vegetable Grill* (page 376) on	75	2 VG
½ cup brown rice	110	1 GR
1 medium orange	80	1 FR
1 cup fat-free milk	85	1 DA
	480	
movie snack		
3 cups light (94% fat-free) microwaved popcorn	**60**	2 GR
daily totals	**1,590**	**3 VG, 2 FR, 6 GR, 2½ DA, 2 PRO, 1 FAT***

*Plus foods from lunch choices.

1,600 calories
day 13: saturday

	Calories	Food Group
breakfast		
1 cup cubed cantaloupe	55	2 FR
1 *Cheesy Florentine Egg Cup* (page 386)	75	1 PRO
2 slices whole-grain bread, toasted, with	140	2 GR
1 tablespoon all-fruit spread	40	
	310	
snack		
1 cup sliced strawberries	**55**	2 FR
lunch		
1 serving *Chicken Minestrone* (page 156)	230	1 PRO, 1 GR, 1 VG
2 whole-wheat breadsticks	80	1 GR
1 cup fat-free milk	85	1 DA
	395	
snack		
8 ounces fat-free yogurt, plain or sugar-free, with	125	1 DA
½ cup sliced peaches	30	1 FR
½ ounce chopped walnuts	95	
	250	
dinner		
1 serving *Stuffed Shells with Arugula and Four Cheeses* (page 324)	280	1 PRO, 1 GR, 1 DA
2 cups leafy greens and 1 cup chopped vegetables with	70	4 VG
2 tablespoons *Sun-Dried Tomato Vinaigrette* (page 163)	45	1 FAT
2 *Pumpkin Oatmeal Cookies* (page 400)	165	1 GR
	560	
daily totals	**1,570**	**5 VG, 5 FR, 6 GR, 3 DA, 3 PRO, 1 FAT**

1,600 calories
day 14: sunday

	Calories	Food Group
breakfast		
1 serving *Crisp French Toast* (page 385) with	170	1½ GR
3 tablespoons sugar-free maple syrup	20	
1 cup fat-free milk	85	1 DA
½ cup sliced strawberries	25	1 FR
	300	
snack		
1 medium apple	95	1 FR
1 *Pumpkin Oatmeal Cookie* (page 400)	85	½ GR
	180	
lunch		
1 serving *Egg Drop Soup with Crabmeat and Vegetables* (page 152)	120	1 PRO, 1 VG
3 crispbreads, choice of flavor	110	1½ GR
2 cups leafy greens with	20	2 VG
2 tablespoons *Sun-Dried Tomato Vinaigrette* (page 163)	45	1 FAT
1 medium orange	80	1 FR
	375	
snack		
1½ ounces fat-free Cheddar or Swiss cheese	70	1 DA
2 cups light (94% fat-free) microwaved popcorn	40	2 GR
	110	
dinner		
1 serving *Beef Stroganoff with Baby Bella Mushrooms* (page 288)	340	1 PRO, 1 GR, 1 VG
1 cup steamed broccoli with salt-free lemon pepper with	45	2 VG
1 teaspoon light tub margarine	15	1 FAT
1 slice *Apple and Pear Strudel* (page 402)	200	1 FR
	600	
daily totals	**1,565**	**6 VG, 4 FR, 6½ GR, 2 DA, 2 PRO, 2 FAT**

2,000 calories
day 1: monday

	Calories	Food Group
breakfast		
1½ cups high-fiber cereal with	225	2 GR
1 cup fat-free milk	85	1 DA
1 cup sliced strawberries	55	2 FR
1 tablespoon chopped walnuts	50	
	415	
snack		
1 medium apple	95	1 FR
2 crispbreads, choice of flavor	75	1 GR
1 tablespoon low-sodium peanut butter	100	
	270	
lunch		
Sandwich of 2 slices whole-grain bread with	140	2 GR
3 ounces grilled chicken breast	140	1 PRO
1 tablespoon light mayonnaise	35	1 FAT
½ cup dark green lettuce and 4 tomato slices	20	1 VG
1 slice *Apple and Dried Cherry Quick Bread* (page 379)	80	
	415	
snack		
8 ounces fat-free yogurt, plain or sugar-free, with	125	1 DA
1 medium banana, sliced	105	2 FR
	230	
dinner		
3 ounces grilled or baked salmon	125	1 PRO
1 cup *Italian Barley and Mushrooms* (page 358)	215	2 GR, 1 VG
1 cup steamed broccoli with salt-free lemon pepper	45	2 VG
1 medium whole-grain roll	95	1 GR
2 cups leafy greens and ½ cup chopped cucumber with	30	3 VG
2 tablespoons *Sun-Dried Tomato Vinaigrette* (page 163)	45	1 FAT
10 animal crackers	110	
	665	
daily totals	**1,995**	**7 VG, 5 FR, 8 GR, 2 DA, 2 PRO, 2 FAT**

2,000 calories
day 2: tuesday

	Calories	Food Group
breakfast		
1 cup *Banana-Blueberry Smoothies* (page 139)	185	1 DA, 1 FR
1 whole-wheat English muffin, toasted, with	135	2 GR
1 tablespoon all-fruit spread	40	
	360	
snack		
4 crispbreads, choice of flavor	145	2 GR
1 ounce fat-free Cheddar or Swiss cheese	45	1 DA
	190	
lunch		
¾ cup *Smoky Roasted Tomato Soup* without optional ingredients (page 148) or 8 ounces low-sodium mixed vegetable juice	80	1 VG
4 whole-wheat crackers	80	1 GR
3 ounces grilled chicken breast on	140	1 PRO
2 cups leafy greens and ½ cup chopped vegetables with	45	3 VG
2 tablespoons *Sun-Dried Tomato Vinaigrette* (page 163)	45	1 FAT
1 cup green grapes	110	2 FR
	500	
snack		
3 cups light (94% fat-free) microwaved popcorn	**60**	2 GR
dinner		
1 serving *Honey-Lime Flank Steak** (page 278; extra steak reserved for *Flank Steak Salad with Sesame-Lime Dressing*—Day 4)	190	1 PRO
1 cup brown rice mixed with ½ cup cooked mushrooms	235	2 GR, 1 VG
1 cup zucchini cooked in 1 teaspoon olive oil	60	2 VG, 1 FAT
1 cup sliced strawberries and blueberries	55	2 FR
1 serving *Cinnamon-Walnut Biscotti* (page 397)	185	
1 cup fat-free milk	85	1 DA
	810	
daily totals	**1,920**	**7 VG, 5 FR, 9 GR, 3 DA, 2 PRO, 2 FAT**

*Prepare the steak in the morning to allow time to marinate.

2,000 calories
day 3: wednesday

	Calories	Food Group
breakfast		
1 serving *Fruit-and-Yogurt Breakfast Parfaits* (page 389)	230	½ DA, 1 FR
1 whole-wheat English muffin, toasted, with	135	2 GR
1 tablespoon all-fruit spread	40	
	405	
snack		
1 medium apple	95	1 FR
6 whole-wheat crackers	120	2 GR
	215	
lunch		
Sandwich of 2 slices whole-grain bread with	140	2 GR
3 ounces very low sodium albacore tuna	90	1 PRO
1 tablespoon light mayonnaise	35	1 FAT
½ cup dark green lettuce	5	½ VG
½ cup raw baby carrots	25	1 VG
1 medium orange	80	1 FR
	375	
snack		
3 medium ribs of celery with	30	1½ VG
3 tablespoons low-sodium peanut butter	300	
	330	
dinner		
1 serving *Fresh Veggie Marinara with Feta* (page 318) Time-Saver: Make extra pasta for tomorrow's dinner.	375	1 PRO, 1 GR, 3 VG
½ cup pineapple chunks	40	1 FR
1 serving *Cinnamon-Walnut Biscotti* (page 397)	185	
1 cup fat-free milk	85	1 DA
	685	
daily totals	**2,010**	**6 VG, 4 FR, 7 GR, 1½ DA, 2 PRO, 1 FAT**

2,000 calories
day 4: thursday

	Calories	Food Group
breakfast		
1½ cups high-fiber cereal with	225	2 GR
1 cup fat-free milk	85	1 DA
1 cup sliced strawberries	55	2 FR
2 tablespoons chopped pecans	95	
	460	
snack		
8 ounces fat-free yogurt, plain or sugar-free, with	125	1 DA
1 medium banana, sliced	105	2 FR
	230	
lunch		
1 serving *Flank Steak Salad with Sesame-Lime Dressing* (page 184) using steak from *Honey-Lime Flank Steak* (Day 2)	230	1 PRO, 2 VG
¾ cup *Smoky Roasted Tomato Soup* without optional ingredients (page 148) or 8 ounces low-sodium mixed vegetable juice	80	1 VG
1 medium orange	80	1 FR
1 slice *Apple and Dried Cherry Quick Bread* (page 379)	80	
	470	
snack		
3 cups light (94% fat-free) microwaved popcorn	**60**	2 GR
dinner		
1 serving *Black-Pepper Chicken* (page 239)	155	1 PRO
1 cup whole-wheat penne with dried basil and	175	2 GR
1 tablespoon Parmesan cheese	20	
2 teaspoons olive oil	80	2 FAT
1 cup broccoli and ½ cup red bell pepper, steamed, with salt-free lemon pepper	65	3 VG
2 *Pumpkin Oatmeal Cookies* (page 400)	165	1 GR
1 cup fat-free milk	85	1 DA
	745	
daily totals	**1,965**	**6 VG, 5 FR, 7 GR, 3 DA, 2 PRO, 2 FAT**

2,000 calories
day 5: friday

	Calories	Food Group
breakfast		
8 ounces fat-free yogurt, plain or sugar-free, with	125	1 DA
½ cup blueberries	40	1 FR
2 slices whole-grain bread, toasted, with	140	2 GR
1 tablespoon all-fruit spread	40	
	345	
snack		
1 cup green grapes	**110**	2 FR
lunch		
Restaurant option or choice of meal less than 600 calories, less than 7 g saturated fat, and less than 600 mg sodium	**600**	1 PRO*
snack		
1 cup chopped raw vegetables of choice	55	2 VG
½ cup *Cucumber and Avocado Dip* (page 127)	110	
4 crispbreads, choice of flavor	145	2 GR
	310	
dinner		
1 serving *Cannellini and Black Bean Salad* (page 185)	210	1 PRO, 3 VG, 1 FR
1 medium whole-grain roll	95	1 GR
1 ear corn on the cob with	80	1 VG
1 teaspoon light tub margarine	15	1 FAT
1 cup fat-free frozen yogurt, choice of flavor	190	1 DA
	590	
daily totals	**1,955**	**6 VG, 4 FR, 5 GR, 2 DA, 2 PRO, 1 FAT***

*Plus foods from lunch choices.

2,000 calories
day 6: saturday

	Calories	Food Group
breakfast		
1 *Cheesy Florentine Egg Cup* (page 386)	75	1 PRO
1 cup mixed fruit, such as sliced pineapple, strawberries, and bananas	70	2 FR
1 whole-wheat English muffin, toasted, with	135	2 GR
1 tablespoon all-fruit spread	40	
1 cup fat-free milk	85	1 DA
	405	
snack		
1 cup *Cran-Raspberry Smoothies* (page 138)	125	1 DA
1 serving *Cinnamon-Walnut Biscotti* (page 397)	185	
	310	
lunch		
1 *Miami Pita Sandwich* (page 336)	325	1 PRO, 2 GR, 1 VG
1 medium apple	95	1 FR
	420	
snack		
4 medium ribs of celery with	40	2 VG
½ cup *Cucumber and Avocado Dip* (page 127)	110	
	150	
dinner		
1 serving *Grilled Sirloin Kebabs with Creamy Herb Dipping Sauce* (page 282)	220	1 PRO, 1 VG
1 cup *Orzo with Tomato and Capers* (page 367)	215	2 GR
½ cup green beans with	20	1 VG
1 teaspoon light tub margarine	15	1 FAT
1 serving *Peach and Pineapple Upside-Down Cake* (page 392) with	100	
½ cup sliced peaches	40	1 FR
1 cup fat-free milk	85	1 DA
	695	
daily totals	**1,980**	**5 VG, 4 FR, 6 GR, 3 DA, 3 PRO, 1 FAT**

2,000 calories
day 7: sunday

	Calories	Food Group
breakfast		
2 *Peach Cornmeal Waffles* (page 384) topped with	385	2 GR, 1 FR
1 cup sliced peaches	80	2 FR
¼ cup sugar-free maple syrup	25	
	490	
snack		
8 ounces fat-free yogurt, plain or sugar-free, with	125	1 DA
½ medium banana	55	1 FR
2 tablespoons chopped pecans	95	
	275	
lunch		
1 serving *Taco Salad with Avocado Dressing* (page 186)	330	1 PRO, 1 GR, 1 VG
1 cup fat-free milk	85	1 DA
	415	
snack		
6 whole-wheat crackers	120	2 GR
1 1-ounce 2% milk mozzarella cheese stick	80	1 DA
1 Roma tomato and fresh basil	10	1 VG
	210	
dinner		
1 serving *Slow-Roasted Sage Turkey Breast** (page 238)	125	1 PRO
¾ cup *Smashed Potatoes with Aromatic Herbs* (page 369)	155	1 VG
½ cup *Stewed Zucchini and Cherry Tomatoes* (page 375)	50	1 VG
1 medium whole-grain roll with	95	1 GR
1 teaspoon light tub margarine	15	1 FAT
2 cups leafy greens with	20	2 VG
2 tablespoons *Sun-Dried Tomato Vinaigrette* (page 163)	45	1 FAT
1 medium orange	80	1 FR
	585	
daily totals	**1,975**	**6 VG, 5 FR, 6 GR, 3 DA, 2 PRO, 2 FAT**

*Use leftovers in meals for Days 9 and 10.

2,000 calories
day 8: monday

	Calories	Food Group

breakfast

1 cup cooked oatmeal with	165	1 GR
¼ cup raisins or other dried fruit	125	1 FR
2 tablespoons chopped pecans	95	
1 cup fat-free milk	85	1 DA
	470	

snack

3 servings *Lemon-Ginger Trail Mix* (page 136)	**365**	1 GR, 1 FR

lunch

Sandwich of 2 slices whole-grain bread with	140	2 GR
1½ ounces (3 slices) fat-free American cheese	65	1 DA
2 teaspoons mustard, if desired	5	
½ cup dark green lettuce and 4 tomato slices	20	1 VG
1 cup raw baby carrots	50	2 VG
1 medium Bartlett pear	105	1 FR
	385	

snack

¾ cup cooked edamame	**150**	1 PRO

dinner

1 95% lean broiled beef patty (3 ounces cooked) with	130	1 PRO
1 tablespoon ketchup (lowest sodium available)	15	
1 cup *Lemon-Herb Brown Rice* (page 371)	180	2 GR
8 spears steamed asparagus with lemon and	30	2 VG
1 teaspoon light tub margarine	15	1 FAT
1 cup fat-free frozen yogurt, choice of flavor, with	160	1 DA
1 cup sliced strawberries	55	2 FR
	585	

	Calories	Food Group
daily totals	**1,955**	**5 VG, 5 FR, 6 GR, 3 DA, 2 PRO, 1 FAT**

2,000 calories
day 9: tuesday

|---|---|---|

breakfast

1 cup *Banana-Blueberry Smoothies* (page 139)	185	1 DA, 1 FR
1 whole-wheat English muffin, toasted, with	135	2 GR
1 tablespoon all-fruit spread	40	
	360	

snack

1 medium apple	95	1 FR
2 crispbreads, choice of flavor	75	1 GR
1 cup fat-free milk	85	1 DA
	255	

lunch

1 serving *Fruit and Spinach Salad with Fresh Mint* (page 165)	135	2 VG, 1 FR
Sandwich of 1 whole-wheat 6-inch pita with	160	2 GR
2 ounces sliced turkey breast*	75	1 PRO
1 ounce (2 slices) fat-free Swiss cheese	40	1 DA
½ cup fat-free frozen yogurt, choice of flavor	80	½ DA
	490	

snack

3 servings *Lemon-Ginger Trail Mix* (page 136)	**365**	1 GR, 1 FR

dinner

1 serving *Tuna and Broccoli with Lemon-Caper Brown Rice* (page 219)	265	1 PRO, 1 GR, 1 VG
1 cup steamed baby carrots with cinnamon and	40	2 VG
1 teaspoon light tub margarine	15	1 FAT
1 medium whole-wheat roll	95	1 GR
1 Bartlett pear	105	1 FR
	520	

daily totals	**1,990**	**5 VG, 5 FR, 8 GR, 3½ DA, 2 PRO, 1 FAT**

*Use leftover *Slow-Roasted Sage Turkey Breast* from Day 7.

2,000 calories
day 10: wednesday

	Calories	Food Group
breakfast		
1 cup cooked oatmeal with	165	1 GR
1 cup blueberries	80	2 FR
1 cup fat-free milk	85	1 DA
	330	
snack		
8 ounces fat-free yogurt, plain or sugar-free, with	125	1 DA
½ cup sliced strawberries	25	1 FR
2 whole-wheat mini bagels	200	2 GR
	350	
lunch		
Sandwich of 2 slices whole-grain bread with	140	2 GR
3 ounces sliced turkey breast* or chicken breast	115	1 PRO
1 tablespoon light mayonnaise	35	1 FAT
½ cup dark green lettuce	5	1 VG
1 serving *Multicolored Marinated Slaw* (page 171)	80	1 VG
	375	
snack		
1 medium banana with	105	2 FR
3 tablespoons low-sodium peanut butter	300	
	405	
dinner		
1 serving *Slow-Cooker Black Bean Chili* (page 332), topped with	325	1 PRO, 2 GR, 1 VG
1 medium tomato, chopped	20	1 VG
½ medium green bell pepper, chopped	10	1 VG
1 6-inch corn tortilla	60	1 GR
1 *Citrus Freeze Bar* (page 412)	135	
	550	
daily totals	**2,010**	**5 VG, 5 FR, 8 GR, 2 DA, 2 PRO, 1 FAT**

*Use leftover *Slow-Roasted Sage Turkey Breast* from Day 7.

2,000 calories
day 11: thursday

	Calories	Food Group
breakfast		
1 slice whole-grain bread, toasted, with	70	1 GR
2 tablespoons low-sodium peanut butter	200	
1 cup cubed cantaloupe	55	2 FR
1 cup fat-free milk	85	1 DA
	410	
snack		
1 medium Bartlett pear	105	1 FR
8 whole-wheat crackers	160	2 GR
	265	
lunch		
1 serving *Spinach and Salmon Salad with Spicy Orange Dressing* (page 179)	210	1 PRO, 1 GR, 2 VG
1 6-inch whole-wheat pita	160	2 GR
1 medium apple	95	1 FR
2 *Pumpkin Oatmeal Cookies* (page 400)	165	1 GR
	630	
snack		
4 medium ribs of celery with	40	2 VG
¼ cup whipped low-fat cream cheese	80	1 DA
	120	
dinner		
1 serving *Pork Tenderloin with Cranberry Salsa* (page 306)	205	1 PRO, 1 FR
½ medium sweet potato, baked, with	50	1 VG
2 tablespoons sugar-free maple syrup and cinnamon	10	
½ cup steamed green beans with lemon	20	1 VG
1 medium whole-grain roll with	95	1 GR
1 teaspoon light tub margarine	15	1 FAT
1 *Citrus Freeze Bar* (page 412)	135	
	530	
daily totals	**1,955**	**6 VG, 5 FR, 8 GR, 2 DA, 2 PRO, 1 FAT**

2,000 calories
day 12: friday

	Calories	Food Group

breakfast

1 cup *Banana-Blueberry Smoothies* (page 139)	185	1 DA, 1 FR
1 whole-wheat English muffin, toasted, with	135	2 GR
1 tablespoon all-fruit spread	40	
½ cup cubed cantaloupe	25	1 FR
	385	

snack

8 whole-wheat crackers	160	2 GR
1 1-ounce 2% milk mozzarella cheese stick	70	1 DA
	230	

lunch

Restaurant option or choice of meal less than 600 calories, less than 7 g saturated fat, and less than 600 mg sodium	**600**	1 PRO*

snack

1 cup raw baby carrots	55	2 VG
1 ounce unsalted almonds	175	
	230	

dinner

1 serving *Tilapia en Papillote* (page 204)	130	1 PRO
1 cup *Mixed Vegetable Grill* (page 376) on	75	2 VG
½ cup brown rice	110	1 GR
1 medium orange	80	1 FR
1 cup fat-free milk	85	1 DA
	480	

movie snack

3 cups light (94% fat-free) microwaved popcorn	**60**	2 GR

	daily totals	**1,985**	**4 VG, 3 FR, 7 GR, 3 DA, 2 PRO***

*Plus foods from lunch choices.

2,000 calories
day 13: saturday

	Calories	Food Group
breakfast		
1 cup cubed cantaloupe	55	2 FR
1 *Cheesy Florentine Egg Cup* (page 386)	75	1 PRO
2 slices whole-grain bread, toasted, with	140	2 GR
1 tablespoon all-fruit spread	40	
	310	
snack		
1 cup sliced strawberries	**55**	2 FR
lunch		
1 serving *Chicken Minestrone* (page 156)	230	1 PRO, 1 GR, 1 VG
2 whole-wheat breadsticks	80	1 GR
1 cup fat-free milk	85	1 DA
1 *Citrus Freeze Bar* (page 412)	135	
	530	
snack		
8 ounces fat-free yogurt, plain or sugar-free, with	125	1 DA
½ cup sliced peaches	30	1 FR
1½ ounces chopped walnuts	275	
	430	
dinner		
1 serving *Stuffed Shells with Arugula and Four Cheeses* (page 324)	280	1 PRO, 1 GR, 1 DA
1 piece (1 ounce) Italian bread with	75	1 GR
1 teaspoon light tub margarine	15	1 FAT
2 cups leafy greens with	20	2 VG
1 cup chopped vegetables of choice	50	2 VG
2 tablespoons *Sun-Dried Tomato Vinaigrette* (page 163)	45	1 FAT
2 *Pumpkin Oatmeal Cookies* (page 400)	165	1 GR
	650	
daily totals	**1,975**	**5 VG, 5 FR, 7 GR, 3 DA, 2 PRO, 2 FAT**

2,000 calories
day 14: sunday

	Calories	Food Group
breakfast		
1 serving *Crisp French Toast* (page 385) with	170	1½ GR
3 tablespoons sugar-free maple syrup	20	
1 cup fat-free milk	85	1 DA
1 cup sliced strawberries	55	2 FR
	330	
snack		
1 medium apple	95	1 FR
2 *Pumpkin Oatmeal Cookies* (page 400)	165	1 GR
	260	
lunch		
1 serving *Egg Drop Soup with Crabmeat and Vegetables* (page 152)	120	1 PRO, 1 VG
3 crispbreads, choice of flavor	110	1½ GR
2 cups leafy greens with	20	2 VG
2 tablespoons *Sun-Dried Tomato Vinaigrette* (page 163)	45	1 FAT
1 medium orange	80	1 FR
1 *Citrus Freeze Bar* (page 412)	135	
	510	
snack		
1 whole-wheat mini bagel with	100	1 GR
2 tablespoons whipped low-fat cream cheese	40	1 DA
	140	
dinner		
1 serving *Beef Stroganoff with Baby Bella Mushrooms* (page 288)	340	1 PRO, 1 GR, 1 VG
1 cup steamed broccoli with salt-free lemon pepper	45	2 VG
1 medium whole-grain roll with 1 teaspoon light tub margarine	110	1 GR, 1 FAT
1 slice *Apple and Pear Strudel* (page 402)	200	1 FR
1 cup fat-free milk	85	1 DA
	780	
daily totals	**2,020**	**6 VG, 5 FR, 7 GR, 3 DA, 2 PRO, 2 FAT**

RECIPES

about the recipes

For every recipe, we provide an analysis of the nutrients included. Because of the many variables involved in analyzing foods, however, the values should be considered approximate.

- Each analysis is based on a single serving, unless otherwise indicated.

- When ingredient options are listed, the first one is analyzed.

- When a range of amounts is given, the average is analyzed.

- Optional ingredients and garnishes are not included in the nutrition analysis.

- The specific ingredients listed in each recipe were analyzed. If you make ingredient substitutions, remember that the nutrition values will change. In most cases, using similar foods (for example, bottled lemon juice for fresh or white onions instead of yellow) won't change the values enough to matter; if you use a low-fat cheese instead of fat-free, however, the calories, fat values, and amount of sodium will be significantly different.

- We use the lowest-sodium products that are widely available, and we encourage you to compare nutrition facts labels and shop for low-sodium products whenever possible. If you have to substitute a high-sodium ingredient, remember to adjust the nutrition values for that recipe. To keep the level of sodium in our recipes low, we call for unprocessed foods or no-salt-added and low-sodium products when possible and add a small amount of table salt sparingly for flavor.

- To keep the cholesterol within reasonable limits, we often use egg substitute instead of whole eggs. For optimal taste and texture, however, we may call for whole eggs or a combination of eggs and egg whites or egg substitute, especially in baked goods.

- Because product labeling in the marketplace can vary and change quickly, we use the generic terms "fat-free" and "low-fat" throughout to avoid confusion.

- We specify canola, corn, and olive oils in these recipes, but you can also use other heart-healthy unsaturated oils, such as safflower, soybean, and sunflower.

- Nutrient values except for fats are rounded to the nearest whole number. Fats are rounded to the nearest half gram; because of the rounding, the amounts for saturated, trans, monounsaturated, and polyunsaturated fats may not add up to the amount of total fat.

- Analyses of meat are based on cooked lean meat with all visible fat discarded.

- For ground beef, we use 95% fat-free meat.

- When meat, poultry, or seafood is marinated and the marinade is discarded, we calculate only the amount of marinade absorbed.

- When alcohol is used in a dish that is cooked, we estimate that most of the alcohol calories evaporate during cooking.

- When no quantity is listed for an ingredient in a recipe (for example, the small amount of flour used to prepare a surface for kneading dough), that ingredient is not included in the analysis.

- We use the abbreviations *g* for "gram" and *mg* for "milligram."

appetizers, snacks, and beverages

Cucumber and Avocado Dip

Artichoke and Spinach Dip

Creamy Cannellini Dip

Kiwi-Banana Dip

Crunchy Cinnamon Chips

Fruit Kebabs with Dipping Sauces

   Yucatán Dipping Sauce

   Maple-Peanut Dipping Sauce

   Poppy Seed Dipping Sauce

Mini Tarts with Cucumber Salsa and Salmon

Lemon-Ginger Trail Mix

Frozen Chocolate Banana Pops

Cran-Raspberry Smoothies

Banana-Blueberry Smoothies

Orange Froth

Green-Tea Lattes

cucumber and avocado dip

serves 6; ¼ cup per serving

So cool and creamy, this jade-green dip is the perfect accompaniment for a platter of raw or grilled vegetables.

- 1 medium cucumber, peeled, cut in half lengthwise, seeded, and cut crosswise into 1-inch slices
- 1 small avocado, diced
- ¼ cup fat-free sour cream
- 1 teaspoon grated lime zest
- 1 tablespoon fresh lime juice
- 2 teaspoons snipped fresh dillweed or ½ teaspoon dried, crumbled
- ¼ teaspoon salt

In a food processor or blender, process the ingredients until smooth. Serve or refrigerate in an airtight container for up to two days.

COOK'S TIP For an interesting side dish, try using this dip on baked potatoes instead of topping them with the more traditional, much-higher-calorie butter and full-fat sour cream and cheese.

····· PER SERVING ·····

calories 55	cholesterol 2 mg	
total fat 3.5 g	sodium 108 mg	
saturated fat 0.5 g	carbohydrates 5 g	
trans fat 0.0 g	fiber 2 g	
polyunsaturated fat 0.5 g	sugars 1 g	
monounsaturated fat 2.5 g	protein 1 g	

100 200 300 400

DIETARY EXCHANGES
1 vegetable, 1 fat

artichoke and spinach dip

serves 15; ¼ cup per serving

Serve raw bell pepper strips of assorted colors, carrot and celery sticks, and broccoli and cauliflower florets with this low-calorie version of a popular dip. It also partners well with steamed vegetables or toasted wedges of whole-grain pita bread.

- 1 15.5-ounce can no-salt-added cannellini beans, rinsed and drained
- 4 medium green onions, chopped
- 2 medium garlic cloves, minced
- 1 14-ounce can quartered artichoke hearts, drained, or 9-ounce package frozen artichoke hearts, thawed and drained
- 1 10-ounce package frozen chopped spinach, thawed and squeezed dry
- 1 cup fat-free plain yogurt
- 1 teaspoon grated lemon zest
- 3 tablespoons fresh lemon juice
- ½ teaspoon ground cumin
- ¼ teaspoon crushed red pepper flakes
- ¼ teaspoon salt
- ¼ teaspoon pepper

In a food processor or blender, process the beans, green onions, and garlic until smooth.

Add the remaining ingredients. Process until smooth. Refrigerate in an airtight container for 2 hours to 4 days before serving.

PER SERVING

calories 48	cholesterol 0 mg
total fat 0.5 g	sodium 123 mg
saturated fat 0.0 g	carbohydrates 8 g
trans fat 0.0 g	fiber 2 g
polyunsaturated fat 0.0 g	sugars 2 g
monounsaturated fat 0.0 g	protein 3 g

100 200 300 400

DIETARY EXCHANGES
½ starch

creamy cannellini dip

serves 8; ¼ cup per serving

Bits of roasted red bell pepper add texture and color to this tantalizing dip, which pairs well with raw veggies. The beans add fiber and protein, making the dip an excellent energy-boosting snack when you need a midday pick-me-up.

1   15.5-ounce can no-salt-added cannellini beans, rinsed and drained

¼   cup fat-free sour cream

2   tablespoons snipped fresh parsley

1   tablespoon fresh lemon juice

1   large garlic clove, minced

½   teaspoon red hot-pepper sauce, or to taste

¼   teaspoon salt

1   7-ounce jar roasted red bell peppers, drained

In a food processor or blender, process the ingredients except the roasted peppers for 15 to 20 seconds, or until almost smooth.

Add the roasted peppers. Pulse until they are distributed throughout the dip but are still large enough to add texture. Refrigerate in an airtight container for 2 to 48 hours. Stir before serving.

COOK'S TIP ON SNIPPING PARSLEY To easily cut parsley down to size, put a small amount in a small measuring cup or custard cup. Point kitchen shears or small, sharp scissors down into the cup. Snip until the parsley pieces are the size you want.

PER SERVING

calories 58	cholesterol 1 mg
total fat 0.5 g	sodium 148 mg
saturated fat 0.0 g	carbohydrates 10 g
trans fat 0.0 g	fiber 2 g
polyunsaturated fat 0.0 g	sugars 1 g
monounsaturated fat 0.0 g	protein 3 g

100   200   300   400

DIETARY EXCHANGES
½ starch

kiwi-banana dip

serves 4; ¼ cup per serving

Be adventurous with this dip by switching to different fruit and all-fruit spreads.

¼ cup fat-free plain yogurt

1 tablespoon sweetened dried cherries or sweetened dried cranberries

1 tablespoon all-fruit orange marmalade

1 small banana, chopped

1 medium kiwifruit, peeled and chopped

In a small bowl, stir together the yogurt, cherries, and marmalade. Gently stir in the banana and kiwifruit.

PER SERVING
calories 60
total fat 0.0 g
  saturated fat 0.0 g
  trans fat 0.0 g
  polyunsaturated fat 0.0 g
  monounsaturated fat 0.0 g
cholesterol 0 mg
sodium 13 mg
carbohydrates 14 g
  fiber 1 g
  sugars 9 g
protein 2 g

100 200 300 400

DIETARY EXCHANGES
1 fruit

crunchy cinnamon chips

serves 4; 4 chips per serving

These tasty chips are a satisfying snack on their own, or try them with Kiwi-Banana Dip on the facing page.

1½ teaspoons sugar

1½ teaspoons firmly packed light brown sugar

¼ teaspoon ground cinnamon

2 8-inch fat-free flour tortillas (lowest sodium available)

Cooking spray

Preheat the oven to 375°F.

In a small bowl, stir together the sugars and cinnamon.

Stack the tortillas and cut them into 8 equal triangles (16 total). Put the triangles in a single layer on a baking sheet. Lightly spray the triangles with cooking spray. Sprinkle with the sugar mixture.

Bake for 6 to 8 minutes, or until the chips are light brown and beginning to crisp. Transfer to a large plate to cool. (As the chips cool, they will become crisper.)

PER SERVING

calories 73
total fat 0.5 g
  saturated fat 0.0 g
  trans fat 0.0 g
  polyunsaturated fat 0.0 g
  monounsaturated fat 0.0 g

cholesterol 0 mg
sodium 171 mg
carbohydrates 15 g
  fiber 1 g
  sugars 4 g
protein 2 g

100 200 300 400

DIETARY EXCHANGES
1 starch

fruit kebabs with dipping sauces

serves 4; ½ cup fruit and 2 tablespoons sauce per serving

Even when you are watching your calories, you can enjoy these attractive kebabs with a choice of three delicious yogurt dipping sauces, all of which could also be great dressings for fruit salad. Substitute in-season fruits when making the kebabs, if you wish.

1 recipe Yucatán, Maple-Peanut, or Poppy Seed Dipping Sauce (recipes follow)

2 medium kiwifruit, peeled and halved lengthwise, then crosswise (8 pieces total)

4 1-inch pineapple cubes

12 seedless red grapes

4 large strawberries, hulled

In a small bowl, stir together the ingredients for your choice of sauce. Cover and refrigerate for at least 1 hour.

Slide the fruit onto four 6-inch wooden skewers, in the following order: kiwifruit, pineapple, grape, strawberry, grape, kiwifruit, grape. (The grapes keep the strawberries from discoloring the other fruits.) Serve the kebabs with the chilled dipping sauce.

yucatán dipping sauce

½ cup fat-free vanilla yogurt

1½ teaspoons fresh lime juice

¼ teaspoon cayenne, or to taste

Scant ⅛ teaspoon salt

maple-peanut dipping sauce

½ cup fat-free plain yogurt

1 tablespoon smooth peanut butter

1 teaspoon maple syrup

Scant ⅛ teaspoon salt

poppy seed dipping sauce

½ cup fat-free vanilla yogurt

1 teaspoon poppy seeds

½ teaspoon very finely grated onion, or to taste

¼ to ½ teaspoon raspberry vinegar

⅛ to ¼ teaspoon dry mustard

Scant ⅛ teaspoon salt

FRUIT KEBABS WITH YUCATÁN DIPPING SAUCE
PER SERVING

calories 75	cholesterol 1 mg
total fat 0.5 g	sodium 58 mg
saturated fat 0.0 g	carbohydrates 17 g
trans fat 0.0 g	fiber 2 g
polyunsaturated fat 0.0 g	sugars 13 g
monounsaturated fat 0.0 g	protein 2 g

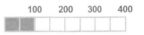

DIETARY EXCHANGES
1 fruit

FRUIT KEBABS WITH MAPLE-PEANUT DIPPING SAUCE
PER SERVING

calories 102	cholesterol 1 mg
total fat 2.5 g	sodium 76 mg
saturated fat 0.5 g	carbohydrates 19 g
trans fat 0.0 g	fiber 2 g
polyunsaturated fat 0.5 g	sugars 15 g
monounsaturated fat 1.0 g	protein 3 g

DIETARY EXCHANGES
1 fruit, ½ fat

FRUIT KEBABS WITH POPPY SEED DIPPING SAUCE
PER SERVING

calories 79	cholesterol 1 mg
total fat 0.5 g	sodium 58 mg
saturated fat 0.0 g	carbohydrates 17 g
trans fat 0.0 g	fiber 2 g
polyunsaturated fat 0.5 g	sugars 13 g
monounsaturated fat 0.0 g	protein 3 g

DIETARY EXCHANGES
1 fruit

mini tarts with cucumber salsa and salmon

serves 5; 3 mini tarts per serving

Light, crisp, and flaky mini phyllo shells are the perfect "nests" for this trendy salmon-and-cucumber appetizer. The shells are already cooked—all you have to do is thaw them.

⅓ cup fat-free plain yogurt

1 tablespoon finely chopped fresh dillweed and 15 sprigs of fresh dillweed, divided use

1½ teaspoons dehydrated minced onion

¼ teaspoon red hot-pepper sauce

salsa

½ cup finely diced unpeeled English, or hothouse, cucumber

2 tablespoons chopped green onions

1 tablespoon diced fresh jalapeño, seeds and ribs discarded

1½ teaspoons plain rice vinegar

1 teaspoon grated peeled gingerroot

½ teaspoon sugar

½ teaspoon toasted sesame oil

1 1.9-ounce package frozen mini phyllo shells (15 mini shells), thawed

1 3-ounce vacuum-sealed pouch boneless, skinless pink salmon, flaked gently

In a small bowl, stir together the yogurt, 1 tablespoon chopped dillweed, dehydrated onion, and hot-pepper sauce. Cover and refrigerate for 30 minutes to 2 hours, stirring occasionally if longer than 30 minutes.

In a small bowl, stir together the salsa ingredients. Cover and refrigerate for 30 minutes to 2 hours.

To assemble the tarts, spoon 1 teaspoon yogurt mixture into each phyllo shell. Top with 1 heaping teaspoon salsa. Spoon 1 heaping teaspoon salmon over the salsa, pressing gently so it adheres to the salsa. Garnish each tart with a dillweed sprig. Serve within 30 minutes of preparation so the phyllo shells remain crisp.

····· PER SERVING ···

calories 85
total fat 4.0 g
  saturated fat 0.5 g
  trans fat 0.0 g
  polyunsaturated fat 0.5 g
  monounsaturated fat 0.5 g

cholesterol 6 mg
sodium 135 mg
carbohydrates 8 g
  fiber 0 g
  sugars 2 g
protein 4 g

100   200   300   400

DIETARY EXCHANGES
½ starch, ½ lean meat,
½ fat

lemon-ginger trail mix

serves 4; ¼ cup plus 2 tablespoons per serving

This trail mix is crunchy, fruity, and nutty, with just a hint of ginger. Store individual servings in resealable snack-size plastic bags so you'll always have a ready-to-go snack to take to work or run errands.

¾ cup high-fiber cereal squares

¼ cup slivered almonds

¼ cup unsalted pumpkin seeds

¼ cup dried apple slices, chopped

2 tablespoons sweetened dried cranberries

1 teaspoon grated lemon zest

½ teaspoon grated peeled gingerroot

In a large nonstick skillet, stir together the ingredients. Cook over medium-high heat for 2 to 3 minutes, or until beginning to lightly brown, separating the bits of lemon zest and gingerroot and stirring frequently. Spread in a single layer over a large plate to cool quickly. Store the cooled mixture in an airtight container for up to two weeks.

PER SERVING

calories 122
total fat 4.5 g
  saturated fat 0.5 g
  trans fat 0.0 g
  polyunsaturated fat 1.5 g
  monounsaturated fat 2.5 g

cholesterol 0 mg
sodium 56 mg
carbohydrates 19 g
  fiber 2 g
  sugars 8 g
protein 3 g

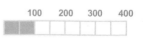

DIETARY EXCHANGES
1 starch, ½ fruit, 1 fat

frozen chocolate banana pops

serves 4; 1 pop per serving

Young children will enjoy helping you prepare this fun after-school snack. Keep a supply handy in the freezer for a filling nibble—for you and for them.

1   cup fat-free plain yogurt

1   very ripe medium banana, mashed (⅓ to ½ cup)

½   teaspoon vanilla extract

2   tablespoons fat-free chocolate syrup and 2 teaspoons fat-free chocolate syrup, divided use

1   tablespoon mini semisweet chocolate chips and 2 teaspoons mini semisweet chocolate chips, divided use

In a small bowl, stir together the yogurt, banana, and vanilla.

Stir in 2 tablespoons chocolate syrup and 1 tablespoon chocolate chips.

Divide the remaining 2 teaspoons chocolate chips into four 4- to 7-ounce paper or plastic juice cups. Spoon 3 tablespoons yogurt mixture over the chips in each cup. Spoon the remaining 2 teaspoons chocolate syrup over the banana mixture. Top with the remaining yogurt mixture.

Insert a wooden craft or Popsicle stick into the center of each filled cup. Cover with plastic wrap or aluminum foil, poking the stick through the covering. Place the cups with the stick side up on a flat surface in the freezer. Freeze for 2 hours, or until frozen. To serve, uncover and peel the frozen pops or gently squeeze them out of the cups.

PER SERVING

calories 120	cholesterol 1 mg
total fat 1.5 g	sodium 56 mg
saturated fat 1.0 g	carbohydrates 23 g
trans fat 0.0 g	fiber 1 g
polyunsaturated fat 0.0 g	sugars 16 g
monounsaturated fat 0.5 g	protein 4 g

100   200   300   400

DIETARY EXCHANGES
½ fruit, ½ fat-free milk,
½ carbohydrate

cran-raspberry smoothies

serves 4; 1 cup per serving

No time to make breakfast before work? Pop these five ingredients into a food processor or blender and you'll have a healthy beverage in just minutes. Pour it into a to-go travel mug and be on your way!

12 ounces fat-free raspberry yogurt

1 cup frozen unsweetened raspberries

1 cup fat-free milk

1 cup light cran-raspberry juice drink

¼ teaspoon vanilla extract

In a food processor or blender, process all the ingredients until thick and smooth. Serve immediately.

···········PER SERVING············

calories 127

total fat 0.0 g

  saturated fat 0.0 g

  trans fat 0.0 g

  polyunsaturated fat 0.0 g

  monounsaturated fat 0.0 g

cholesterol 5 mg

sodium 101 mg

carbohydrates 26 g

  fiber 1 g

  sugars 21 g

protein 6 g

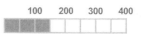

100 200 300 400

DIETARY EXCHANGES

1 fat-free milk, 1 fruit

banana-blueberry smoothies

serves 2; 1 cup per serving

Start your day off right with this fruit-laden smoothie for breakfast or enjoy it as a cold, refreshing mid-morning or mid-afternoon snack.

8 ounces fat-free milk

6 ounces fat-free plain yogurt

1 cup fresh or frozen blueberries

1 medium banana, cut into large chunks

In a food processor or blender, process the ingredients until smooth.

····· PER SERVING ··········

calories 184
total fat 0.5 g
  saturated fat 0.0 g
  trans fat 0.0 g
  polyunsaturated fat 0.0 g
  monounsaturated fat 0.0 g

cholesterol 4 mg
sodium 118 mg
carbohydrates 37 g
  fiber 3 g
  sugars 27 g
protein 10 g

100   200   300   400

DIETARY EXCHANGES
1½ fruit, 1 fat-free milk

orange froth

serves 4; ½ cup per serving

To replace a calorie-laden soft drink, try this light, fizzy fruit-based beverage.

2 cups crushed ice
1 6-ounce can frozen orange juice concentrate
6 ounces lime-flavored sparkling water

In a food processor or blender, process the crushed ice and orange juice concentrate until smooth.

Pour in the sparkling water. Process just long enough to combine. Serve immediately.

PER SERVING

calories 68
total fat 0.0 g
  saturated fat 0.0 g
  trans fat 0.0 g
  polyunsaturated fat 0.0 g
  monounsaturated fat 0.0 g

cholesterol 0 mg
sodium 9 mg
carbohydrates 16 g
  fiber 0 g
  sugars 16 g
protein 1 g

100   200   300   400

DIETARY EXCHANGES
1 fruit

green-tea lattes

serves 4; 1 cup per serving

This frothy beverage—garnished with festive fruit—is a nice complement at breakfast or a refreshing weekend snack as you do chores around the house. Keep chilled green tea and a variety of fruit juices on hand so you can make it anytime.

- 1 cup water
- 4 single-serving green-tea bags
- 1 cup fruit nectar or fruit juice, such as apricot, mango, guava, or tropical blend
- 1 cup fat-free milk
- 1 cup ice cubes
- ½ star fruit, cut crosswise into 4 slices (optional)

In a small saucepan, bring the water to a boil over high heat. Remove from the heat. Put the tea bags in the water and let steep, covered, for 5 minutes. Discard the tea bags.

In a blender, process the tea, nectar, milk, and ice cubes until smooth. Pour into tall glasses.

Cut a small slit in each slice of star fruit. Place a slice over the rim of each glass.

COOK'S TIP ON STAR FRUIT Also called carambola, star fruit looks like a star when cut crosswise. Do not peel it before slicing. Look for star fruit from August through February. If it is not available when you prepare this recipe, you can substitute 4 large strawberries or orange, lemon, or lime slices.

PER SERVING

calories 56	cholesterol 1 mg
total fat 0.0 g	sodium 29 mg
saturated fat 0.0 g	carbohydrates 12 g
trans fat 0.0 g	fiber 0 g
polyunsaturated fat 0.0 g	sugars 3 g
monounsaturated fat 0.0 g	protein 2 g

100 200 300 400

DIETARY EXCHANGES
1 fruit

soups

Quick Mexican-Style Soup

Cream of Triple-Mushroom Soup

Artichoke and Spinach Soup

Creamy Broccoli Soup with Sour Cream and Cheddar

Smoky Roasted Tomato Soup

Chilled Blueberry Soup

Egg Drop Soup with Crabmeat and Vegetables

Wild Rice and Chicken Chowder

Market-Fresh Fish and Vegetable Soup

Chicken Minestrone

Bayou Andouille and Chicken Chowder

Vegetable Beef Soup

Slow-Cooker Lentil Soup

quick mexican-style soup

serves 4; ¾ cup per serving

Super fast and super low in calories—only 35 per serving—this soup abounds in south-of-the-border flavors. Try it as an accompaniment to Southwest Lime Chicken (page 240) or Chicken Fajitas (page 262), or serve it before your meal to help curb your appetite.

1¾ cups fat-free, low-sodium chicken broth
1 large tomato, diced
1 4-ounce can chopped mild green chiles
¼ cup snipped fresh cilantro
1 to 2 tablespoons fresh lime juice
1½ teaspoons olive oil (extra-virgin preferred)
¾ teaspoon ground cumin

In a medium saucepan, bring the broth to a boil over high heat. Stir in the tomato and green chiles. Return to a boil. Remove from the heat.

Stir in the remaining ingredients. Let stand, covered, for 5 minutes so the flavors blend.

PER SERVING

calories 35	cholesterol 0 mg	
total fat 2.0 g	sodium 132 mg	
saturated fat 0.0 g	carbohydrates 3 g	
trans fat 0.0 g	fiber 1 g	
polyunsaturated fat 0.0 g	sugars 1 g	
monounsaturated fat 1.0 g	protein 1 g	

100 200 300 400

DIETARY EXCHANGES
½ fat

cream of triple-mushroom soup

serves 6; 1 cup per serving

This impressive soup combines dried and fresh mushrooms in a rich-tasting starter for family or guests.

½ ounce dried morel mushrooms

½ ounce dried chanterelle mushrooms

2 cups low-sodium vegetable broth

1 cup chopped onion

¾ cup chopped button mushrooms

2 tablespoons soy sauce (lowest sodium available)

½ cup whole-wheat flour

½ cup water

1 teaspoon sugar

1 cup low-fat buttermilk

½ cup fat-free evaporated milk

Paprika to taste

In a small bowl, soak the dried mushrooms in enough warm water to cover for 20 to 30 minutes, or until soft. In a small sieve, rinse and drain the mushrooms, discarding the soaking water. Squeeze any remaining water from the mushrooms. Chop the mushrooms.

In a large saucepan, stir together the broth, onion, button mushrooms, soy sauce, and dried mushrooms. Bring to a boil over high heat. Reduce the heat and simmer, covered, for several minutes while you proceed.

In a small bowl, whisk the flour, water, and sugar into a smooth paste. Whisk in 1 tablespoon soup until blended. Whisk in 2 tablespoons soup until blended. Pour the flour mixture through a sieve into the soup, stirring until blended. Simmer, uncovered, for 3 minutes, stirring occasionally.

Pour in the milks. Return to a simmer. Remove from the heat.

In a food processor or blender, process the soup in batches until smooth. Return the soup to the pan. Cook over medium heat until the soup just begins to simmer, stirring constantly. Serve sprinkled with the paprika.

···· **PER SERVING** ··

calories 102
total fat 1.0 g
  saturated fat 0.5 g
  trans fat 0.0 g
  polyunsaturated fat 0.0 g
  monounsaturated fat 0.0 g

cholesterol 3 mg
sodium 210 mg
carbohydrates 18 g
  fiber 2 g
  sugars 7 g
  protein 7 g

100   200   300   400

DIETARY EXCHANGES
½ starch, ½ fat-free milk,
1 vegetable

artichoke and spinach soup

serves 4; 1 cup per serving

Baby spinach leaves provide the vibrant green color of this thick, smooth soup, and artichokes give it a mellow flavor. The navy beans and cheeses provide fiber and protein, helping make the soup hearty and filling. Round out the meal with crusty multigrain rolls.

1 teaspoon olive oil

8 ounces baby spinach

4 medium green onions, chopped

1 15.5-ounce can no-salt-added navy beans, rinsed and drained

1 9-ounce package frozen artichoke hearts, thawed and drained

1 cup fat-free, low-sodium chicken broth

½ cup fat-free half-and-half

1 teaspoon dried dillweed, crumbled

¼ teaspoon salt

¼ teaspoon pepper

¼ cup crumbled low-fat feta cheese

2 tablespoons shredded or grated Parmesan cheese

In a medium saucepan, heat the oil over medium heat, swirling to coat the bottom. Cook the spinach and green onions for 1 to 2 minutes, or until the spinach is wilted, stirring occasionally.

In a food processor or blender, process the spinach mixture with the beans, artichokes, and broth until smooth. Return the mixture to the pan.

Stir in the half-and-half, dillweed, salt, and pepper. Cook over medium heat for 6 to 8 minutes, or until the mixture is heated through, stirring occasionally.

Stir in the feta and Parmesan. Cook for 1 minute, or until the feta is melted, stirring occasionally.

··············**PER SERVING**··················

calories 214	cholesterol 5 mg	
total fat 3.0 g	sodium 478 mg	
saturated fat 1.5 g	carbohydrates 35 g	
trans fat 0.0 g	fiber 12 g	
polyunsaturated fat 0.0 g	sugars 7 g	
monounsaturated fat 1.0 g	protein 14 g	

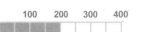

100   200   300   400

DIETARY EXCHANGES
1½ starch, 3 vegetable,
1 very lean meat

creamy broccoli soup with sour cream and cheddar

serves 6; ¾ cup soup per serving

This calorie-cut version of a classic soup is comfort in a bowl! Try making it with yellow summer squash or cauliflower instead of broccoli to suit your own taste or for some variety.

1 teaspoon olive oil
¾ cup diced onion
½ cup matchstick-size carrot strips
2 medium garlic cloves, minced
1¾ cups fat-free, low-sodium chicken broth
1 14-ounce package frozen broccoli florets
¾ teaspoon dried thyme, crumbled
⅛ to ¼ teaspoon cayenne
1½ cups fat-free milk
⅛ teaspoon salt
¼ cup plus 2 tablespoons fat-free sour cream
¼ cup plus 2 tablespoons shredded fat-free sharp Cheddar cheese

In a large saucepan, heat the oil over medium-high heat, swirling to coat the bottom. Cook the onion and carrot for about 3 minutes, or until the onion is soft, stirring frequently.

Stir in the garlic. Cook for 15 seconds, stirring constantly.

Stir in the broth, broccoli, thyme, and cayenne. Increase the heat to high and bring to a boil. Reduce the heat and simmer, covered, for 8 to 10 minutes, or until the broccoli is tender. Remove from the heat.

In a food processor or blender, process the soup in batches until smooth. Return the soup to the pan.

Stir the milk and salt into the soup. Cook over medium heat for 1 minute, or until heated. Serve topped with the sour cream and Cheddar.

PER SERVING

calories 88	cholesterol 5 mg
total fat 1.0 g	sodium 199 mg
saturated fat 0.0 g	carbohydrates 12 g
trans fat 0.0 g	fiber 3 g
polyunsaturated fat 0.0 g	sugars 6 g
monounsaturated fat 0.5 g	protein 8 g

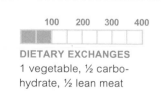

100 200 300 400

DIETARY EXCHANGES
1 vegetable, ½ carbohydrate, ½ lean meat

smoky roasted tomato soup

serves 4; ¾ cup per serving

Although this soup is low in calories, it definitely isn't low in flavor. Roasted vegetables and chipotle peppers packed in adobo sauce make it wonderfully spicy and intense.

      Cooking spray
4   medium tomatoes, halved crosswise
1   medium red bell pepper, coarsely chopped
1   medium onion, coarsely chopped
1   or 2 chipotle peppers canned in adobo sauce with
    2 teaspoons sauce
½   cup water and 1 cup water, divided use
1   tablespoon cider vinegar
1   tablespoon olive oil (extra-virgin preferred)
⅛   teaspoon salt
¼   cup fat-free sour cream (optional)
1   tablespoon plus 1 teaspoon finely chopped green onions
    (optional)

Preheat the broiler. Line a baking sheet with aluminum foil. Lightly spray the foil with cooking spray.

Arrange the tomatoes with the cut side down, bell pepper, and onion in a single layer on the baking sheet. Lightly spray the vegetables with cooking spray.

Broil about 4 inches from the heat for 10 minutes. Turn the tomatoes over and stir the bell pepper and onion. Broil for 8 minutes, or until the vegetables are richly browned on the edges. Transfer to a food processor or blender.

Stir the chipotle pepper(s), adobo sauce, and ½ cup water into the boiled vegetables. Process until smooth. Transfer to a medium saucepan.

Stir the vinegar and remaining 1 cup water into the vegetable mixture. Bring to a boil over high heat. Remove from the heat. Stir in the oil and salt. Serve topped with the sour cream and green onions.

COOK'S TIP ON CHIPOTLE PEPPERS IN ADOBO SAUCE Check the ethnic section of your supermarket for chipotle peppers, which are smoked jalapeños, canned in adobo sauce—a robust combination of chiles, vinegar, herbs, and spices.

SMOKY ROASTED TOMATO SOUP
PER SERVING

calories 81	cholesterol 0 mg
total fat 4.0 g	sodium 179 mg
saturated fat 0.5 g	carbohydrates 10 g
trans fat 0.0 g	fiber 3 g
polyunsaturated fat 0.5 g	sugars 7 g
monounsaturated fat 2.5 g	protein 2 g

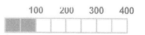

DIETARY EXCHANGES
2 vegetable, 1 fat

SMOKY ROASTED TOMATO SOUP WITH OPTIONAL INGREDIENTS
PER SERVING

calories 97	cholesterol 3 mg
total fat 4.0 g	sodium 192 mg
saturated fat 0.5 g	carbohydrates 13 g
trans fat 0.0 g	fiber 3 g
polyunsaturated fat 0.5 g	sugars 8 g
monounsaturated fat 2.5 g	protein 3 g

DIETARY EXCHANGES
2 vegetable, 1 fat

chilled blueberry soup

serves 6; ¾ cup soup per serving

This is a perfect soup to take to work for lunch. After it has chilled, pour it into an insulated container so it will keep cold—no microwave required!

- ¼ cup sugar
- 2 tablespoons cornstarch
- 1½ cups unsweetened apple juice
- 4 cups blueberries
- 1 teaspoon ground cardamom
- ¾ teaspoon ground cinnamon
- 1 cup fat-free plain yogurt and ¼ cup plus 2 tablespoons fat-free plain yogurt, divided use
- 6 sprigs of fresh mint (optional)

In a medium saucepan, stir together the sugar and cornstarch. Gradually whisk in the apple juice until smooth. Stir in the blueberries, cardamom, and cinnamon. Bring to a boil over medium-high heat, stirring frequently. Boil for 1 minute, stirring constantly. Reduce the heat and simmer for 5 minutes, stirring occasionally.

In a food processor or blender, process the soup in batches until smooth. Pour into a medium bowl. Cover and refrigerate for 4 hours, or until chilled.

At serving time, stir 1 cup yogurt into the chilled soup. Ladle into wine glasses or cups (to serve without spoons) or into soup bowls. Top each serving with 1 tablespoon of the remaining ¼ cup plus 2 table-spoons yogurt. Using a wooden toothpick, swirl the yogurt into an attractive pattern, if desired. Garnish each serving with the mint.

COOK'S TIP ON CARDAMOM Cardamom, a member of the ginger family, adds a wonderfully sweet and pungent flavor to foods. Because cardamom is one of the more expensive spices, and one that you may not use on a regular basis, you can assure a fresh product and probably save money by purchasing a small quantity at a store that sells spices in bulk.

TIME-SAVER An ice bath is a quick and easy method for rapidly cooling hot liquids, such as this soup. To make an ice bath, fill a large container or your sink with ice. Add a small amount of water. Place the bowl with the liquid to be cooled in the ice bath and stir the contents occasionally. Instead of chilling the blueberry soup for 4 hours, let it cool for about 20 minutes using the ice-bath method, then add the 1 cup yogurt and proceed as directed.

···· **PER SERVING** ···

calories 161	cholesterol 1 mg
total fat 0.5 g	sodium 47 mg
saturated fat 0.0 g	carbohydrates 37 g
trans fat 0.0 g	fiber 3 g
polyunsaturated fat 0.0 g	sugars 29 g
monounsaturated fat 0.0 g	protein 4 g

100 200 300 400

DIETARY EXCHANGES
2 fruit, ½ fat-free milk

egg drop soup with crabmeat and vegetables

serves 4; 1 cup per serving

Experiment with this versatile soup by adding different vegetables, such as broccoli, broccoli slaw, bok choy, or bell peppers. You can replace the crabmeat with low-sodium canned tuna, salmon from a can or pouch, or lean chicken, pork, or beef cooked without salt.

3 cups fat-free, low-sodium chicken broth

2 tablespoons cornstarch

2 medium carrots, shredded

4 ounces snow peas, trimmed and cut into matchstick-size strips

2 medium green onions, chopped

1 teaspoon toasted sesame oil

⅛ teaspoon pepper

6 ounces canned crabmeat, drained, cartilage discarded

½ cup egg substitute

In a medium saucepan, whisk together the broth and cornstarch. Bring to a simmer over medium-high heat. Reduce the heat and simmer for 2 to 3 minutes, or until thickened, stirring occasionally.

Stir in the carrots, snow peas, green onions, oil, and pepper. Simmer for 1 to 2 minutes, or until the carrots and snow peas are tender-crisp, stirring occasionally.

Stir in the crabmeat. Simmer for 1 minute, or until the crabmeat is heated through.

Pour the egg substitute in a thin stream and circular pattern into the simmering soup. Wait for 10 seconds, then gently stir until the egg substitute is cooked (it will appear shredded or resemble egg threads).

PER SERVING

calories 122	cholesterol 38 mg
total fat 2.0 g	sodium 172 mg
saturated fat 0.5 g	carbohydrates 11 g
trans fat 0.0 g	fiber 2 g
polyunsaturated fat 0.5 g	sugars 4 g
monounsaturated fat 0.5 g	protein 14 g

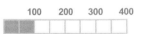

100 200 300 400

DIETARY EXCHANGES
½ starch, 1 vegetable,
2 very lean meat

wild rice and chicken chowder

serves 4; 1½ cups per serving

This hearty soup will fill you up *and* warm you up on a cold winter day.

- 1 teaspoon canola or corn oil
- 8 ounces chicken tenders or boneless, skinless chicken breasts, all visible fat discarded, cut into ½-inch cubes
- 1 medium carrot, sliced crosswise
- ½ medium onion, thinly sliced
- 3 cups fat-free, low-sodium chicken broth
- ½ 6- to 7-ounce box quick-cooking white and wild rice, seasoning packet discarded
- ½ teaspoon dried thyme, crumbled
- ¼ teaspoon dried sage
- ¼ teaspoon salt
- ⅛ teaspoon pepper
- 8 ounces broccoli florets
- ½ cup fat-free half-and-half
- ¼ cup shredded or grated Parmesan cheese

In a large saucepan, heat the oil over medium-high heat, swirling to coat the bottom. Cook the chicken for 4 minutes, stirring occasionally.

Stir in the carrot and onion. Cook for 2 to 3 minutes, or until they are tender-crisp, stirring occasionally.

Pour in the broth. Bring to a simmer. Stir in the rice, thyme, sage, salt, and pepper. Return to a simmer. Reduce the heat and simmer, covered, for 20 minutes, stirring occasionally.

Stir in the broccoli. Simmer, covered, for 5 minutes, or until tender.

Stir in the half-and-half and Parmesan. Cook over low heat for 1 to 2 minutes, or until the Parmesan is melted, stirring occasionally.

PER SERVING

calories 243	cholesterol 37 mg
total fat 3.5 g	sodium 377 mg
saturated fat 1.0 g	carbohydrates 31 g
trans fat 0.0 g	fiber 3 g
polyunsaturated fat 0.5 g	sugars 5 g
monounsaturated fat 1.5 g	protein 23 g

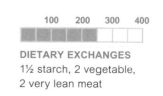

100   200   300   400

DIETARY EXCHANGES
1½ starch, 2 vegetable,
2 very lean meat

market-fresh fish and vegetable soup

serves 4; 1½ cups per serving

Stroll through your local market and select the freshest available seafood and seasonal vegetables for this versatile soup. Managing your weight doesn't need to be monotonous—use different fish and veggies to suit your individual taste and to introduce plenty of variety.

1   teaspoon olive oil

4   ounces shiitake mushrooms, stems discarded, halved

4   medium green onions (green part only), chopped

1   medium garlic clove, minced

3   cups fat-free, low-sodium chicken broth

2   medium Italian plum (Roma) tomatoes, diced

½   cup dried whole-grain macaroni or small shell pasta

¼   teaspoon salt

⅛   teaspoon pepper

8   ounces salmon fillets, rinsed and cut into 1-inch cubes

8   ounces halibut fillets, rinsed and cut into 1-inch cubes

8   ounces asparagus, trimmed and cut into 1-inch pieces

4   ounces broccoli florets, cut into 1-inch pieces

1   tablespoon chopped fresh oregano or 1 teaspoon dried, crumbled

In a large saucepan, heat the oil over medium-high heat, swirling to coat the bottom. Cook the mushrooms, green onions, and garlic for 3 to 4 minutes, or until soft, stirring occasionally.

Stir in the broth and tomatoes. Bring to a simmer, stirring occasionally.

Stir in the pasta, salt, and pepper. Reduce the heat and simmer for 5 to 6 minutes, or until the pasta is almost tender, stirring occasionally.

Stir in the remaining ingredients. Simmer for 5 to 6 minutes, or until the pasta is tender and the fish flakes easily when tested with a fork, gently stirring occasionally. (Try to keep the cubes of fish intact.)

COOK'S TIP For variety, try some of these tasty substitutions:

- Vegetables: shredded carrots; sliced bok choy, celery, zucchini, yellow summer squash; halved snow peas, sugar snap peas; baby corn
- Herbs: rosemary, basil, marjoram, thyme, dill, tarragon
- Fish: tuna, cod, tilapia, haddock, red snapper

····· **PER SERVING** ··

calories 239	cholesterol 48 mg
total fat 5.0 g	sodium 276 mg
saturated fat 0.5 g	carbohydrates 19 g
trans fat 0.0 g	fiber 5 g
polyunsaturated fat 1.5 g	sugars 4 g
monounsaturated fat 2.0 g	protein 29 g

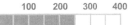

100   200   300   400

DIETARY EXCHANGES
½ starch, 2 vegetable,
3 lean meat

chicken minestrone

serves 8; 1¼ cups per serving

Bring a bit of Italian restaurant dining, minus most of the calories, sodium, and saturated fat, into your home with this flavorful soup. It's perfect for a lunch or dinner entrée; for a side dish, leave out the chicken.

Cooking spray
1 small onion, chopped
4 medium garlic cloves, minced
2 cups fat-free, low-sodium chicken broth
2 cups no-salt-added tomato juice
1 15.5-ounce can no-salt-added chickpeas, rinsed and drained
1 14.5-ounce can no-salt-added stewed tomatoes, undrained
½ cup frozen green peas and carrots
½ cup dry red wine (regular or nonalcoholic)
1 medium rib of celery, chopped
1½ teaspoons dried basil, crumbled
¼ teaspoon dried oregano, crumbled
Dash of pepper
10 ounces boneless, skinless chicken breasts, cubed
1 cup dried whole-grain rotini or small or medium shell pasta
1 to 2 ounces baby spinach
3 tablespoons shredded or grated Parmesan cheese

Lightly spray a Dutch oven with cooking spray. Cook the onion and garlic over medium-high heat for about 3 minutes, or until soft, stirring frequently.

Stir in the broth, tomato juice, chickpeas, tomatoes with liquid, peas and carrots, wine, celery, basil, oregano, and pepper. Break the tomatoes into smaller pieces with a spoon. Bring to a boil, still on medium high. Reduce the heat and simmer, covered, for 45 minutes, stirring occasionally.

Stir in the chicken, pasta, and spinach. Increase the heat to medium high and bring to a boil. Reduce the heat and simmer, uncovered, for 10 to 15 minutes, or until the chicken and pasta are tender, stirring occasionally. Serve sprinkled with the Parmesan.

COOK'S TIP This soup will thicken as it cools. You can thin it with water, if needed.

····· PER SERVING ·········

calories 228
total fat 3.0 g
  saturated fat 1.0 g
  trans fat 0.0 g
  polyunsaturated fat 0.5 g
  monounsaturated fat 1.0 g

cholesterol 31 mg
sodium 148 mg
carbohydrates 29 g
  fiber 6 g
  sugars 6 g
protein 18 g

100   200   300   400

DIETARY EXCHANGES
1½ starch, 2 vegetable,
1½ very lean meat

bayou andouille and chicken chowder

serves 4; 1½ cups per serving

Andouille (*an-DOO-ee*) sausage, a smoky Cajun favorite with a nice bit of heat, revs up the flavor in this chowder.

Cooking spray
2 ounces andouille sausage, cut into ½-inch pieces
2 ounces boneless, skinless chicken breast, all visible fat discarded, cut into ½-inch pieces
1¾ cups fat-free, low-sodium chicken broth
8 ounces baking potatoes (russet preferred), cut into ½-inch pieces
1½ medium green bell peppers, chopped
1 large onion, chopped
¾ cup frozen whole-kernel corn
½ teaspoon dried thyme, crumbled
1 4-ounce jar diced pimientos, drained
½ cup finely snipped fresh parsley
½ cup fat-free half-and-half
¼ teaspoon salt
¼ teaspoon pepper
2 ounces shredded fat-free sharp Cheddar cheese

Lightly spray a Dutch oven with cooking spray. Heat over medium-high heat. Cook the sausage for 3 minutes, or until beginning to richly brown on the edges, stirring constantly. Transfer to a small plate.

Lightly respray the Dutch oven with cooking spray. Cook the chicken for 3 minutes, stirring frequently.

Stir in the broth, potatoes, bell peppers, onion, corn, and thyme. Bring to a boil, still on medium high. Reduce the heat and simmer, covered, for 20 minutes, or until the potatoes are tender. Remove from the heat.

Stir in the sausage and remaining ingredients except the Cheddar. Let stand, covered, for 15 minutes so the flavors blend and the soup thickens slightly. (Don't skip this step.) Reheat the chowder over medium heat for 2 to 3 minutes if needed. Serve sprinkled with the Cheddar.

····· PER SERVING ···

calories 196
total fat 3.0 g
  saturated fat 1.0 g
  trans fat 0.0 g
  polyunsaturated fat 0.0 g
  monounsaturated fat 0.0 g

cholesterol 19 mg
sodium 424 mg
carbohydrates 29 g
  fiber 4 g
  sugars 8 g
  protein 16 g

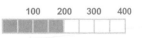

DIETARY EXCHANGES
1½ starch, 2 vegetable,
2 very lean meat

vegetable beef soup

serves 4; 1½ cups per serving

Yellow-skinned potatoes and exotic mushrooms update this one-dish-meal classic.

Cooking spray

1 pound eye-of-round steak, all visible fat discarded, cut into ½-inch cubes

4 ounces shiitake mushrooms, stems discarded, halved

1 medium carrot, cut crosswise into ½-inch slices

3 cups fat-free, no-salt-added beef broth

2 medium yellow-skinned potatoes, such as Yukon Gold (about 8 ounces total), cut into 1-inch cubes

4 ounces baby bella mushrooms, halved

¼ cup no-salt-added tomato paste

1 teaspoon dried marjoram, crumble

1 teaspoon dried thyme, crumbled

1 teaspoon onion powder

¼ teaspoon salt

¼ teaspoon pepper

½ cup frozen green peas

Lightly spray a Dutch oven with cooking spray. Heat over medium-high heat. Cook the beef for 3 to 4 minutes, or until browned, stirring occasionally.

Stir in the shiitake mushrooms and carrot. Cook for 3 to 4 minutes, or until the mushrooms are soft and the carrot is tender-crisp, stirring occasionally.

Stir in the remaining ingredients except the peas. Bring to a simmer. Reduce the heat and simmer, covered, for 30 to 40 minutes, or until the beef and vegetables are tender (no stirring needed).

Stir in the peas. Simmer, covered, for 4 minutes.

PER SERVING

calories 240
total fat 3.0 g
  saturated fat 1.0 g
  trans fat 0.0 g
  polyunsaturated fat 0.5 g
  monounsaturated fat 1.5 g

cholesterol 54 mg
sodium 353 mg
carbohydrates 21 g
  fiber 4 g
  sugars 5 g
protein 32 g

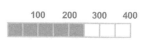

DIETARY EXCHANGES
1 starch, 1 vegetable,
3 very lean meat

slow-cooker lentil soup

serves 6; 1⅔ cups per serving

After this soup slow cooks, thicken it by pureeing part, then returning it to the rest of the soup.

Cooking spray
1 teaspoon olive oil
1 medium onion, chopped
1 large carrot, cut crosswise into pieces about ⅛ inch thick
1 small parsnip, peeled and cut crosswise into pieces about ⅛ inch thick
1 large rib of celery, sliced crosswise
1½ tablespoons curry powder
3 medium garlic cloves, minced
6 cups low-sodium vegetable broth
1 14.5-ounce can no-salt-added diced tomatoes, undrained
1½ cups dried lentils, sorted for stones and shriveled lentils and rinsed
1 teaspoon pepper
¾ teaspoon salt
2 tablespoons fresh lemon juice

Lightly spray a 3½- or 4-quart slow cooker with cooking spray. Set aside.

In a large skillet, heat the oil over medium-high heat, swirling to coat the bottom. Cook the onion, carrot, parsnip, and celery for 6 to 8 minutes, or until tender-crisp, stirring frequently.

Stir in the curry powder and garlic. Cook for 1 to 2 minutes, or until fragrant, stirring frequently. Transfer to the slow cooker.

Stir in the remaining ingredients except the juice. Cook, covered, on low for 7 to 8 hours or on high for 3½ to 4 hours. Stir in the juice.

Transfer 2 cups soup to a food processor or blender and process until smooth. Stir into the remaining soup to thicken it.

PER SERVING

calories 229	cholesterol 0 mg
total fat 1.5 g	sodium 343 mg
saturated fat 0.0 g	carbohydrates 41 g
trans fat 0.0 g	fiber 14 g
polyunsaturated fat 0.5 g	sugars 8 g
monounsaturated fat 0.5 g	protein 15 g

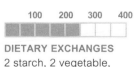

DIETARY EXCHANGES
2 starch, 2 vegetable,
1 very lean meat

salads

Greek Salad with Sun-Dried Tomato Vinaigrette

Baby Greens with Spiced Cranberry Vinaigrette

Fruit and Spinach Salad with Fresh Mint

Asparagus and Cucumber Salad with Lemon and Mint

Vegetable Salad Vinaigrette

Broccoli and Edamame Salad with Dill

Zingy Carrot Salad

Carrot-Pineapple Slaw with Ginger

Multicolored Marinated Slaw

Mango-Avocado Salad

Asian Citrus Salad

Tabbouleh

Black-Eyed Pea Salad

Grilled Veggie and Quinoa Chopped Salad

Lemony Rice and Bean Salad with Feta

Spinach and Salmon Salad with Spicy Orange Dressing

Tuna Pasta Provençal

Chicken and Toasted Walnut Salad

Grilled Chicken and Raspberry Salad

Flank Steak Salad with Sesame-Lime Dressing

Cannellini and Black Bean Salad

Taco Salad with Avocado Dressing

greek salad with sun-dried tomato vinaigrette

serves 4; 2 cups per serving

Jam-packed with assertive ingredients, this is a salad to remember.

sun-dried tomato vinaigrette

- 4 dry-packed sun-dried tomato halves (about ½ ounce)
- ¼ cup dry white wine (regular or nonalcoholic)
- 2 tablespoons finely snipped fresh parsley
- 2 tablespoons fresh lemon juice
- 1 tablespoon cider vinegar
- 1 tablespoon olive oil (extra-virgin preferred)
- 1½ teaspoons dried oregano, crumbled
- 1 medium garlic clove, minced
- ¼ teaspoon ground cumin
- ⅛ teaspoon salt
- ¼ teaspoon pepper

salad

- 8 ounces lettuce leaves, any variety, torn into bite-size pieces
- ¼ to ½ cup thinly sliced red onion
- 2 tablespoons crumbled low-fat feta cheese with sun-dried tomatoes and basil

Put the tomatoes in a small bowl. Pour in boiling water to cover. Let stand for 15 minutes, or until very soft. Drain the tomatoes, discarding the water. Finely chop the tomatoes.

In a small bowl, whisk together the vinaigrette ingredients.

In a large bowl, combine the lettuce and onion. Add the vinaigrette and feta, tossing gently to coat.

PER SERVING

calories 85	cholesterol 1 mg
total fat 4.0 g	sodium 164 mg
saturated fat 0.5 g	carbohydrates 7 g
trans fat 0.0 g	fiber 2 g
polyunsaturated fat 0.5 g	sugars 2 g
monounsaturated fat 2.5 g	protein 3 g

100 200 300 400

DIETARY EXCHANGES
1 vegetable, 1 fat

baby greens with spiced cranberry vinaigrette

serves 4; 2 cups per serving

You don't have to wait until the winter holidays to enjoy the flavor of cranberries. Cool and refreshing, this salad with cranberry vinaigrette is just right with grilled foods in the heat of summer.

spiced cranberry vinaigrette

- ¼ cup sweetened cranberry juice
- 2 tablespoons red wine vinegar
- 1½ tablespoons honey
- 1 teaspoon grated peeled gingerroot
- ½ teaspoon ground cinnamon
- ⅛ teaspoon ground cloves
- ⅛ teaspoon salt

salad

- 8 ounces mixed salad greens (baby or spring greens preferred), torn into bite-size pieces
- ½ cup thinly sliced onion
- ½ medium Gala or Jonathan apple, unpeeled and sliced into thin wedges
- 2 ounces crumbled soft goat cheese

In a small bowl, whisk together the vinaigrette ingredients.

Put the greens on plates. Arrange the onion and apple on top.

Pour the vinaigrette over the salad. Sprinkle with the goat cheese.

COOK'S TIP ON SALAD DRESSING Salad dressing clings better to thoroughly dried greens, allowing you to use less dressing and save calories.

PER SERVING

calories 108	cholesterol 7 mg
total fat 3.5 g	sodium 155 mg
saturated fat 2.0 g	carbohydrates 17 g
trans fat 0.0 g	fiber 3 g
polyunsaturated fat 0.0 g	sugars 12 g
monounsaturated fat 0.5 g	protein 5 g

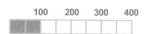

100 200 300 400

DIETARY EXCHANGES
1 carbohydrate, ½ lean meat, ½ fat

fruit and spinach salad with fresh mint

serves 6; 2 cups per serving

Savor this jewel-toned salad as a side dish or top it with grilled chicken, salmon, or tuna to turn it into a light meal.

salad

8 ounces baby spinach

2 cups strawberries, hulled and halved

4 medium kiwifruit, peeled and sliced crosswise

1 medium mango, cubed

dressing

1 cup fat-free plain yogurt

¼ cup finely snipped fresh mint

2 tablespoons honey

1 tablespoon fresh orange juice

1 tablespoon fresh lemon juice

2 sprigs of mint (optional)

Put the spinach on plates. Arrange the strawberries, kiwifruit, and mango on the spinach.

In a small bowl, whisk together the dressing ingredients. Pour over the salad, tossing gently to coat. Garnish with the mint.

COOK'S TIP ON MEASURING HONEY Lightly spray your measuring cup or spoon with cooking spray before you measure honey. The honey will easily slide out of the measuring implement without sticking.

PER SERVING

calories 133	cholesterol 1 mg
total fat 0.5 g	sodium 97 mg
saturated fat 0.0 g	carbohydrates 31 g
trans fat 0.0 g	fiber 5 g
polyunsaturated fat 0.0 g	sugars 21 g
monounsaturated fat 0.0 g	protein 5 g

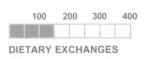

DIETARY EXCHANGES
1½ fruit, ½ carbohydrate

asparagus and cucumber salad with lemon and mint

serves 4; ½ cup per serving

You'll be tempted to eat this unusual salad with a spoon so you can catch all the great flavors!

4 ounces asparagus spears (4 to 5 medium), trimmed and cut into
  ½-inch pieces
1 medium cucumber, peeled, seeded, and diced
½ cup finely chopped red onion
¼ cup chopped fresh mint or snipped fresh cilantro
1 tablespoon sugar
1½ teaspoons grated lemon zest
2 tablespoons fresh lemon juice
⅛ teaspoon salt

In a medium saucepan, steam the asparagus for 1½ to 2 minutes, or until just tender-crisp. Immediately drain in a colander and run under cold water to cool completely. Drain well. Pat dry with paper towels.

In a medium bowl, gently toss together all the ingredients. Let stand for 10 minutes so the flavors blend.

PER SERVING

calories 37	cholesterol 0 mg
total fat 0.0 g	sodium 78 mg
saturated fat 0.0 g	carbohydrates 8 g
trans fat 0.0 g	fiber 2 g
polyunsaturated fat 0.0 g	sugars 5 g
monounsaturated fat 0.0 g	protein 1 g

100 200 300 400

DIETARY EXCHANGES
1 vegetable

vegetable salad vinaigrette

serves 4; ½ cup per serving

Need a new twist on a side salad? This crunchy combination is it!

salad

½ medium cucumber, peeled and diced

1 medium rib of celery, sliced crosswise

3 ounces button mushrooms, coarsely chopped

¼ cup chopped red onion

¼ cup snipped fresh parsley

vinaigrette

1 tablespoon olive oil (extra-virgin preferred)

1 tablespoon red wine vinegar

1 teaspoon sugar

½ teaspoon Dijon mustard (stone-ground preferred)

⅛ teaspoon salt

⅛ teaspoon crushed red pepper flakes

In a medium bowl, toss together all the ingredients. Serve immediately for peak flavor.

COOK'S TIP To prepare in advance, combine the salad ingredients in a medium bowl and the vinaigrette ingredients in a small bowl. Cover the bowls and refrigerate separately for up to 8 hours. At serving time, whisk the vinaigrette. Pour over the salad and toss.

PER SERVING

calories 50
total fat 3.5 g
  saturated fat 0.5 g
  trans fat 0.0 g
  polyunsaturated fat 0.5 g
  monounsaturated fat 2.5 g

cholesterol 0 mg
sodium 98 mg
carbohydrates 4 g
  fiber 1 g
  sugars 2 g
protein 1 g

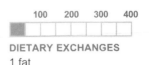

DIETARY EXCHANGES
1 fat

broccoli and edamame salad with dill

serves 6; ½ cup per serving

Buy some fresh baby dillweed and make this salad when you want something unusual to perk up your dinner menu. You can turn the salad into an entrée by adding slices of skinless chicken breast cooked without salt.

salad

- 1 cup frozen shelled edamame (green soybeans)
- 2 cups broccoli florets, cut into bite-size pieces
- ⅓ cup chopped red onion or sweet onion, such as Vidalia, Maui, or Oso Sweet
- ¼ cup sweetened dried cranberries
- 2 tablespoons finely snipped dillweed (baby dillweed preferred)

dressing

- ⅓ cup plain rice vinegar
- 1 tablespoon honey
- 1 teaspoon olive oil (extra-virgin preferred)

Cook the edamame using the package directions, omitting the salt. Drain well.

Meanwhile, in a large bowl, toss together the remaining salad ingredients.

In a small bowl, whisk together the dressing ingredients.

Add the edamame to the salad. Pour the dressing over the salad, tossing to coat. Cover and refrigerate for about 1 hour so the flavors blend, tossing occasionally.

PER SERVING

calories 88	cholesterol 0 mg
total fat 2.5 g	sodium 15 mg
saturated fat 0.5 g	carbohydrates 13 g
trans fat 0.0 g	fiber 3 g
polyunsaturated fat 1.0 g	sugars 8 g
monounsaturated fat 1.0 g	protein 4 g

100 200 300 400

DIETARY EXCHANGES
1 carbohydrate,
½ lean meat

zingy carrot salad

Double or triple this quick and easy dish to ensure having leftovers for a low-calorie snack or to serve again in a few days.

- 2 medium carrots, cut crosswise into ⅛-inch pieces
- ½ medium green bell pepper (cut lengthwise), cut into thin strips
- ½ cup thinly sliced onion
- 3 tablespoons balsamic vinegar
- 2 tablespoons firmly packed dark brown sugar
- ⅛ teaspoon salt

In a small saucepan, steam the carrots for 3 to 4 minutes, or until just tender. Drain well.

In a medium bowl, toss together all the ingredients. Cover and refrigerate for about 1 hour so the flavors blend.

PER SERVING

calories 60
total fat 0.0 g
  saturated fat 0.0 g
  trans fat 0.0 g
  polyunsaturated fat 0.0 g
  monounsaturated fat 0.0 g

cholesterol 0 mg
sodium 103 mg
carbohydrates 15 g
  fiber 2 g
  sugars 12 g
  protein 1 g

100 200 300 400

DIETARY EXCHANGES
1 vegetable,
½ carbohydrate

carrot-pineapple slaw with ginger

serves 4; ½ cup per serving

This modernized version of the classic 1950s carrot-raisin salad is bursting with fresh citrus and ginger.

1½ cups shredded carrots
1 8-ounce can crushed pineapple in its own juice, drained
3 ounces dried apricots, finely chopped
1 teaspoon grated lemon zest
2 tablespoons fresh lemon juice
1 teaspoon grated peeled gingerroot

In a medium bowl, toss together all the ingredients. Let stand for 10 minutes so the flavors blend.

PER SERVING

calories 88
total fat 0.0 g
  saturated fat 0.0 g
  trans fat 0.0 g
  polyunsaturated fat 0.0 g
  monounsaturated fat 0.0 g

cholesterol 0 mg
sodium 31 mg
carbohydrates 23 g
  fiber 3 g
  sugars 18 g
protein 1 g

100   200   300   400

DIETARY EXCHANGES
1½ fruit

multicolored marinated slaw

serves 8; ½ cup per serving

Marinated slaw provides a change of pace from the usual mixed green salad. Prepare at least 12 hours in advance so the flavors can blend.

dressing

⅓ cup white wine vinegar

¼ cup water

¼ cup sugar

1 tablespoon canola or corn oil

½ teaspoon garlic powder

½ teaspoon celery seeds

¼ teaspoon dry mustard

⅛ teaspoon salt

⅛ teaspoon pepper

slaw

½ medium head green cabbage, coarsely shredded (about 4 cups)

1 medium red bell pepper, cut into strips

1 medium cucumber, peeled, cut in half lengthwise, seeded, and thinly sliced crosswise

1 medium rib of celery, thinly sliced crosswise

1 large carrot, thinly sliced crosswise

1 small sweet onion, such as Vidalia, Maui, or Oso Sweet, thinly sliced and cut into bite-size pieces

In a large bowl, whisk together the dressing ingredients.

Add the slaw ingredients, tossing to coat. Cover and refrigerate for at least 12 hours so the flavors blend, tossing occasionally. The slaw will keep for several days in the refrigerator.

PER SERVING

calories 82	cholesterol 0 mg
total fat 2.0 g	sodium 67 mg
saturated fat 0.0 g	carbohydrates 15 g
trans fat 0.0 g	fiber 3 g
polyunsaturated fat 0.5 g	sugars 11 g
monounsaturated fat 1.0 g	protein 1 g

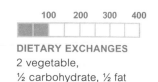

DIETARY EXCHANGES
2 vegetable,
½ carbohydrate, ½ fat

mango-avocado salad

serves 6; ½ cup per serving

The addition of avocado gives this salad a creamy touch. It's the perfect match for Black-Pepper Chicken (page 239) or simply-seasoned grilled sirloin.

1½ cups diced fresh or bottled mango or fresh or frozen unsweetened peaches, thawed if frozen (fresh preferred)

1 medium avocado, cut into ½-inch cubes

¼ cup finely chopped red onion

¼ cup snipped fresh cilantro

¼ cup fresh lime juice

1 teaspoon sugar

In a medium bowl, gently toss together all the ingredients. Serve or cover and refrigerate for up to 2 hours so the flavors blend.

COOK'S TIP For fruit salsa, finely chop the avocado and mango.

COOK'S TIP ON CHOPPING MANGOES Here's one good way to chop a mango. Place an unpeeled mango on its side. Making one lengthwise cut, cut off a piece that is about one-third of the mango. Turn the mango over and repeat. The pit will be in the middle third. Without cutting through the skin, score those two outer pieces lengthwise. Give the scored pieces a one-quarter turn and, again without cutting through the skin, score to create small squares. Turn the mango inside out and cut the small squares from the skin.

PER SERVING

calories 89
total fat 5.0 g
 saturated fat 0.5 g
 trans fat 0.0 g
 polyunsaturated fat 0.5 g
 monounsaturated fat 3.5 g

cholesterol 0 mg
sodium 4 mg
carbohydrates 12 g
 fiber 3 g
 sugars 8 g
 protein 1 g

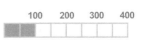

DIETARY EXCHANGES
1 fruit, 1 fat

asian citrus salad

serves 6; ½ cup per serving

Experimenting with produce and seasonings can be interesting and fun. This salad uses a large pomelo—similar to a grapefruit but sweeter—and honey infused with Chinese five-spice powder and fresh mint.

- 3 tablespoons honey
- 1 tablespoon chopped fresh mint
- ½ teaspoon five-spice powder
- 1 teaspoon pomelo zest or a combination of pomelo, orange, and tangerine zest
- 1 large pomelo, peeled, seeded, and divided into segments
- 1 medium orange, peeled, seeded, and divided into segments
- 1 small tangerine, peeled, seeded, and divided into segments

In a small saucepan, stir together the honey, mint, five-spice powder, and zest. Cook over medium-low heat for 1 to 2 minutes, or until heated through, stirring occasionally.

In a medium bowl, combine the pomelo, orange, and tangerine. Pour in the honey mixture, tossing gently to coat. Serve or cover and refrigerate to serve chilled.

COOK'S TIP ON POMELO Choose a pomelo that is heavy for its size, smells sweet, and is bright yellow, pinkish, or light green. To segment a pomelo, cut both ends from the fruit and cut away all the remaining thick peel. Using a knife with a thin blade, cut each segment of fruit from the tough white membrane.

COOK'S TIP ON FIVE-SPICE POWDER Five-spice powder usually can be found in the spice section of your grocery and Asian markets. It is a fragrant blend of star anise, cloves, fennel, cinnamon, and Szechuan peppercorns.

PER SERVING

calories 93	cholesterol 0 mg
total fat 0.0 g	sodium 2 mg
saturated fat 0.0 g	carbohydrates 24 g
trans fat 0.0 g	fiber 2 g
polyunsaturated fat 0.0 g	sugars 21 g
monounsaturated fat 0.0 g	protein 1 g

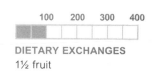

DIETARY EXCHANGES
1½ fruit

tabbouleh

serves 10; ½ cup per serving

This Middle Eastern favorite incorporates a whole grain into your meal, helping make you feel full. Although you won't need to spend much time preparing this salad, it does take time for the bulgur to reconstitute and for the salad to chill. If you want to serve fewer people, cut the ingredients by half.

¾ cup uncooked bulgur

¾ cup boiling water

¼ cup fresh lemon juice

1 tablespoon olive oil (extra-virgin preferred)

2 medium tomatoes, chopped

1 cup diced unpeeled English, or hothouse, cucumber

½ cup chopped red onion

½ cup snipped fresh parsley

2 medium green onions, chopped (green and white parts)

2 tablespoons chopped fresh mint

3 medium garlic cloves, minced

¼ teaspoon salt

¼ teaspoon pepper

In a large bowl, stir together the bulgur and boiling water. Let stand for 1 hour. If needed, drain well, discarding any remaining water.

In a small bowl, whisk together the lemon juice and oil. Pour over the reconstituted bulgur.

Gently stir in the remaining ingredients. Cover and refrigerate for at least 1 hour so the flavors blend (will keep up to three days). Serve chilled or let the tabbouleh return to room temperature before serving.

PER SERVING

calories 64
total fat 1.5 g
  saturated fat 0.0 g
  trans fat 0.0 g
  polyunsaturated fat 0.0 g
  monounsaturated fat 1.0 g

cholesterol 0 mg
sodium 66 mg
carbohydrates 12 g
  fiber 3 g
  sugars 2 g
  protein 2 g

100	200	300	400

DIETARY EXCHANGES
1 starch

black-eyed pea salad

serves 10; ½ cup per serving

An old southern tradition suggests that eating black-eyed peas on New Year's Day brings good luck for the coming year. This salad is so tasty that you won't want to wait for the holiday to prepare it.

salad

1 15.5-ounce can no-salt-added black-eyed peas, rinsed and drained
1 medium cucumber, cut in half lengthwise, seeded, and cut into ¼-inch pieces
1 medium red bell pepper, chopped
1 medium rib of celery, chopped
4 medium green onions, chopped
1 tablespoon chopped fresh basil
2 ounces fat-free feta cheese, crumbled

dressing

3 tablespoons fresh lemon juice
2 tablespoons coarsely chopped fresh oregano
1½ tablespoons olive oil (extra-virgin preferred)
½ teaspoon red hot-pepper sauce
⅛ teaspoon pepper

In a large bowl, toss together the salad ingredients.

In a small bowl, whisk together the dressing ingredients. Pour over the salad, tossing to coat. Serve or cover and refrigerate to serve chilled.

PER SERVING

calories 75	cholesterol 0 mg
total fat 2.0 g	sodium 98 mg
saturated fat 0.5 g	carbohydrates 10 g
trans fat 0.0 g	fiber 3 g
polyunsaturated fat 0.0 g	sugars 3 g
monounsaturated fat 1.5 g	protein 4 g

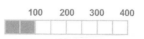

100 200 300 400

DIETARY EXCHANGES
½ starch, ½ lean meat

grilled veggie and quinoa chopped salad

serves 6; ½ cup per serving

Combine grilled veggies with quinoa (*KEEN-wah*), then spoon over slices of tomato for layers of flavor and texture in every bite. If you grill the veggies a day ahead, you'll be able to put this light and healthy salad together in no time at all.

Cooking spray
½ medium onion
½ medium green bell pepper
1 medium zucchini or yellow summer squash, halved lengthwise
1 cup water
¼ cup uncooked quinoa, rinsed and drained
1 tablespoon olive oil (extra-virgin preferred)
1 tablespoon balsamic vinegar
1 medium garlic clove, minced
⅛ teaspoon salt
⅛ teaspoon pepper
2 medium tomatoes, each cut into 6 slices

Lightly spray a grilling rack with cooking spray. Preheat the grill on medium high.

Lightly spray both sides of the onion, bell pepper, and zucchini with cooking spray. Put them on the grilling rack.

Grill for 4 minutes on each side, or until just tender-crisp. Transfer to a cutting board and let stand until cool enough to handle. Coarsely chop.

Meanwhile, in a small saucepan, bring the water to a boil over high heat. Stir in the quinoa. Reduce the heat and simmer, covered, for 10 to 12 minutes, or until the water is absorbed and the quinoa is tender. Transfer to a fine-mesh strainer. Run under cold water to cool quickly. Drain well. Shake off any excess liquid. Transfer to a medium bowl.

Stir the grilled vegetables and remaining ingredients except the tomatoes into the quinoa.

Arrange the tomatoes in a single layer on a serving plate. Spoon the quinoa mixture over the tomatoes.

···· PER SERVING ···

calories 67
total fat 3.0 g
  saturated fat 0.5 g
  trans fat 0.0 g
  polyunsaturated fat 0.5 g
  monounsaturated fat 2.0 g

cholesterol 0 mg
sodium 57 mg
carbohydrates 9 g
  fiber 2 g
  sugars 3 g
protein 2 g

100 200 300 400

DIETARY EXCHANGES
½ starch, ½ fat

lemony rice and bean salad with feta

serves 4; ½ cup per serving

Turn this filling salad into a meatless entrée for four by doubling the recipe.

⅔ cup water

½ cup uncooked instant brown rice

½ 15.5-ounce can no-salt-added navy beans, rinsed and drained

¼ cup finely chopped red onion

¾ ounce fat-free feta cheese with sun-dried tomatoes and basil, crumbled

2 teaspoons olive oil (extra-virgin preferred)

1 teaspoon dried dillweed, crumbled

1 teaspoon grated lemon zest

2 to 3 teaspoons fresh lemon juice

½ teaspoon dried oregano, crumbled

½ medium garlic clove, minced (optional)

¼ teaspoon salt

In a small saucepan, bring the water to a boil over high heat. Stir in the rice. Reduce the heat and simmer, covered, for about 10 minutes, or until the rice is tender. Spoon the rice in a single layer onto a baking sheet. Let stand for 5 to 7 minutes, or until completely cooled. Transfer the rice to a medium bowl.

Add the remaining ingredients, tossing gently to coat. Serve or cover and refrigerate for up to 8 hours.

PER SERVING

calories 125	cholesterol 2 mg
total fat 3.0 g	sodium 222 mg
saturated fat 0.5 g	carbohydrates 19 g
trans fat 0.0 g	fiber 3 g
polyunsaturated fat 0.5 g	sugars 2 g
monounsaturated fat 2.0 g	protein 5 g

100 200 300 400

DIETARY EXCHANGES
1 starch, ½ lean meat

spinach and salmon salad with spicy orange dressing

serves 4; 2½ cups per serving

Fresh orange zest and a small amount of juice add big flavor but only very few calories to the dressing for this elegant entrée salad.

½ cup dried whole-grain rotini

spicy orange dressing

1½ to 2 tablespoons grated orange zest

⅓ to ½ cup fresh orange juice

2 tablespoons sugar

2 tablespoons balsamic vinegar

1 tablespoon canola or corn oil

¼ teaspoon crushed red pepper flakes or 1 medium fresh jalapeño, seeds and ribs discarded, finely chopped

⅛ teaspoon salt

4 to 5 ounces baby spinach

½ medium red onion, thinly sliced

2 medium oranges, peeled and sectioned

1 5-ounce vacuum-sealed pouch pink salmon, flaked

Prepare the pasta using the package directions, omitting the salt. Drain in a colander. Rinse under cold water until cool. Drain well.

Meanwhile, in a small bowl, whisk together the orange zest, orange juice, sugar, vinegar, oil, red pepper flakes, and salt.

Arrange the spinach on plates. Top, in order, with the pasta, onion, orange dressing, and orange sections. Sprinkle with the salmon.

PER SERVING

calories 212	cholesterol 13 mg
total fat 5.5 g	sodium 304 mg
saturated fat 1.0 g	carbohydrates 34 g
trans fat 0.0 g	fiber 5 g
polyunsaturated fat 1.5 g	sugars 17 g
monounsaturated fat 2.5 g	protein 10 g

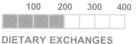

DIETARY EXCHANGES
1 starch, 1 fruit, 1 vegetable, 1 very lean meat, ½ fat

tuna pasta provençal

serves 4; 1½ cups per serving

With its blend of tuna, black olives, and red bell pepper, along with garlic, tarragon, and Dijon mustard, this dish is typical of flavors found in the south of France. This is an ideal salad to make the night before and take to work the next day.

4   ounces dried whole-grain or spinach rotini or small pasta shells
1   teaspoon olive oil
1   large sweet onion, such as Vidalia, Maui, or Oso Sweet, chopped
1   large red bell pepper, chopped
1   medium garlic clove, minced
12 ounces canned very low sodium albacore tuna, packed in water, drained and flaked
¼   cup chopped black olives
⅓   cup fat-free plain yogurt
¼   cup light mayonnaise
1½ tablespoons snipped fresh tarragon or 1½ teaspoons dried, crumbled
2   teaspoons Dijon mustard
½   teaspoon pepper

Prepare the pasta using the package directions, omitting the salt. Drain in a colander. Rinse under cold water. Drain well. Transfer to a large bowl.

Meanwhile, in a large nonstick skillet, heat the oil over medium-high heat, swirling to coat the bottom. Cook the onion, bell pepper, and garlic for about 3 minutes, or until the onion is soft, stirring frequently.

Stir the onion mixture, tuna, and olives into the pasta.

In a small bowl, whisk together the remaining ingredients. Pour over the pasta mixture, tossing to coat. Cover and refrigerate for at least 1 hour so the flavors blend. (You can refrigerate the salad, covered, for up to one day before serving.)

PER SERVING

calories 329
total fat 10.5 g
  saturated fat 2.0 g
  trans fat 0.0 g
  polyunsaturated fat 4.0 g
  monounsaturated fat 3.5 g

cholesterol 41 mg
sodium 288 mg
carbohydrates 32 g
  fiber 5 g
  sugars 8 g
  protein 26 g

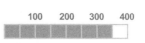

100   200   300   400

DIETARY EXCHANGES
1½ starch, 2 vegetable, 3 lean meat

chicken and toasted walnut salad

serves 4; ½ cup per serving

Serve this sweet and crunchy chicken salad as is or bump up your veggie, fruit, or grain servings by spooning it over a bed of spring greens or slices of cantaloupe or using it to stuff hollowed-out apples or whole-grain pita pockets.

1 teaspoon canola or corn oil

12 ounces chicken tenders, all visible fat discarded

¼ cup fat-free sour cream

2 tablespoons light mayonnaise

2 tablespoons fat-free half-and-half or fat-free milk

½ teaspoon curry powder (optional)

¼ teaspoon salt

¼ teaspoon pepper

¾ cup halved green or red seedless grapes

1 medium rib of celery, thinly sliced

½ cup finely chopped red onion

¼ cup finely chopped dried apricots

¼ cup finely chopped walnuts, dry-roasted

In a large nonstick skillet, heat the oil over medium heat, swirling to coat the bottom. Cook the chicken for 5 minutes on each side, or until no longer pink in the center. Transfer to a cutting board to cool slightly.

Meanwhile, in a medium bowl, whisk together the sour cream, mayonnaise, half-and-half, curry powder, salt, and pepper. Stir in the remaining ingredients except the chicken.

Chop the chicken into bite-size pieces. Stir into the salad. Serve or cover and refrigerate for up to 24 hours.

PER SERVING

calories 246	cholesterol 55 mg
total fat 9.5 g	sodium 282 mg
saturated fat 1.0 g	carbohydrates 18 g
trans fat 0.0 g	fiber 2 g
polyunsaturated fat 5.5 g	sugars 12 g
monounsaturated fat 2.5 g	protein 23 g

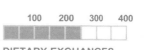

DIETARY EXCHANGES
1 fruit, 3 lean meat

grilled chicken and raspberry salad

serves 4; 3 ounces chicken and 1½ cups salad per serving

A tangy but slightly sweet raspberry vinaigrette does double duty as marinade and dressing for this very attractive salad.

⅓ cup all-fruit seedless red raspberry spread
¼ cup plus 2 tablespoons balsamic vinegar
2 teaspoons olive oil (extra-virgin preferred)
4 boneless, skinless chicken breast halves (about 4 ounces each), all visible fat discarded
Cooking spray
8 ounces mixed greens or mixed field greens
¼ cup crumbled fat-free feta cheese
2 medium green onions, finely chopped
6 ounces red raspberries
¼ cup slivered almonds, dry-roasted

In a small bowl, whisk together the raspberry spread, vinegar, and oil. Pour ¼ cup of the mixture into a large shallow glass dish to use as the marinade. Cover the remaining mixture (about ½ cup) and refrigerate to use as the salad dressing.

Add the chicken to the marinade, turning to coat. Cover and refrigerate for 30 minutes to 12 hours, turning occasionally.

Lightly spray the grill rack with cooking spray. Preheat the grill on medium high.

Drain the chicken, discarding the marinade.

Grill the chicken for 6 minutes. Turn over. Grill for 5 to 6 minutes, or until no longer pink in the center. Transfer to a cutting board. Cut on the diagonal into thick slices.

In a large bowl, toss together the mixed greens, feta, and green onions. Pour in the ½ cup reserved salad dressing, tossing to coat. Gently stir in the raspberries. Arrange on plates. Fan the sliced chicken over the salads. Sprinkle with the almonds. Serve immediately for the best texture.

····· PER SERVING ··

calories 305
total fat 7.5 g
  saturated fat 1.0 g
  trans fat 0.0 g
  polyunsaturated fat 1.5 g
  monounsaturated fat 4.0 g

cholesterol 66 mg
sodium 247 mg
carbohydrates 28 g
  fiber 5 g
  sugars 19 g
protein 31 g

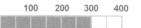

DIETARY EXCHANGES
2 fruit, 3½ lean meat

flank steak salad with sesame-lime dressing

serves 4; 1½ cups salad and 2 ounces steak per serving

The dressing in this recipe is a fine complement for the Honey-Lime Flank Steak (page 278) or other grilled steak saved from a previous meal.

salad

3   cups shredded napa cabbage (about ½ medium)

2   ounces mixed salad greens (spring greens preferred), torn into bite-size pieces

1   8-ounce can sliced water chestnuts, drained

1   7-ounce jar pickled baby corn, drained

4   medium green onions, sliced

8   grape tomatoes or cherry tomatoes

sesame-lime dressing

¼   teaspoon grated lime zest

⅓   cup fresh lime juice

2   tablespoons honey

1   tablespoon plain rice vinegar

2   teaspoons sesame seeds, dry-roasted

Dash of cayenne

8   ounces grilled flank steak (such as reserved from Honey-Lime Flank Steak), thinly sliced on the diagonal and warmed if desired

¼   cup slivered almonds, dry-roasted

In a large bowl, toss together the salad ingredients.

In a small bowl, whisk together the dressing ingredients. Add to the salad, tossing to coat. Place the beef on top. Sprinkle with the almonds.

PER SERVING

calories 231	cholesterol 18 mg
total fat 7.5 g	sodium 198 mg
saturated fat 1.5 g	carbohydrates 25 g
trans fat 0.0 g	fiber 6 g
polyunsaturated fat 1.5 g	sugars 16 g
monounsaturated fat 3.5 g	protein 17 g

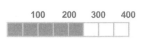

100   200   300   400

DIETARY EXCHANGES
3 vegetable,
½ carbohydrate, 2 lean meat

cannellini and black bean salad

serves 4; 1½ cups bean salad and 1 cup spinach per serving

This colorful salad has it all—smooth and crunchy textures; tart, sweet, and hot flavors; and protein, fruit, and vegetables.

2 cups grape tomatoes or chopped tomatoes
1 cup no-salt-added cannellini beans, rinsed and drained
1 cup no-salt-added black beans, rinsed and drained
1 cup peeled jícama in 1-inch-long strips (about 10 ounces)
1 large mango, chopped
1 small onion, chopped
2 small fresh jalapeños, seeds and ribs discarded, diced
¼ cup snipped fresh cilantro
3 tablespoons fresh lime juice
1 tablespoon white wine vinegar
½ teaspoon salt
¼ teaspoon pepper
4 ounces baby spinach

In a large bowl, toss together all the ingredients except the spinach. (You can refrigerate the mixture, covered, for up to one day before serving.)

Put the spinach on plates. Top with the bean mixture.

TIME-SAVER For a shortcut, substitute 3 cups of refrigerated pico de gallo for the tomatoes, onion, jalapeños, cilantro, and 1 tablespoon of the lime juice. You can find pico de gallo in the produce section of your grocery store.

PER SERVING

calories 212
total fat 1.0 g
  saturated fat 0.0 g
  trans fat 0.0 g
  polyunsaturated fat 0.0 g
  monounsaturated fat 0.0 g

cholesterol 0 mg
sodium 364 mg
carbohydrates 45 g
  fiber 11 g
  sugars 18 g
protein 9 g

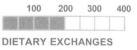

DIETARY EXCHANGES
1 starch, 1 fruit,
3 vegetable

taco salad
with avocado dressing

serves 4; 2 cups per serving

Dressed with a luscious mix of rich avocado, fat-free milk and sour cream, and fresh lime juice, this vegetarian taco salad has a kick of flavor and packs enough protein to fill you up.

avocado dressing

1	medium ripe avocado, peeled
½	cup fat-free milk
¼	cup fat-free sour cream
2	tablespoons fresh lime juice
2	medium garlic cloves, peeled
1	teaspoon red hot-pepper sauce

salad

8	ounces shredded lettuce, such as romaine (about 3½ cups)
1	15.5-ounce can no-salt-added pinto beans, rinsed and drained
¼	medium red onion, finely chopped
1	cup frozen whole-kernel corn, thawed
¼	teaspoon salt
1½	ounces baked tortilla chips (lowest sodium available), coarsely crumbled
2	ounces shredded fat-free sharp Cheddar cheese (about ½ cup)
¼	cup snipped fresh cilantro
1	medium tomato, diced
1	medium lime, quartered

In a food processor or blender, process the dressing ingredients until smooth.

In an 11 x 7 x 2-inch glass casserole dish, make one layer each of lettuce, beans, onion, and corn. Spoon the dressing on top, spreading to cover. Sprinkle with the salt. Make one layer each of the remaining salad ingredients except the lime wedges. Serve or cover and refrigerate for up to 1 hour. Serve with the lime wedges to squeeze over the salad.

COOK'S TIP You can make the creamy avocado dressing up to 48 hours in advance. Cover and refrigerate it until needed. The lime juice not only livens up the flavors but also keeps the avocado from discoloring. Once you've tasted the dressing, you'll want to use it frequently, on other salads, as a dip for raw vegetables, or even as a quick sauce for grilled chicken, seafood, or pork.

PER SERVING

calories 328	cholesterol 6 mg
total fat 8.5 g	sodium 333 mg
saturated fat 1.0 g	carbohydrates 50 g
trans fat 0.0 g	fiber 11 g
polyunsaturated fat 1.0 g	sugars 10 g
monounsaturated fat 5.0 g	protein 17 g

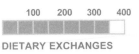

DIETARY EXCHANGES
3 starch, 1 vegetable,
1 very lean meat, 1 fat

seafood

Cornmeal-Crusted Catfish with Lemon-Ginger Tartar Sauce

Baked Almond-Crunch Halibut

Grilled Fish with Cucumber Salsa

Pasta with Salmon, Roasted Mushrooms, and Asparagus

Salmon-and-Veggie Patties with Mustard Cream

Salmon Florentine

Salmon with Creamy Caper Sauce

Skillet-Poached Salmon with Wasabi Soy Sauce

Tilapia Champignon

Tilapia en Papillote

Tilapia and Spinach Roll-Ups with Shallot and White Wine Sauce

Fish Tacos with Tomato and Avocado Salsa

Lime-Cilantro Swordfish with Mixed Bean and Pineapple Salsa

Hazelnut-Crusted Trout with Balsamic Glaze

Grilled Trout with Horseradish Sour Cream

Sweet-Heat Broiled Trout

Gourmet Tuna-Noodle Casserole

Tuna Lettuce Wraps with Asian Sauce

Tuna and Broccoli with Lemon-Caper Brown Rice

Orange-Ginger Tuna Steaks

Tuna Steaks with Tarragon Sour Cream

Scallop and Spinach Sauté

Tomato-Caper Shrimp with Herbed Feta

Cumin Shrimp and Rice Toss

cornmeal-crusted catfish with lemon-ginger tartar sauce

serves 4; 3 ounces fish and 1 tablespoon tartar sauce per serving

Catfish goes from common to chic with this classy dish. The fillets are dusted with a figure-friendly lemon-pepper cornmeal coating, pan-seared until crisp, and topped with a zesty, low-calorie tartar sauce. A good choice for a side dish is either Carrot-Pineapple Slaw with Ginger (page 170) or Multicolored Marinated Slaw (page 171).

tartar sauce

¼ cup light mayonnaise

1 tablespoon sweet pickle relish

1 teaspoon grated peeled gingerroot

1 teaspoon grated lemon zest

1 teaspoon fresh lemon juice

fish

¼ cup low-fat buttermilk

½ teaspoon salt-free lemon pepper

4 catfish fillets (about 4 ounces each), rinsed and patted dry

¼ cup whole-wheat flour

¼ cup yellow cornmeal

1 teaspoon canola or corn oil

Cooking spray

In a small bowl, stir together the tartar sauce ingredients. Cover and refrigerate until ready to serve. (The tartar sauce will keep for up to three days in the refrigerator.)

In a large shallow dish, stir together the buttermilk and lemon pepper. Add the fish, turning to coat. Let the fish soak for 10 minutes at room temperature or cover and refrigerate for up to 4 hours.

In a medium shallow dish, stir together the flour and cornmeal. Dip one piece of fish in the cornmeal mixture, turning to coat and gently shaking off any excess. Using your fingertips, gently press the coating so it adheres to the fish. Transfer to a large plate. Repeat with the remaining fish.

In a large nonstick skillet, heat the oil over medium-high heat, swirling to coat the bottom. Cook the fish for 4 to 5 minutes, or until browned on one side. Remove the pan from the heat and lightly spray the top of the fish with cooking spray. Turn the fish over. Cook for 4 to 5 minutes, or until the fish is golden brown and flakes easily when tested with a fork. Serve with the tartar sauce.

······ **PER SERVING** ···

calories 235
total fat 10.0 g
  saturated fat 2.0 g
  trans fat 0.0 g
  polyunsaturated fat 4.0 g
  monounsaturated fat 3.0 g

cholesterol 72 mg
sodium 198 mg
carbohydrates 16 g
  fiber 2 g
  sugars 3 g
protein 21 g

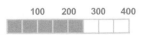

DIETARY EXCHANGES
1 starch, 3 lean meat

baked almond-crunch halibut

serves 4; 3 ounces fish, ½ cup carrots, and ½ potato per serving

Simplify dinnertime by baking your fish and vegetables in one pan. Add Asparagus and Cucumber Salad with Lemon and Mint (page 166) or a simple tossed salad for a delicious meal.

Cooking spray

2   medium baking potatoes, such as russet, unpeeled, cut lengthwise into ½-inch-thick strips

2   cups baby carrots

⅛   teaspoon salt and ⅛ teaspoon salt, divided use

Pepper to taste

4   halibut steaks or fillets (about 4 ounces each), rinsed and patted dry

Pepper to taste

2   tablespoons Dijon mustard

2   tablespoons light tub margarine, melted

1   tablespoon plus 1 teaspoon honey

¼   cup plain dry bread crumbs (lowest sodium available)

¼   cup sliced almonds

2   tablespoons snipped fresh parsley or 1 teaspoon dried, crumbled

2   tablespoons snipped fresh cilantro or 1 teaspoon dried, crumbled

Preheat the oven to 375°F. Lightly spray a large baking sheet with cooking spray.

Place the potatoes and carrots in a single layer on the baking sheet. Lightly spray with cooking spray. Sprinkle with ⅛ teaspoon salt and the pepper.

Bake for 15 minutes.

Meanwhile, sprinkle the fish with the remaining ⅛ teaspoon salt and pepper.

In a small bowl, stir together the mustard, margarine, and honey. Brush on both sides of the fish.

In another small bowl, stir together the remaining ingredients. Using your fingertips, gently press the mixture on both sides so it adheres to the fish.

Remove the baking sheet from the oven. Increase the temperature to 450°F. Using a spatula, turn the potatoes and carrots over, making room in the middle for the fish. Without disturbing the crumb coating, gently place the fish on the baking sheet.

Bake for 10 minutes for each inch of thickness, or until the fish flakes easily when tested with a fork.

······ **PER SERVING** ······

calories 319
total fat 9 g
  saturated fat 0.5 g
  trans fat 0.0 g
  polyunsaturated fat 2.5 g
  monounsaturated fat 4 g

cholesterol 36 mg
sodium 481 mg
carbohydrates 32 g
  fiber 4 g
  sugars 11 g
  protein 28 g

100   200   300   400

DIETARY EXCHANGES
1½ starch, 1 vegetable,
3 lean meat

grilled fish
with cucumber salsa

serves 4; 3 ounces fish and ½ cup salsa per serving

Serve this on a summer night when you don't want to heat up the kitchen.

Cooking spray

salsa

1 medium cucumber, finely chopped

½ medium green bell pepper, finely chopped

½ medium avocado, finely chopped

⅓ cup snipped fresh parsley

½ teaspoon grated lemon zest

1 to 2 tablespoons fresh lemon juice

¼ teaspoon salt

¼ teaspoon red hot-pepper sauce

fish

4 firm-fleshed fish fillets, such as halibut (about 4 ounces each), rinsed and patted dry

½ teaspoon chili powder

¼ teaspoon salt

1 medium lemon, cut into 4 wedges

Lightly spray the grill rack with cooking spray. Preheat the grill on medium high.

In a medium bowl, gently stir together the salsa ingredients. Set aside.

Sprinkle the fish on both sides with the chili powder and remaining ¼ teaspoon salt. Using your fingertips, gently press the seasonings so they adhere to the fish. Lightly spray both sides of the fish with cooking spray.

Grill for 3 minutes on each side, or until the fish flakes easily when tested with a fork. Spoon the salsa over the fish. Place the lemon wedges on the side to squeeze over the fish.

······ **PER SERVING** ··

calories 183
total fat 6.5 g
  saturated fat 1.0 g
  trans fat 0.0 g
  polyunsaturated fat 1.5 g
  monounsaturated fat 3.5 g

cholesterol 36 mg
sodium 362 mg
carbohydrates 6 g
  fiber 3 g
  sugars 2 g
protein 25 g

100	200	300	400

DIETARY EXCHANGES
1 vegetable, 3 lean meat

pasta with salmon, roasted mushrooms, and asparagus

serves 4; 1½ cups per serving

·····

While the vegetables are roasting, the pasta is cooking for this all-in-one meal featuring salmon in a pouch. Fit in some extra veggies with a tossed salad or add some fruit with Asian Citrus Salad (page 173).

Cooking spray

3 tablespoons red wine vinegar or balsamic vinegar

1 tablespoon soy sauce or teriyaki sauce (lowest sodium available)

2 teaspoons sugar

2 medium garlic cloves, minced

1 teaspoon minced peeled gingerroot

¼ teaspoon pepper

8 ounces baby bella or other mushrooms, thickly sliced

8 ounces asparagus, trimmed and cut diagonally into 1-inch pieces

2 tablespoons sesame seeds

6 ounces whole-grain or spinach elbow macaroni

1 7-ounce vacuum-sealed pouch pink salmon, coarsely flaked

2 teaspoons toasted sesame oil

2 medium green onions, chopped

Preheat the oven to 425°F. Lightly spray a rimmed baking sheet with cooking spray. Set aside.

In a large bowl, stir together the vinegar, soy sauce, sugar, garlic, gingerroot, and pepper.

Add the mushrooms and asparagus, stirring to coat. Place in a single layer on the baking sheet. Spoon the vinegar mixture remaining in the bowl over them. Sprinkle with the sesame seeds.

Bake for 10 minutes. Stir. Bake for 5 minutes, or until the mushrooms and asparagus are beginning to caramelize or become richly browned.

Meanwhile, prepare the pasta using the package directions, omitting the salt. Drain well in a colander. Transfer to a large bowl.

Gently stir the fish, mushroom mixture with accumulated pan juices, and oil into the pasta. Sprinkle with the green onions.

COOK'S TIP ON GINGERROOT When purchasing gingerroot, look for firm, unwrinkled pieces with thin skin. Peel the gingerroot with a sharp paring knife or a vegetable peeler, then grate, mince, chop, or slice.

····· PER SERVING ··

calories 301
total fat 8.5 g
  saturated fat 1.5 g
  trans fat 0.0 g
  polyunsaturated fat 3.0 g
  monounsaturated fat 2.5 g

cholesterol 18 mg
sodium 350 mg
carbohydrates 41 g
  fiber 8 g
  sugars 7 g
protein 18 g

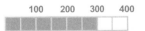

DIETARY EXCHANGES
2 starch, 2 vegetable,
1 very lean meat, 1 fat

salmon-and-veggie patties with mustard cream

serves 4; 2 patties and 2 tablespoons sauce per serving

Add red bell pepper, corn, and green onions to salmon patties for color, texture, and the fiber that helps fill you up.

1 teaspoon canola or corn oil, 1 teaspoon canola or corn oil, and 1 teaspoon canola or corn oil, divided use

patties

½ medium red bell pepper, diced

4 medium green onions, finely chopped

1 5-ounce vacuum-sealed pouch pink salmon, flaked

½ cup frozen whole-kernel corn, thawed

¼ cup snipped fresh parsley

¼ cup cornmeal

2 large egg whites

2 tablespoons light mayonnaise

2 tablespoons fat-free milk

1½ teaspoons yellow mustard

sauce

⅓ cup fat-free sour cream

2 tablespoons light mayonnaise

1 tablespoon fat-free milk

1 teaspoon yellow mustard

⅛ teaspoon salt

In a large nonstick skillet, heat 1 teaspoon oil over medium heat, swirling to coat the bottom. Cook the bell pepper for 4 minutes, or until tender, stirring frequently. Remove from the heat.

In a medium bowl, stir together the bell pepper and remaining salmon patty ingredients.

In the same skillet, heat 1 teaspoon oil over medium heat, swirling to coat the bottom. Using about half the mixture, spoon four mounds of the salmon mixture, about ¼ cup each, into the skillet. Using the back of a fork or spoon, slightly flatten each mound to make patties. Cook for 2 to 3 minutes on each side, or until golden brown and cooked through, turning the patties gently so they don't break up. Transfer to a large plate. Cover to keep warm. Repeat with the final 1 teaspoon oil and remaining salmon mixture. Transfer all the patties to plates.

Meanwhile, in a small bowl, whisk together the sauce ingredients. Spoon next to the patties.

····· PER SERVING ···

calories 205
total fat 9.0 g
  saturated fat 1.0 g
  trans fat 0.0 g
  polyunsaturated fat 4.0 g
  monounsaturated fat 3.5 g

cholesterol 21 mg
sodium 474 mg
carbohydrates 20 g
  fiber 3 g
  sugars 5 g
protein 12 g

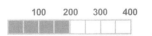

DIETARY EXCHANGES
1½ starch, 1 lean meat, 1 fat

salmon florentine

serves 4; 3 ounces fish and ½ cup spinach per serving

The large amount of spinach in this entrée cooks down into a colorful bed for the salmon—and a veggie serving for you.

    Cooking spray
1   tablespoon salt-free all-purpose seasoning blend
1   teaspoon pepper
1   teaspoon paprika
1   teaspoon olive oil
1   teaspoon water
2   medium garlic cloves, minced
¼   teaspoon salt
4   salmon fillets (about 4 ounces each), rinsed and patted dry
8   ounces baby spinach
1   6-ounce jar marinated artichoke hearts, drained and chopped

Preheat the oven to 375°F. Lightly spray a 13 x 9 x 2-inch baking pan with cooking spray.

In a small bowl, stir together the seasoning blend, pepper, paprika, oil, water, garlic, and salt. Brush over both sides of the fish.

Put the spinach in the baking pan, covering the bottom. Put the fish and artichokes on the spinach. Lightly spray with cooking spray.

Bake for 15 to 20 minutes, or to the desired doneness.

PER SERVING

calories 189
total fat 8.5 g
  saturated fat 1.0 g
  trans fat 0.0 g
  polyunsaturated fat 2.0 g
  monounsaturated fat 2.0 g

cholesterol 59 mg
sodium 385 mg
carbohydrates 6 g
  fiber 3 g
  sugars 0 g
  protein 24 g

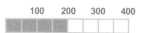

DIETARY EXCHANGES
1 vegetable, 3 lean meat

salmon with creamy caper sauce

serves 4; 3 ounces fish and 2 tablespoons sauce per serving

If you need a fast entrée for a busy night, you can depend on this dish. Combine the sauce ingredients while the salmon cooks, then steam some broccoli and whole-wheat couscous for a complete meal that keeps the calories in check.

Cooking spray

4 salmon fillets with skin (about 5 ounces each), rinsed and patted dry

¼ teaspoon pepper

sauce

⅓ cup fat-free plain yogurt

2 tablespoons capers, drained

2 teaspoons fat-free milk

1 teaspoon dried dillweed, crumbled

¾ teaspoon Dijon mustard (stone-ground preferred)

½ medium garlic clove, minced

¼ teaspoon pepper (coarsely ground preferred)

Preheat the oven to 350°F. Line a baking sheet with aluminum foil. Lightly spray with cooking spray.

Put the fish with the skin side down on the baking sheet. Sprinkle with ¼ teaspoon pepper.

Bake for 18 to 20 minutes, or to the desired doneness.

Meanwhile, in a small bowl, stir together the sauce ingredients. Serve with the fish.

PER SERVING

calories 148
total fat 4.0 g
  saturated fat 0.5 g
  trans fat 0.0 g
  polyunsaturated fat 1.5 g
  monounsaturated fat 1.0 g

cholesterol 59 mg
sodium 240 mg
carbohydrates 3 g
  fiber 0 g
  sugars 2 g
  protein 24 g

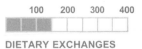

DIETARY EXCHANGES
3 lean meat

skillet-poached salmon with wasabi soy sauce

serves 4; 3 ounces fish and ½ cup sugar snap peas per serving

A pungent blend of wasabi, soy sauce, and fresh ginger makes an unusual poaching liquid for salmon. With sugar snap peas added, the sauce is then reduced to a tempting glaze. Serve with soba noodles and fresh orange slices.

½ cup fat-free, low-sodium chicken broth

2 medium green onions, chopped

2 tablespoons light brown sugar

2 tablespoons soy sauce (lowest sodium available)

1 teaspoon grated peeled gingerroot

1 teaspoon wasabi paste

1 teaspoon toasted sesame oil

1 medium garlic clove, minced

4 salmon fillets (about 4 ounces each), rinsed and patted dry

8 ounces sugar snap peas, trimmed

In a large skillet, bring the broth, green onions, brown sugar, soy sauce, gingerroot, wasabi paste, oil, and garlic to a simmer over medium-high heat.

Add the fish. Spoon the sauce mixture over the fish to coat. Reduce the heat and simmer, covered, for 8 to 9 minutes, or until the fish is almost the desired doneness.

Stir in the peas. Increase the heat to medium high. Occasionally spooning the sauce over the fish, cook, uncovered, for 2 to 3 minutes, or until the fish is the desired doneness, the peas are tender, and the sauce is slightly reduced, to the consistency of a glaze.

PER SERVING

calories 205
total fat 5.5 g
  saturated fat 1.0 g
  trans fat 0.0 g
  polyunsaturated fat 2.0 g
  monounsaturated fat 1.5 g

cholesterol 59 mg
sodium 310 mg
carbohydrates 13 g
  fiber 2 g
  sugars 9 g
  protein 25 g

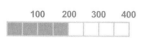

DIETARY EXCHANGES
1 carbohydrate, 3 lean meat

tilapia champignon

serves 4; 3 ounces fish per serving

Mushrooms and wine combine magnificently with tilapia to create a delicate entrée. It will transform an ordinary weeknight meal into a special occasion.

Olive oil spray

8 ounces button mushrooms, sliced

¼ cup dry white wine and ¼ cup dry white wine (regular or nonalcoholic), divided use

2 medium garlic cloves, minced

2½ tablespoons plain dry bread crumbs (lowest sodium available)

2 tablespoons shredded or grated Romano cheese

2 teaspoons salt-free all-purpose seasoning blend

1 teaspoon dried parsley, crumbled

1 teaspoon paprika

4 tilapia fillets (about 4 ounces each), rinsed and patted dry

1 medium lemon, cut into 4 wedges

Preheat the oven to 375°F. Lightly spray a 13 x 9 x 2-inch baking pan with olive oil spray. Set aside.

In a large nonstick skillet, cook the mushrooms and ¼ cup wine over medium-high heat for 7 to 10 minutes, or until the mushrooms are soft, stirring occasionally.

Stir in the garlic. Cook for 1 minute.

Meanwhile, in a small bowl, stir together the bread crumbs, Romano, seasoning blend, parsley, and paprika.

Put the fillets side by side in the baking pan. Pour in the mushroom mixture. Pour the remaining ¼ cup wine around, not over, the fish. Sprinkle the fish with the bread-crumb mixture.

Bake for 15 to 18 minutes, or until the fish flakes easily when tested with a fork. Serve with the lemon wedges.

PER SERVING

calories 170	cholesterol 58 mg	
total fat 3.0 g	sodium 113 mg	
saturated fat 1.0 g	carbohydrates 7 g	
trans fat 0.0 g	fiber 1 g	
polyunsaturated fat 0.5 g	sugars 2 g	
monounsaturated fat 0.5 g	protein 26 g	

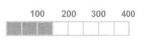

DIETARY EXCHANGES
½ starch, 3 very lean meat

tilapia en papillote

serves 4; 3 ounces fish and ¼ cup pico de gallo per serving

For tender, moist fish, steam it in parchment paper (*en papillote*). Serving each diner a puffed parchment pouch, with the top split open to release the aromatic steam, makes a dramatic presentation.

pico de gallo

- ½ cup chopped tomato
- ½ cup chopped onion
- ¼ cup snipped fresh cilantro
- ½ medium fresh jalapeño, seeds and ribs discarded, diced
- 1 tablespoon fresh lime juice

....

- Cooking spray
- 4 tilapia fillets (about 4 ounces each), rinsed and patted dry
- ⅛ teaspoon salt
- ⅛ teaspoon pepper
- 2 medium limes, each cut into 4 or 8 slices

Preheat the oven to 450°F.

In a small bowl, stir together the pico de gallo ingredients. Set aside.

Fold four pieces of cooking parchment, each about 14 x 12 inches, in half lengthwise. Cut each piece into a heart shape using the fold as the center of the heart and cutting half a heart. Open the paper hearts and set them on a flat surface with the point of each heart toward you. Lightly spray the center of one half of each with cooking spray. Place the fish lengthwise on the sprayed area. Sprinkle with salt and pepper. Top with pico de gallo. Cover with slices of lime. For each serving, fold the half without the fish over. Starting at the top of the heart, seal the packets by rolling the edges together. When you reach the bottom of the heart, turn the last fold under the parchment pouch. Transfer with the smooth side up to a baking sheet.

Bake for 8 minutes. Transfer the pouches to plates. Cut into the pouches at the top, being careful to avoid a steam burn.

COOK'S TIP Try different types of fish and vegetables to create your own signature dishes. Sole, cod, and catfish are just a few fish that would work well. Instead of the pico de gallo, experiment with slices of mushrooms, zucchini, carrots, or shallots placed under the fillet, and top with dill, thyme, or basil and lemon slices. Prepare as directed above.

TIME-SAVER Use store-bought pico de gallo instead of making your own. You'll need 1 cup for this recipe.

···· PER SERVING ···

calories 128
total fat 2.0 g
  saturated fat 1.0 g
  trans fat 0.0 g
  polyunsaturated fat 0.5 g
  monounsaturated fat 0.5 g

cholesterol 57 mg
sodium 135 mg
carbohydrates 5 g
  fiber 1 g
  sugars 2 g
protein 23 g

100   200   300   400

DIETARY EXCHANGES
1 vegetable,
3 very lean meat

tilapia and spinach roll-ups with shallot and white wine sauce

serves 4; 3 ounces fish per serving

Mild-flavored tilapia, which blends so nicely with other foods, is complemented here with baby spinach and a topping of crushed walnuts. Don't worry about the calories in the wine; most of the alcohol calories evaporate during the cooking process.

- 4 tilapia fillets (about 4 ounces each), rinsed and patted dry
- ¼ teaspoon salt
   Pepper to taste
- 5 ounces baby spinach
- ½ cup shredded or grated Parmesan cheese
- 1 cup dry white wine (regular or nonalcoholic), plus more as needed
- ½ cup fat-free, low-sodium chicken broth or low-sodium vegetable broth, plus more as needed
- 1 medium shallot, minced
- 2 tablespoons walnuts, crushed

Preheat the oven to 375°F.

Place the fish on a flat work surface. Sprinkle the fish with the salt and pepper. Place the spinach on the fish. Sprinkle with the Parmesan. Starting at a short end, roll each fillet jelly-roll style and secure with a wooden toothpick. Transfer the roll-ups to a 13 x 9 x 2-inch glass baking dish.

Pour the wine and broth over the fish. If the dish isn't filled to a depth of about ½ inch, add more wine and broth, using twice as much wine as broth.

Sprinkle the roll-ups with the shallot.

Bake, covered, for 30 minutes, or until the fish flakes easily when tested with a fork.

Using a slotted pancake turner or spatula, transfer the roll-ups to plates. Sprinkle with the walnuts.

···· PER SERVING ··
calories 234	cholesterol 64 mg	
total fat 7.0 g	sodium 441 mg	
saturated fat 2.5 g	carbohydrates 6 g	
trans fat 0.0 g	fiber 2 g	
polyunsaturated fat 2.5 g	sugars 0 g	
monounsaturated fat 2.0 g	protein 28 g	

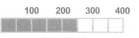

100   200   300   400

1 vegetable, 3½ lean meat

fish tacos with tomato and avocado salsa

serves 4; 1 taco per serving

Finely chopped fresh vegetables absorb flavor—lime and cilantro here— more evenly than larger pieces would, giving you a very tasty salsa.

salsa

1 medium tomato, finely chopped

1 medium avocado, chopped

½ medium green bell pepper, finely chopped

⅓ cup snipped fresh cilantro

¼ cup finely chopped red onion

1 to 2 tablespoons fresh lime juice

¼ teaspoon salt

tacos

4 thin mild fish fillets, such as tilapia (about 4 ounces each), rinsed and patted dry

½ teaspoon ground cumin

Paprika to taste

1 teaspoon canola or corn oil

Cooking spray

4 8-inch fat-free flour tortillas (lowest sodium available)

2 cups shredded lettuce

In a medium bowl, stir together the salsa ingredients. Set aside.

Sprinkle the fish on both sides with the cumin and paprika. Using your fingertips, gently press the seasonings so they adhere to the fish.

In a large nonstick skillet, heat the oil over medium-high heat, swirling to coat the bottom. Remove the skillet from the heat and lightly spray the fish with cooking spray. Cook for 3 minutes on each side, or until the fish flakes easily when tested with a fork.

Meanwhile, warm the tortillas using the package directions.

Top each tortilla with lettuce, fish, and salsa. Serve either open-face or as a wrap.

···· **PER SERVING** ···

calories 340

total fat 11.0 g

  saturated fat 2.0 g

  trans fat 0.0 g

  polyunsaturated fat 2.0 g

  monounsaturated fat 6.5 g

cholesterol 57 mg

sodium 555 mg

carbohydrates 33 g

  fiber 7 g

  sugars 3 g

  protein 29 g

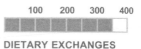

DIETARY EXCHANGES

1½ starch, 2 vegetable,

3 lean meat

lime-cilantro swordfish with mixed bean and pineapple salsa

serves 4; 3 ounces fish and ¾ cup salsa per serving

This dish is inspired by the tropics and Mexico. Prepare the salsa several hours in advance, if possible, to allow the flavors to blend.

marinade

3 to 4 tablespoons fresh lime juice

1 tablespoon olive oil (extra-virgin preferred)

1 tablespoon honey

¼ teaspoon salt

Pepper to taste

4 swordfish steaks (about 4 ounces each), rinsed and patted dry

salsa

1 cup canned no-salt-added black beans, rinsed and drained

1 cup canned no-salt-added pink or pinto beans, rinsed and drained

1 cup finely diced pineapple

½ cup snipped fresh cilantro

3 to 4 tablespoons fresh lime juice

2 tablespoons minced red onion

1 tablespoon olive oil (extra-virgin preferred)

½ teaspoon ground cumin

⅛ teaspoon salt

Dash of pepper

1 tablespoon snipped fresh cilantro (optional)

In a large shallow glass dish, stir together the marinade ingredients. Add the fish, turning to coat. Cover and refrigerate for 20 minutes to 2 hours, turning occasionally.

Meanwhile, stir together the salsa ingredients. Set aside.

Preheat the grill on high.

Drain the fish, discarding the marinade.

Grill for about 3 minutes on each side, or until seared and the desired doneness. Serve topped with the salsa. Garnish with the remaining 1 tablespoon cilantro.

COOK'S TIP ON SEA SALT Sea salt is the least processed salt and therefore contains the most natural nutrients. It is very flavorful, so when substituting it for table salt, use slightly less sea salt.

···· **PER SERVING** ··

calories 296

total fat 8.0 g

  saturated fat 1.5 g

  trans fat 0.0 g

  polyunsaturated fat 1.5 g

  monounsaturated fat 4.0 g

cholesterol 41 mg

sodium 316 mg

carbohydrates 27 g

  fiber 6 g

  sugars 9 g

protein 28 g

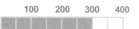

100   200   300   400

DIETARY EXCHANGES

1½ starch, ½ fruit,

3½ lean meat

hazelnut-crusted trout with balsamic glaze

serves 4; 3 ounces fish and 1 tablespoon glaze per serving

An almost-effortless, intense balsamic glaze is the crowning touch to pan-seared trout fillets coated with crunchy hazelnut breading.

3   tablespoons all-purpose flour

¼   cup low-fat buttermilk

¼   cup plain dry bread crumbs (lowest sodium available)

2   tablespoons finely chopped hazelnuts

4   trout fillets with skin (about 5 ounces each), rinsed and patted dry

1   teaspoon olive oil

    Olive oil spray

½   cup balsamic vinegar

2   medium shallots, finely chopped

1   tablespoon light brown sugar

Put the flour and buttermilk in separate shallow dishes. In a third shallow dish, stir together the bread crumbs and hazelnuts. Set the dishes in a row, assembly-line fashion. Dip one fillet in the flour, turning to coat and gently shaking off any excess. Dip only the flesh side of the fillet in the buttermilk, letting the excess drip off. Dip the flesh side in the bread crumb mixture. Using your fingertips, lightly press the mixture so it adheres to the fish. Transfer to a large plate. Repeat with the remaining fish.

In a large nonstick skillet, heat the oil over medium-high heat, swirling to coat the bottom. Cook the fish with the flesh side down for 3 to 4 minutes, or until the crust is golden brown. Remove the pan from the heat. Lightly spray the skin side of the fish with olive oil spray. Turn the fish over and cook with the skin side down for 3 to 4 minutes, or until the fish flakes easily when tested with a fork.

Meanwhile, in a small saucepan, stir together the vinegar and shallots. Bring to a simmer over medium-high heat. Reduce the heat and simmer without stirring for 5 minutes, or until the mixture is reduced by half (to about ¼ cup).

Stir in the brown sugar. Simmer without stirring for 1 minute, or until the sugar is dissolved.

Using tongs, remove and discard the fish skin. Serve the fish with the crust side up. Drizzle with the glaze.

···· PER SERVING ··

calories 267
total fat 8.0 g
  saturated fat 1.5 g
  trans fat 0.0 g
  polyunsaturated fat 2.0 g
  monounsaturated fat 4.0 g

cholesterol 68 mg
sodium 110 mg
carbohydrates 22 g
  fiber 1 g
  sugars 12 g
protein 26 g

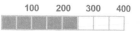

DIETARY EXCHANGES
1 starch, ½ carbohydrate,
3 lean meat

grilled trout with horseradish sour cream

serves 4; 3 ounces fish and 2 tablespoons sauce per serving

One surprise in this mouthwatering dish is the use of steak seasoning blend in the rub mixture. Another is the cream sauce's low calorie count, which lets you enjoy rich taste without feeling guilty.

Cooking spray

sauce

½ cup fat-free sour cream

2 teaspoons olive oil (extra-virgin preferred)

1½ teaspoons bottled white horseradish, drained

½ teaspoon Worcestershire sauce (lowest sodium available)

¼ teaspoon pepper

¼ teaspoon salt

fish

4 trout fillets (about 4 ounces each), rinsed and patted dry

1 teaspoon olive oil and 1 teaspoon olive oil, divided use

½ teaspoon salt-free steak seasoning blend and ½ teaspoon salt-free steak seasoning blend, divided use

1 medium lemon, cut into 4 wedges

Lightly spray the grill rack with cooking spray. Preheat the grill on medium high.

In a small bowl, whisk together the sauce ingredients. Cover and refrigerate.

Place the fish on a cutting board or other flat surface. Lightly brush 1 teaspoon oil over the tops. Sprinkle ½ teaspoon seasoning blend over the fish. Using your fingertips, gently press the mixture so it adheres to the fish. Turn over. Repeat with the remaining 1 teaspoon oil and remaining ½ teaspoon seasoning blend.

Grill the fish for 4 to 5 minutes on each side, or until it flakes easily when tested with a fork. Serve with the sauce and lemon wedges to squeeze over the fish.

···· PER SERVING ·······

calories 209
total fat 8.5 g
  saturated fat 1.5 g
  trans fat 0.0 g
  polyunsaturated fat 2.0 g
  monounsaturated fat 4.5 g

cholesterol 72 mg
sodium 213 mg
carbohydrates 6 g
  fiber 0 g
  sugars 3 g
protein 25 g

100	200	300	400

DIETARY EXCHANGES
½ carbohydrate,
3 lean meat

sweet-heat broiled trout

serves 4; 3 ounces fish per serving

It takes only three ingredients to provide a touch of sweetness and heat for mild-tasting trout. With this simple-to-prepare dish, you'll have dinner on the table in minutes—it's as easy as 1-2-3!

Cooking spray

4 trout fillets with skin (about 5 ounces each), rinsed and patted dry

2 tablespoons firmly packed light brown sugar

1 teaspoon ground cumin

⅛ teaspoon cayenne

Place a broiler rack on the top level, about 2 inches from the heat. Preheat the broiler.

Lightly spray a large baking sheet (not nonstick) with cooking spray. Place the fish with the skin side down on the baking sheet.

In a small bowl, stir together the brown sugar, cumin, and cayenne. Sprinkle over the flesh side of the fish. Using your fingertips, firmly press the mixture so it adheres to the fish.

Broil the fish for 4 to 5 minutes, or until it flakes easily when tested with a fork. Remove the baking sheet from the broiler. Turn the fish over so the skin side is up.

Using tongs, remove and discard the fish skin. Carefully place the fish with the seasoned side up on plates.

PER SERVING

calories 163	cholesterol 70 mg
total fat 4.0 g	sodium 38 mg
saturated fat 1.0 g	carbohydrates 7 g
trans fat 0.0 g	fiber 0 g
polyunsaturated fat 1.5 g	sugars 7 g
monounsaturated fat 1.5 g	protein 23 g

100   200   300   400

DIETARY EXCHANGES
½ carbohydrate,
3 lean meat

gourmet tuna-noodle casserole

serves 6; 1½ cups per serving

This creamy casserole uses fat-free and low-fat ingredients to cut calories as well as saturated fat and cholesterol.

- 8 ounces dried whole-grain pasta, such as rotini
- Cooking spray
- 12 ounces canned very low sodium albacore tuna, packed in water, drained and flaked
- 1 10.75-ounce can low-fat condensed cream of chicken soup (lowest sodium available)
- 1 10-ounce package frozen chopped spinach, thawed and squeezed dry
- 1 8-ounce can sliced water chestnuts, drained, coarsely chopped
- ½ cup fat-free milk
- ½ cup fat-free sour cream
- 2 medium green onions, thinly sliced
- 1 tablespoon snipped fresh dillweed
- 2 teaspoons grated lemon zest
- ¼ teaspoon salt
- ½ cup cornflake crumbs (about 1¼ cups cornflakes)

Prepare the pasta using the package directions, omitting the salt. Drain well in a colander. Transfer to a large bowl.

Meanwhile, preheat the oven to 350°F. Lightly spray a 13 x 9 x 2-inch baking pan with cooking spray.

Stir the remaining ingredients except the crumbs into the pasta. Spoon into the baking pan. Sprinkle with the crumbs.

Bake for 30 minutes, or until heated through.

PER SERVING

calories 323
total fat 4.0 g
  saturated fat 1.0 g
  trans fat 0.0 g
  polyunsaturated fat 1.0 g
  monounsaturated fat 1.0 g

cholesterol 30 mg
sodium 432 mg
carbohydrates 49 g
  fiber 8 g
  sugars 6 g
protein 23 g

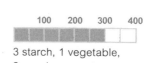

3 starch, 1 vegetable, 2 very lean meat

tuna lettuce wraps with asian sauce

serves 4; 3 wraps per serving

This version of tuna salad sandwiches cuts calories by using lettuce leaves instead of bread and adds nutrients by including extra veggies and nuts.

sauce

- ¼ cup sugar
- ¼ cup fresh lime juice
- 1½ tablespoons canola or corn oil

wraps

- 8 ounces packaged shredded cabbage and carrot coleslaw mix
- ½ cup matchstick-size carrot strips
- ¼ cup sliced almonds, dry-roasted
- ¼ cup snipped fresh cilantro
- 1 medium fresh jalapeño, seeds and ribs discarded, finely chopped
- 2 tablespoons snipped fresh basil
- 12 Bibb lettuce leaves
- 1 5-ounce can very low sodium albacore tuna, packed in water, drained and flaked

In a small bowl, whisk together the sauce invgredients until the sugar is dissolved. Set aside.

In a medium bowl, toss together the coleslaw mix, carrot, almonds, cilantro, jalapeño, and basil.

Just before serving, place the lettuce leaves on a platter. Spoon the coleslaw mixture and sauce into each "cup." Top with the tuna. Roll up for wraps or leave unwrapped to serve as a salad.

PER SERVING

calories 196	cholesterol 15 mg
total fat 9.0 g	sodium 51 mg
saturated fat 0.5 g	carbohydrates 21 g
trans fat 0.0 g	fiber 3 g
polyunsaturated fat 2.0 g	sugars 16 g
monounsaturated fat 5.0 g	protein 12 g

100   200   300   400

DIETARY EXCHANGES
1 vegetable, 1 carbohydrate, 1½ very lean meat, 1½ fat

tuna and broccoli with lemon-caper brown rice

serves 4; 1 cup tuna mixture and ½ cup rice per serving

This dish has all you need in a healthy meal—protein, a veggie, and a whole grain.

1¼ cups fat-free, low-sodium chicken broth and 1½ cups fat-free, low-sodium chicken broth, divided use

1 tablespoon capers, drained

1 teaspoon grated lemon zest

1 cup uncooked instant brown rice

3 tablespoons all-purpose flour

½ teaspoon salt-free all-purpose seasoning blend

¼ teaspoon salt

½ cup fat-free half-and-half

2 cups frozen broccoli florets, thawed

10 ounces canned very low sodium albacore tuna, packed in water, drained and flaked

¼ cup shredded or grated Parmesan cheese

In a medium saucepan, bring 1¼ cups broth, capers, and lemon zest to a simmer over medium-high heat. Stir in the rice. Reduce the heat and simmer, covered, for 8 to 10 minutes, or until tender. Set aside.

Meanwhile, in a separate medium saucepan, whisk together the remaining 1½ cups broth, flour, seasoning blend, and salt until smooth. Bring to a simmer over medium-high heat. Reduce the heat and simmer for 2 minutes, or until thickened, whisking occasionally. Whisk in the half-and-half. Increase the heat to medium. Cook for 2 minutes, whisking occasionally.

Stir in the broccoli, tuna, and Parmesan. Cook for 2 to 3 minutes, or until heated through. Serve over the rice.

PER SERVING

calories 266	cholesterol 33 mg
total fat 4.5 g	sodium 424 mg
saturated fat 1.5 g	carbohydrates 30 g
trans fat 0.0 g	fiber 4 g
polyunsaturated fat 1.5 g	sugars 3 g
monounsaturated fat 1.5 g	protein 27 g

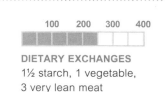

100 200 300 400

DIETARY EXCHANGES
1½ starch, 1 vegetable,
3 very lean meat

orange-ginger tuna steaks

serves 4; 3 ounces fish per serving

Eating this tuna will make you feel as if you're dining in a white-tablecloth restaurant—it's that good! Serve it with soba noodles and Stir-Fried Sugar Snap Peas with Shallots and Walnuts (page 368).

marinade

½ cup fresh orange juice

¼ cup sliced green onions

2 large garlic cloves, minced

1 tablespoon grated peeled gingerroot

1 tablespoon soy sauce (lowest sodium available)

2 teaspoons honey

¼ teaspoon toasted sesame oil

⅛ teaspoon pepper (white preferred)

4 tuna steaks, about 1 inch thick (about 4 ounces each), rinsed and patted dry

Cooking spray

In a large shallow glass dish, stir together the marinade ingredients. Add the fish, turning to coat. Cover and refrigerate for at least 30 minutes (up to several hours), turning occasionally.

Meanwhile, lightly spray the grill rack with cooking spray. Preheat the grill on medium high.

Drain the fish, discarding the marinade.

Grill for 3 to 5 minutes on each side, or to the desired doneness.

PER SERVING

calories 119	cholesterol 53 mg
total fat 1.0 g	sodium 140 mg
saturated fat 0.5 g	carbohydrates 0 g
trans fat 0.0 g	fiber 0 g
polyunsaturated fat 0.5 g	sugars 0 g
monounsaturated fat 0.0 g	protein 25 g

100 200 300 400

DIETARY EXCHANGES

3 very lean meat

tuna steaks with tarragon sour cream

serves 4; 3 ounces fish and 2 tablespoons sauce per serving

The rich flavor of tuna blends perfectly with this bold tarragon-lime sauce.

sauce

⅓ cup fat-free sour cream

2 tablespoons light mayonnaise

2 teaspoons fresh lime juice

¾ teaspoon dried tarragon, crumbled

½ teaspoon pepper

¼ teaspoon salt

fish

¼ teaspoon paprika

⅛ teaspoon garlic powder

⅛ teaspoon salt

4 tuna steaks (about 4 ounces each), rinsed and patted dry

1 teaspoon canola or corn oil

1 medium lime, cut into 4 wedges (optional)

In a small bowl, whisk together the sauce ingredients. Set aside.

In a separate small bowl, stir together the paprika, garlic powder, and remaining ⅛ teaspoon salt. Sprinkle over both sides of the fish. Using your fingertips, gently press the mixture so it adheres to the fish.

In a large nonstick skillet, heat the oil over medium-high heat, swirling to coat the bottom. Cook the fish for 2 minutes on each side, or to the desired doneness. Serve drizzled with the sauce. Place the lime wedges on the side to squeeze over the fish.

PER SERVING

calories 175
total fat 5.0 g
  saturated fat 1.0 g
  trans fat 0.0 g
  polyunsaturated fat 2.0 g
  monounsaturated fat 1.5 g

cholesterol 59 mg
sodium 328 mg
carbohydrates 5 g
  fiber 0 g
  sugars 2 g
  protein 27 g

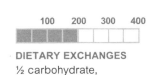

DIETARY EXCHANGES
½ carbohydrate,
3 lean meat

scallop and spinach sauté

serves 4; 3 ounces scallops and ½ cup spinach per serving

Seafood is ideal for busy days because it cooks so fast. Here, tender scallops are combined with vitamin- and mineral-rich leeks and baby spinach for a super-quick meal. Instant or frozen brown rice is an excellent complement to this dish.

1 teaspoon olive oil

2 medium leeks (white part only), thinly sliced

1 pound bay or sea scallops, rinsed and patted dry, quartered if large

1 tablespoon snipped fresh dillweed or 1 teaspoon dried, crumbled

1 teaspoon grated lemon zest

1 pound baby spinach

1 2-ounce jar diced pimientos, drained

1 tablespoon capers, drained

In a large nonstick skillet, heat the oil over medium-high heat, swirling to coat the bottom. Cook the leeks for 1 to 2 minutes, or until tender-crisp, stirring occasionally.

Add the scallops, dillweed, and lemon zest. Cook for 30 seconds. Stir. Cook for 1 minute, stirring occasionally. (If the scallops have ever been frozen, they may need to cook for an additional 1 to 2 minutes to evaporate the extra liquid they may release.)

Stir in the spinach, pimientos, and capers. Cook for 1 to 2 minutes, or until the spinach is wilted, stirring occasionally.

PER SERVING

calories 188	cholesterol 37 mg
total fat 2.0 g	sodium 437 mg
saturated fat 0.5 g	carbohydrates 22 g
trans fat 0.0 g	fiber 7 g
polyunsaturated fat 0.5 g	sugars 2 g
monounsaturated fat 1.0 g	protein 23 g

100 200 300 400

DIETARY EXCHANGES
4 vegetable,
3 very lean meat

tomato-caper shrimp with herbed feta

serves 4; 1½ cups per serving

Try this Greek-inspired dish when you need dinner in a hurry. Boiling the shrimp with the pasta is a definite time-saver, plus the tomato sauce cooks in only five minutes.

3 quarts water

6 ounces dried whole-grain bow-tie pasta

1 pound raw medium shrimp, peeled, rinsed, and patted dry

3 medium tomatoes, diced

1 teaspoon dried basil, crumbled

½ teaspoon dried oregano, crumbled

1 medium garlic clove, minced

⅛ teaspoon crushed red pepper flakes

2 tablespoons capers, drained

1 tablespoon olive oil (extra-virgin preferred)

⅛ teaspoon salt

1 ounce fat-free tomato-basil feta cheese, crumbled

In a large saucepan, bring the water to a boil over high heat. Stir in the pasta. Boil for 6 minutes.

Stir in the shrimp. Return to a boil. Boil for 3 to 5 minutes, or until the shrimp are pink on the outside and the pasta is tender. Drain well in a colander.

Meanwhile, in a large nonstick skillet stir together the tomatoes, basil, oregano, garlic, and red pepper flakes. Cook over medium-high heat for 5 minutes, or until the tomatoes are tender, stirring frequently. Remove from the heat. Stir in the capers, oil, and salt.

Spoon the pasta mixture onto plates. Spoon the tomato sauce on top. Sprinkle with the feta.

PER SERVING

calories 300
total fat 6.5 g
  saturated fat 1.5 g
  trans fat 0.0 g
  polyunsaturated fat 1.0 g
  monounsaturated fat 3.0 g

cholesterol 171 mg
sodium 481 mg
carbohydrates 36 g
  fiber 6 g
  sugars 4 g
protein 26 g

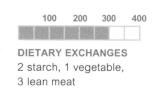

DIETARY EXCHANGES
2 starch, 1 vegetable,
3 lean meat

cumin shrimp and rice toss

serves 4; 1½ cups per serving

....

Squeeze a generous amount of fresh lime over this dish to raise it from good to great.

Cooking spray

1   medium poblano or green bell pepper, seeds and ribs discarded, cut into 1-inch pieces

1   medium yellow summer squash, cut crosswise into ¼-inch slices

1   medium onion, cut into ½-inch wedges

12 cherry tomatoes

1   cup uncooked instant brown rice

1   pound raw medium shrimp, peeled, rinsed, and patted dry

1½ teaspoons chili powder

1   teaspoon ground cumin

¼   teaspoon cayenne

⅛   teaspoon salt and ¼ teaspoon salt, divided use

1   tablespoon olive oil (extra-virgin preferred)

⅓   cup snipped fresh cilantro

2   medium limes, each cut into 4 wedges

Preheat the broiler. Line a broiler pan with aluminum foil. Lightly spray with cooking spray.

Place the poblano, squash, onion, and tomatoes in a single layer on the broiler pan. Lightly spray with cooking spray.

Broil about 4 inches from the heat for 10 minutes. Stir gently. Broil for 2 minutes, or until the poblano, squash, and onion are tender-crisp and beginning to richly brown on the edges. Transfer to a medium bowl. Cover and let stand so the flavors blend.

Meanwhile, prepare the rice using the package directions, omitting the salt and margarine.

In a large skillet, stir together the shrimp, chili powder, cumin, cayenne, and ⅛ teaspoon salt. Cook over medium heat for 5 minutes, or until the shrimp are pink on the outside, stirring frequently.

Stir the rice, oil, and remaining ¼ teaspoon salt into the poblano mixture. Spoon onto plates. Top with the shrimp and any accumulated juices. Sprinkle with the cilantro. Serve with the lime wedges.

COOK'S TIP ON CHERRY TOMATOES Enjoy cherry tomatoes for a low-calorie snack by themselves or dipped in just a bit of light ranch dressing.

····· **PER SERVING** ·····

calories 245	cholesterol 168 mg
total fat 5.5 g	sodium 438 mg
saturated fat 1.0 g	carbohydrates 28 g
trans fat 0.0 g	fiber 4 g
polyunsaturated fat 1.0 g	sugars 6 g
monounsaturated fat 3.0 g	protein 22 g

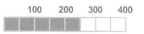

100 200 300 400

DIETARY EXCHANGES
1 starch, 2 vegetable,
3 lean meat

poultry

Turkey Cutlets with Chutney Sauce

Turkey Burgers with Mediterranean Tomato Relish

Turkish Meatballs

Turkey Sausage and Lentils with Brown Rice

Artichoke and Bell Pepper Lasagna

Slow-Roasted Sage Turkey Breast

Black-Pepper Chicken

Southwest Lime Chicken

Chicken with Zesty Apricot Sauce

Bistro Chicken with Fresh Asparagus

Grilled Honey Mustard Chicken with Pineapple Salsa

Salsa Chicken

Slow-Cooker White Chili

Chicken with Herbed Mustard and Green Onion Sauce

Chicken Breasts with Spinach, Apricots,
and Pine Nuts

Chicken Breasts Stuffed with Goat Cheese, Dates,
and Spinach

*Chicken Breasts Stuffed with Fresh Basil
and Red Bell Pepper*

Stuffed Chicken Breasts in Lemon-Oregano Tomato Sauce

Chicken and Snow Pea Stir-Fry

Chicken and Bow-Ties with Green Beans

Cheesy Chicken and Quinoa Stir-Fry

Chicken Fajitas

Risotto with Porcini Mushrooms and Chicken

Chicken and Veggies with Noodles

Chicken Enchiladas

Chicken Pot Pie with Mashed Potato Crust

Mashed Potatoes

turkey cutlets
with chutney sauce

serves 4; 3 ounces turkey per serving

Tired of chicken? A quick-and-easy chutney sauce adds a bit of foreign flair to turkey cutlets.

    3 tablespoons all-purpose flour and 1 tablespoon all-purpose flour, divided use
    1 teaspoon curry powder and ½ teaspoon curry powder, divided use
    ½ teaspoon garlic powder
    ¼ teaspoon ground cumin
    ⅛ teaspoon salt
    4 turkey cutlets (about 4 ounces each), all visible fat discarded, flattened to ¼-inch thickness
    2 teaspoons olive oil
    ¼ cup fresh orange juice
    ½ cup fat-free, low-sodium chicken broth
    ¼ cup raisins (regular or golden)
    ¼ cup mango chutney
  1½ tablespoons plain rice vinegar
    2 medium green onions, sliced (optional)

In a medium shallow dish, stir together 3 tablespoons flour, 1 teaspoon curry powder, the garlic powder, cumin, and salt. Dip one turkey cutlet in the flour mixture, turning to coat and gently shaking off any excess. Using your fingertips, gently press the coating so it adheres to the turkey. Transfer to a large plate. Repeat with the remaining turkey.

In a large nonstick skillet, heat the oil over medium-high heat, swirling to coat the bottom. Cook the turkey for 4 minutes on each side, or until no longer pink in the center. Transfer to a separate large plate. Cover to keep warm.

Put the remaining 1 tablespoon flour in a small bowl. Add the orange juice, whisking until the flour is dissolved. Whisk in the broth, raisins, chutney, vinegar, and remaining ½ teaspoon curry powder. Pour into the skillet. Bring to a boil, still on medium high, scraping the skillet to dislodge any browned bits. Reduce the heat and simmer for 1 minute, stirring constantly.

Return the turkey to the skillet, spooning the sauce over the turkey. Heat for 1 to 2 minutes, or until warmed through, stirring constantly. Serve the turkey topped with the sauce. Garnish with the green onions.

····· **PER SERVING** ··

calories 242

total fat 3.5 g

  saturated fat 0.5 g

  trans fat 0.0 g

  polyunsaturated fat 0.5 g

  monounsaturated fat 2.0 g

cholesterol 70 mg

sodium 172 mg

carbohydrates 24 g

  fiber 1 g

  sugars 14 g

protein 30 g

100 200 300 400

DIETARY EXCHANGES

½ starch, 1 fruit,

3 very lean meat

turkey burgers with mediterranean tomato relish

serves 4; 1 turkey burger and 2 tablespoons relish per serving

Satisfy your cravings for a good burger with these Mediterranean-style turkey burgers, grilled outdoors or in a grill pan. Kalamata olives and feta cheese enhance the flavor of the relish topping. Serve the burgers with Mixed Vegetable Grill (page 376) and grilled corn on the cob.

relish

1 tablespoon white wine vinegar

1 teaspoon olive oil (extra virgin preferred)

½ teaspoon dried Italian seasoning, crumbled

½ teaspoon honey

½ cup chopped Italian plum (Roma) tomato

¼ cup chopped cucumber

2 tablespoons crumbled fat-free feta cheese

6 kalamata olives, finely chopped

burgers

1 teaspoon canola or corn oil

¾ cup chopped button mushrooms

¼ cup chopped sweet onion, such as Vidalia, Maui, or Oso Sweet

1 medium garlic clove, minced

1 pound ground skinless turkey breast

2 tablespoons panko (Japanese bread crumbs)

1 teaspoon dried oregano, crumbled

¼ teaspoon pepper

⅛ teaspoon salt

Cooking spray

If using an outdoor grill (rather than a ridged stovetop grill pan), preheat on medium high.

In a small bowl, whisk together the vinegar, olive oil, Italian seasoning, and honey.

Stir in the remaining relish ingredients. Set aside.

In a small nonstick skillet, heat the canola oil over medium-high heat, swirling to coat the bottom. Cook the mushrooms and onion for about 3 minutes, or until both are soft, stirring frequently. Remove from the heat. Stir in the garlic.

In a medium bowl, using your hands or a spoon, combine the turkey, panko, oregano, pepper, salt, and mushroom mixture just until blended. Shape into 4 burgers, each about ½ inch thick. Lightly spray the tops with cooking spray.

Grill the burgers with the sprayed side down on the grill or grill pan over medium-high heat for 5 to 7 minutes on each side, or until no longer pink in the center.

Drain and discard any accumulated liquid from the relish. Serve over the burgers.

···· **PER SERVING** ···

calories 192	cholesterol 70 mg
total fat 4.5 g	sodium 300 mg
saturated fat 0.5 g	carbohydrates 6 g
trans fat 0.0 g	fiber 1 g
polyunsaturated fat 1.0 g	sugars 2 g
monounsaturated fat 3.0 g	protein 30 g

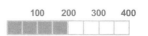

DIETARY EXCHANGES
1 vegetable, 3 lean meat

turkish meatballs

serves 4; 4 meatballs and ¼ cup sauce per serving

These meatballs and their tomato-wine sauce partner well with Lemon-Herb Brown Rice (page 371). Add a green salad, and dinner is served.

Cooking spray

1 pound ground skinless turkey breast

⅓ cup fat-free, low-sodium chicken broth

¼ cup plain dry bread crumbs (lowest sodium available)

¼ cup finely chopped onion

½ medium rib of celery, finely chopped

¼ cup snipped fresh Italian (flat-leaf) parsley

½ teaspoon ground cinnamon

¼ teaspoon ground allspice

¼ teaspoon ground turmeric or curry powder

¼ teaspoon pepper

1 teaspoon canola or corn oil

1 small onion, thinly sliced crosswise

2 medium garlic cloves, minced

1 cup low-sodium mixed-vegetable juice or no-salt-added tomato sauce

⅓ cup dry red wine (regular or nonalcoholic)

¼ teaspoon crushed red pepper flakes

Preheat the oven to 400°F. Lightly spray a large cooling rack with cooking spray. Place the rack on a 15 x 10 x 1-inch rimmed baking sheet.

In a large bowl, using your hands or a spoon, combine the turkey, broth, bread crumbs, chopped onion, celery, parsley, cinnamon, allspice, turmeric, and pepper. Shape into 16 meatballs. Place the meatballs on the rack on the baking sheet.

Bake for 12 to 15 minutes, or until the meatballs are light golden, turning occasionally. Using tongs or a spatula, transfer the meatballs to paper towels to drain. Set aside.

In a large nonstick skillet, heat the oil over medium-high heat, swirling to coat the bottom. Cook the sliced onion and garlic for about 3 minutes, or until the onion is soft, stirring frequently.

Stir in the vegetable juice, wine, and red pepper flakes. Bring to a boil. Gently add the meatballs, spooning the sauce over them. Reduce the heat and simmer, covered, for 10 to 12 minutes, or until the meatballs are cooked through, turning them once about halfway through.

COOK'S TIP ON TURMERIC Turmeric is a spice often used in place of very expensive saffron—not for the flavor, which is quite different, but rather because of the similarity in their yellow-orange color. Turmeric also is a component in many prepared curry powder blends.

···· **PER SERVING** ···

calories 220
total fat 3.5 g
  saturated fat 1.0 g
  trans fat 0.0 g
  polyunsaturated fat 1.0 g
  monounsaturated fat 1.0 g

cholesterol 68 mg
sodium 173 mg
carbohydrates 13 g
  fiber 2 g
  sugars 5 g
protein 29 g

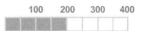

DIETARY EXCHANGES
½ starch, 1 vegetable,
3 very lean meat

turkey sausage and lentils with brown rice

serves 4; ¾ cup lentil mixture and ½ cup rice per serving

Bay leaves, fresh parsley, and thyme add zip to a traditionally mild dish. Eating high-fiber foods and whole grains, such as the lentils and brown rice in this dish, keeps you satiated and helps you manage your weight.

1 teaspoon olive oil, 1 teaspoon olive oil, and 2 teaspoons olive oil (extra-virgin preferred), divided use

4 ounces smoked turkey sausage ring, thinly sliced

1 medium onion, finely chopped

2 medium garlic cloves, minced

2 cups water and 1½ cups water, divided use

½ cup dried lentils, sorted for stones and shriveled lentils and rinsed

2 medium dried bay leaves

¾ cup uncooked quick-cooking brown rice

¼ cup snipped fresh parsley

1½ teaspoons fresh thyme or ½ teaspoon dried, crumbled

¼ teaspoon salt

In a medium nonstick skillet, heat 1 teaspoon oil over medium-high heat, swirling to coat the bottom. Cook the sausage for about 3 minutes, or until browned on the edges, stirring frequently. Transfer to a medium plate.

In the same skillet, heat 1 teaspoon oil over medium-high heat, swirling to coat the bottom. Cook the onion for about 3 minutes, or until soft, stirring frequently.

Stir in the garlic. Cook for 10 seconds, stirring constantly.

Stir in 2 cups water, the lentils, bay leaves, and sausage with any accumulated juices. Bring to a boil, still on medium high. Reduce the heat and simmer, covered, for 25 to 30 minutes, or until the lentils are tender, stirring occasionally. Remove from the heat. Discard the bay leaves.

Meanwhile, prepare the rice using the package directions for time and stove setting, but omitting the salt and margarine and using the remaining 1½ cups water instead of what is called for.

Stir the parsley, thyme, salt, and remaining 2 teaspoons oil into the sausage mixture. Spoon over the rice.

COOK'S TIP Adding the parsley and thyme at the end of the cooking time allows the flavors to be more pronounced.

···· PER SERVING ····································

calories 253
total fat 8.0 g
  saturated fat 1.5 g
  trans fat 0.0 g
  polyunsaturated fat 1.5 g
  monounsaturated fat 4.5 g

cholesterol 19 mg
sodium 427 mg
carbohydrates 34 g
  fiber 5 g
  sugars 5 g
protein 13 g

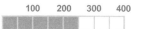

DIETARY EXCHANGES
2 starch, 1 lean meat, ½ fat

artichoke and bell pepper lasagna

serves 4; 1 5½ x 3½-inch piece per serving

You can still include typically high calorie dishes, such as lasagna, in your eating plan when you make healthier choices. Turkey pepperoni adds an unexpected element to this vegetable-laden version.

Cooking spray
4 dried whole-grain lasagna noodles
3 medium green bell peppers, finely chopped
1 small zucchini, finely chopped
½ cup spaghetti sauce (lowest sodium available)
1½ teaspoons dried basil, crumbled
1 teaspoon dried oregano, crumbled
16 turkey pepperoni slices, quartered (lowest sodium available)
1 14.5-ounce can artichokes, drained and finely chopped
2 ounces shredded low-fat mozzarella cheese
1 tablespoon shredded or grated Parmesan cheese

Preheat the oven to 350°F. Lightly spray an 11 x 7 x 2-inch baking dish and a large skillet with cooking spray. Set aside.

Prepare the noodles using the package directions, omitting the salt. Drain well in a colander.

Meanwhile, in the large skillet, cook the bell peppers and zucchini over medium-high heat for 5 minutes, or until beginning to brown, stirring frequently. Remove from the heat.

Place 2 noodles in the baking dish. Make sure the edges of the noodles are tucked under to keep them from drying out. Spoon 2 tablespoons spaghetti sauce over each noodle. Sprinkle with half of each of the following, in order: basil, oregano, pepperoni, artichokes, bell-pepper mixture, and mozzarella. Repeat the layers.

Lightly spray a sheet of aluminum foil with cooking spray. Cover the baking dish with the foil with the sprayed side down.

Bake for 25 minutes, or until the mozzarella has melted. Remove from the oven. Sprinkle with the Parmesan. Let stand for 10 minutes before cutting so the flavors blend.

PER SERVING

calories 212
total fat 4.5 g
  saturated fat 1.0 g
  trans fat 0.0 g
  polyunsaturated fat 1.0 g
  monounsaturated fat 1.5 g

cholesterol 16 mg
sodium 562 mg
carbohydrates 31 g
  fiber 7 g
  sugars 7 g
protein 14 g

100 200 300 400

DIETARY EXCHANGES
1 starch, 3 vegetable,
1 lean meat

slow-roasted sage turkey breast

serves 4; 3 ounces turkey per serving (plus 1 pound reserved)

A thin coating of seasoning mixture and a squeeze of fresh lemon between the breast meat and the skin impart flavor that permeates the turkey as it slowly roasts. Prepare the turkey for a weekend dinner, then you and your family can enjoy leftovers on a green salad, as a sandwich filling on whole-grain bread, or in place of the chicken in Chicken Minestrone (page 156).

   Cooking spray
1½ teaspoons dried sage
 1 teaspoon paprika
 ¾ teaspoon dried rosemary, crushed
 ¼ teaspoon onion powder
 ¼ teaspoon garlic powder
 ¼ teaspoon pepper
 1 3-pound boneless turkey breast with skin
 1 medium lemon, halved crosswise

Preheat the oven to 325°F. Lightly spray a baking rack and roasting pan with cooking spray. Set aside.

   In a small bowl, combine the sage, paprika, rosemary, onion powder, garlic powder, and pepper.

   Carefully pull back the skin from the turkey, leaving it attached at one end and trying not to tear the skin. Squeeze the lemon over the breast meat. Sprinkle with the sage mixture. Using your fingertips, gently press the seasonings so they adhere to the turkey. Pull the skin back in place. Put the turkey on the rack in the pan.

   Roast for 1 hour 45 minutes, or until the turkey registers 170°F on an instant-read thermometer. Transfer the turkey to a cutting board. Let stand for 10 minutes. Discard the skin before slicing the turkey.

PER SERVING

calories 125
total fat 1.0 g
  saturated fat 0.5 g
  trans fat 0.0 g
  polyunsaturated fat 0.5 g
  monounsaturated fat 0.0 g

cholesterol 74 mg
sodium 49 mg
carbohydrates 1 g
  fiber 0 g
  sugars 0 g
  protein 26 g

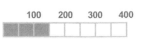

| 100 | 200 | 300 | 400 |

DIETARY EXCHANGES
3 very lean meat

black-pepper chicken

serves 4; 3 ounces chicken per serving

Sear chicken coated with black pepper over high heat, then quickly reduce the sauce. That's all it takes to get these chicken tenders ready to serve. Make extra to add flavor, but not many calories, to soups, salads, sandwiches, and casseroles.

1 pound chicken tenders, all visible fat discarded
½ teaspoon black pepper, or to taste
1½ teaspoons olive oil and 1½ teaspoons olive oil, divided use
½ cup water
¼ teaspoon salt

Sprinkle both sides of the chicken with the pepper.

In a 12-inch nonstick skillet, heat 1½ teaspoons oil over medium-high heat, swirling to coat the bottom. Cook the chicken for 2 minutes. Reduce the heat to medium. Pour in the remaining 1½ teaspoons oil, swirling to coat the bottom as well as possible. Turn the chicken over. Cook for 2 minutes, or until no longer pink in the center. Transfer to a large plate.

Add the water and salt to the skillet. Increase the heat to high and bring the water to a boil. Boil for 1½ to 2 minutes, or until reduced to 2 tablespoons, scraping to dislodge any browned bits. Pour over the chicken, turning to coat.

COOK'S TIP If you don't have a 12-inch skillet, cook the chicken in two batches. Otherwise, you will crowd the chicken, causing it to simmer, not brown.

PER SERVING

calories 155
total fat 5.0 g
  saturated fat 1.0 g
  trans fat 0.0 g
  polyunsaturated fat 0.5 g
  monounsaturated fat 3.0 g

cholesterol 66 mg
sodium 220 mg
carbohydrates 0 g
  fiber 0 g
  sugars 0 g
  protein 26 g

100   200   300   400

DIETARY EXCHANGES
3 lean meat

southwest lime chicken

serves 4; 3 ounces chicken per serving

The combination of hot pepper and lime provides just the right balance of spiciness in this dish.

- 2 tablespoons all-purpose flour
- 1 tablespoon snipped fresh parsley
- 2 teaspoons grated lime zest
- 1 teaspoon salt-free all-purpose seasoning blend
- ½ teaspoon garlic powder
- ¼ teaspoon salt
- ⅛ to ¼ teaspoon cayenne
- ⅛ teaspoon paprika
- 4 boneless, skinless chicken breast halves (about 4 ounces each), all visible fat discarded, flattened to ¼-inch thickness
- 1 tablespoon olive oil
- 1½ to 2 tablespoons fresh lime juice

In a small shallow dish, stir together the flour, parsley, lime zest, seasoning blend, garlic powder, salt, cayenne, and paprika. Dip one piece of chicken in the mixture, turning to coat and gently shaking off any excess. Using your fingertips, gently press the coating so it adheres to the chicken. Transfer to a large plate. Repeat with the remaining chicken.

In a large nonstick skillet, heat the oil over medium-high heat, swirling to coat the bottom. Cook the chicken for 3 to 5 minutes on each side, or until lightly browned on the outside and no longer pink in the center.

Sprinkle with the lime juice. Cook for 5 to 10 seconds on each side.

PER SERVING

calories 173
total fat 5.0 g
  saturated fat 1.0 g
  trans fat 0.0 g
  polyunsaturated fat 0.5 g
  monounsaturated fat 3.0 g

cholesterol 66 mg
sodium 218 mg
carbohydrates 4 g
  fiber 0 g
  sugars 0 g
  protein 27 g

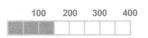

DIETARY EXCHANGES
3 lean meat

chicken with zesty apricot sauce

serves 4; 3 ounces chicken and 2 tablespoons sauce per serving

Whole-wheat couscous tossed with sliced green onions and slivers of sweet red bell pepper would make a colorful side for this sweet-tart entrée.

- 1 teaspoon chili powder
- ¼ teaspoon ground cumin
- ⅛ teaspoon salt and ⅛ teaspoon salt, divided use
- 4 boneless, skinless chicken breast halves (about 4 ounces each), all visible fat discarded
- 1 teaspoon canola or corn oil
- ½ cup all-fruit apricot spread
- 2 tablespoons cider vinegar
- 2 teaspoons sugar
- ⅛ teaspoon crushed red pepper flakes
- 1 medium lemon, cut into 4 wedges

In a small bowl, stir together the chili powder, cumin, and ⅛ teaspoon salt. Sprinkle over the smooth side of the chicken. Using your fingertips, gently press so the seasonings adhere to the chicken.

In a large skillet, heat the oil over medium-high heat, swirling to coat the bottom. Cook the chicken with the seasoned side down for 3 minutes. Turn the chicken over. Reduce the heat to medium and cook for 3 to 5 minutes, or until the chicken is no longer pink in the center.

Meanwhile, in a small saucepan, stir together the apricot spread, vinegar, sugar, and red pepper flakes. Cook over medium heat for 2 minutes, or until the spread is melted and the sugar is dissolved, stirring frequently. Spoon onto each plate. Spread to a 6-inch diameter. Sprinkle the remaining ⅛ teaspoon salt over the chicken. Place the chicken on the apricot mixture. Squeeze the lemon over the chicken.

PER SERVING

calories 230	cholesterol 66 mg	
total fat 2.5 g	sodium 226 mg	
saturated fat 0.5 g	carbohydrates 24 g	
trans fat 0.0 g	fiber 0 g	
polyunsaturated fat 0.5 g	sugars 19 g	
monounsaturated fat 1.0 g	protein 26 g	

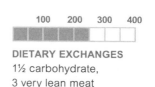

DIETARY EXCHANGES
1½ carbohydrate,
3 very lean meat

bistro chicken
with fresh asparagus

serves 4; 3 ounces chicken, ⅓ cup mushroom mixture, and 2 asparagus spears per serving

The next time you have dinner guests, serve this easy-to-prepare chicken dish.

½ cup plain dry bread crumbs (lowest sodium available)

1 tablespoon shredded or grated Parmesan cheese

½ teaspoon salt-free lemon pepper

½ teaspoon salt-free all-purpose seasoning blend

½ teaspoon garlic powder

½ teaspoon dried oregano, crumbled

2 tablespoons Dijon honey mustard

4 boneless, skinless chicken breast halves (about 4 ounces each), all visible fat discarded, flattened to ¼-inch thickness

1 teaspoon canola or corn oil

2 tablespoons dry white wine, 2 tablespoons dry white wine, and ¼ cup dry white wine (regular or nonalcoholic), divided use

8 ounces button mushrooms, sliced

1 small onion, chopped

8 medium asparagus spears, trimmed

1 medium tomato, seeded and chopped

1 tablespoon capers, drained

In a medium shallow dish, stir together the bread crumbs, Parmesan, lemon pepper, seasoning blend, garlic powder, and oregano.

Spread the mustard on both sides of the chicken. Dip one piece of chicken in the bread-crumb mixture, turning to coat and gently shaking off any excess. Using your fingertips, gently press so the coating adheres to the chicken. Transfer to a large plate. Repeat with the remaining chicken.

In a large nonstick skillet, heat the oil over medium-high heat. Put the chicken in the skillet. Pour 2 tablespoons wine over the chicken. Cook for 2 minutes. Turn the chicken over. Pour in the second 2 tablespoons wine. Cook for 1 to 2 minutes, or until the chicken is no longer pink in the center. Transfer the chicken to a separate large plate, leaving the remaining wine in the skillet. Cover the chicken to keep warm. Set aside.

In the same skillet, cook the mushrooms and onion over medium-high heat for 3 minutes, or until lightly browned, stirring frequently.

Stir in the asparagus and remaining ¼ cup wine. Cook, covered, for 2 to 4 minutes, or until the asparagus is tender-crisp. Stir in the tomato. Serve over the chicken. Sprinkle with the capers.

··· PER SERVING ···

calories 268
total fat 4.0 g
  saturated fat 1.0 g
  trans fat 0.0 g
  polyunsaturated fat 1.0 g
  monounsaturated fat 1.5 g

cholesterol 67 mg
sodium 272 mg
carbohydrates 21 g
  fiber 3 g
  sugars 5 g
  protein 32 g

100 200 300 400

DIETARY EXCHANGES
1 starch, 1 vegetable,
3 very lean meat

grilled honey mustard chicken with pineapple salsa

serves 4; 3 ounces chicken and ⅓ cup salsa per serving

The low-effort prep, grilling, and clean-up of this dish will please you almost as much as the fact that it is low in calories.

Cooking spray

½ medium green bell pepper (halved lengthwise), flattened with the palm of your hand

2 pineapple slices, about ½ inch thick

4 medium green onions

1 teaspoon dried tarragon, crumbled

¼ teaspoon salt

¼ teaspoon pepper (coarsely ground preferred)

4 boneless, skinless chicken breast halves (about 4 ounces each), all visible fat discarded, flattened to ½-inch thickness

1 tablespoon honey mustard and 1 tablespoon honey mustard, divided use

1 tablespoon balsamic vinegar

Lightly spray a grilling rack with cooking spray. Preheat the grill on medium high.

Lightly spray both sides of the bell pepper, pineapple, and green onions with cooking spray.

Grill them for 3 to 4 minutes on each side, or until the bell pepper is tender-crisp. Transfer to a cutting board. Set aside until cool enough to handle.

In a small bowl, stir together the tarragon, salt, and pepper. Sprinkle over both sides of the chicken. Using your fingertips, gently press so the seasonings adhere to the chicken.

Grill for 4 minutes on each side, or until no longer pink in the center. Brush one side of the chicken with 1 tablespoon mustard. Grill with that side down for 30 seconds. Brush the other side with the remaining 1 tablespoon mustard. Grill with that side down for 30 seconds.

Meanwhile, chop the bell pepper, pineapple, and green onions. Transfer to a small bowl. Stir in the vinegar. Spoon the salsa over the chicken or serve on the side.

COOK'S TIP Flattening the bell pepper makes for quicker, more even cooking.

····· **PER SERVING** ·······
calories 168
total fat 1.5 g
  saturated fat 0.5 g
  trans fat 0.0 g
  polyunsaturated fat 0.5 g
  monounsaturated fat 0.5 g

cholesterol 66 mg
sodium 235 mg
carbohydrates 9 g
  fiber 2 g
  sugars 4 g
protein 27 g

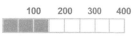

DIETARY EXCHANGES
½ carbohydrate,
3 very lean meat

salsa chicken

serves 4; 3 ounces chicken and 2 tablespoons salsa per serving

Tomato-based salsa tops citrus- and cilantro-enhanced chicken for a spicy combo that goes well with brown rice and a combination of steamed zucchini and yellow summer squash.

salsa

1 small tomato, chopped

⅓ cup snipped fresh cilantro or Italian (flat-leaf) parsley

2 medium green onions, chopped

1 small fresh jalapeño, seeds and ribs discarded, minced,
  or ½ teaspoon bottled pickled jalapeño juice

¼ cup low-sodium mixed-vegetable juice or low-sodium tomato juice

2 medium garlic cloves, minced

1 teaspoon grated lemon or lime zest

1 tablespoon fresh lemon or lime juice

½ teaspoon ground cumin

chicken

4 boneless, skinless chicken breast halves (about 4 ounces each),
  all visible fat discarded, flattened to ¼-inch thickness

2 tablespoons fresh lemon or lime juice

½ cup yellow cornmeal

2 tablespoons snipped fresh cilantro or Italian (flat-leaf) parsley

1 teaspoon grated lemon or lime zest

¼ teaspoon crushed red pepper flakes

2 teaspoons canola or corn oil

In a small bowl, stir together the salsa ingredients. Set aside.

Sprinkle both sides of the chicken with the remaining 2 tablespoons lemon juice.

In a medium shallow dish, stir together the remaining ingredients except the oil. Dip one piece of chicken in the mixture, turning to coat and gently shaking off any excess. Using your fingertips, gently press so the coating adheres to the chicken. Transfer to a large plate. Repeat with the remaining chicken.

In a large nonstick skillet, heat the oil over medium-high heat, swirling to coat the bottom. Cook the chicken for 3 to 5 minutes on each side, or until lightly browned on the outside and no longer pink in the center. Serve topped with the salsa.

····· **PER SERVING** ·····

calories 227
total fat 4.0 g
  saturated fat 0.5 g
  trans fat 0.0 g
  polyunsaturated fat 1.0 g
  monounsaturated fat 2.0 g

cholesterol 66 mg
sodium 89 mg
carbohydrates 19 g
  fiber 2 g
  sugars 2 g
  protein 28 g

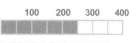

DIETARY EXCHANGES
1 starch, 1 vegetable,
3 very lean meat

slow-cooker white chili

serves 5; 1½ cups per serving

All but the two topping ingredients are combined and cooked right in the slow cooker, making this dish an ideal meal for busy days. If you like your food really spicy, you may want to increase the amount of jalapeño or hot-pepper sauce in this hearty chili.

    Cooking spray

chili

2	cups chopped sweet onion, such as Vidalia, Maui, or Oso Sweet
1	14.5-ounce can no-salt-added diced tomatoes, undrained
1¼	cups fat-free, low-sodium chicken broth
1½	tablespoons ground cumin
2	teaspoons diced fresh jalapeño, seeds and ribs discarded, or to taste
3	medium garlic cloves, minced
1	teaspoon dried oregano, crumbled
½	teaspoon red hot-pepper sauce, or to taste
¼	teaspoon salt
1	pound boneless, skinless chicken breasts, all visible fat discarded
1	15.5-ounce can no-salt-added cannellini or white kidney beans, rinsed and drained
1	15.25-ounce can no-salt-added whole-kernel corn, drained
¼	cup snipped fresh cilantro
2	tablespoons fresh lime juice

topping

¼	cup plus 1 tablespoon fat-free sour cream
¼	cup plus 1 tablespoon grated low-fat Cheddar cheese

Lightly spray a 3½- or 4-quart slow cooker with cooking spray.

In the slow cooker, stir together the onion, tomatoes with liquid, broth, cumin, jalapeño, garlic, oregano, hot-pepper sauce, and salt. Add the chicken, spooning some of the sauce on top. Cook, covered, on low for 5 to 6 hours, or on high for 2½ to 3 hours, or until the chicken is no longer pink in the center.

Transfer the chicken to a cutting board. Using two forks, shred the chicken. Return to the slow cooker.

Stir in the remaining chili ingredients. Cook, covered, on low for 15 minutes, or until heated through. Serve topped with the sour cream and Cheddar.

···· PER SERVING ···

calories 322
total fat 3.5 g
  saturated fat 0.5 g
  trans fat 0.0 g
  polyunsaturated fat 1.0 g
  monounsaturated fat 0.5 g

cholesterol 57 mg
sodium 292 mg
carbohydrates 41 g
  fiber 7 g
  sugars 11 g
protein 32 g

100   200   300   400

DIETARY EXCHANGES
2 starch, 2 vegetable,
3 very lean meat

chicken with herbed mustard and green onion sauce

serves 4; 3 ounces chicken and 2 tablespoons sauce per serving

This dish features chicken breasts smothered in a delicate creamy Dijon sauce seasoned with fragrant tarragon, rosemary, and green onions.

2 medium green onions

4 boneless, skinless chicken breast halves (about 4 ounces each), all visible fat discarded, flattened to ¼-inch thickness

¼ teaspoon dried rosemary, crushed

¼ teaspoon dried tarragon, crumbled

¼ teaspoon salt and ¼ teaspoon salt, divided use

Cooking spray

1 teaspoon canola or corn oil

½ cup dry white wine (regular or nonalcoholic)

¼ cup fat-free half-and-half

¼ cup fat-free sour cream

1 tablespoon Dijon mustard

2 teaspoons olive oil (extra-virgin preferred)

Pepper to taste

1 medium lemon or lime, cut into 4 wedges (optional)

Chop the green part of the onions. Finely chop the white part, keeping separate from the green part. Set aside.

Sprinkle both sides of the chicken with the rosemary, tarragon, and ¼ teaspoon salt. Using your fingertips, gently press so the seasonings adhere to the chicken.

Lightly spray a large skillet with cooking spray. Add the canola oil, swirling to coat the bottom. Cook the chicken over medium heat for 5 minutes on each side, or until no longer pink in the center. Transfer to a large plate. Cover to keep warm.

In the same skillet, bring the wine and white part of the green onions to a boil over high heat. Boil for 1½ to 3 minutes, or until most of the liquid has evaporated, scraping the skillet frequently. Remove the skillet from the heat.

Meanwhile, in a small bowl, whisk together the half-and-half, sour cream, and mustard.

Pour the half-and-half mixture into the reduced wine mixture, stirring to combine. Set over medium-low heat. Cook the mixture for 1 to 2 minutes, or until heated through. (Be careful not to boil, or the sauce will break down.) Remove from the heat.

Stir in the olive oil and remaining ¼ teaspoon salt. Spoon over the chicken. Sprinkle with the pepper and green onion tops. Serve with the lemon wedges on the side.

····· PER SERVING ···

calories 211
total fat 5.0 g
  saturated fat 1.0 g
  trans fat 0.0 g
  polyunsaturated fat 1.0 g
  monounsaturated fat 2.5 g

cholesterol 68 mg
sodium 473 mg
carbohydrates 6 g
  fiber 1 g
  sugars 3 g
protein 29 g

100   200   300   400

DIETARY EXCHANGES
½ carbohydrate,
3 lean meat

chicken breasts with spinach, apricots, and pine nuts

serves 4; 3 ounces chicken, scant ½ cup apricots, and ¼ cup spinach per serving

This elegant dish is a feast for your eyes as well as your taste buds. If you thought you had to sacrifice while dieting, this dish will prove you wrong.

- 3 large egg whites
- ¾ cup plain dry bread crumbs (lowest sodium available)
- 3 tablespoons pine nuts, crushed or finely chopped
- ¼ teaspoon salt
  Pepper to taste
- 4 boneless, skinless chicken breast halves (about 4 ounces each), all visible fat discarded, flattened to ¼-inch thickness
- 2 teaspoons olive oil
- 1 10-ounce can apricot halves in extra-light syrup, drained, with liquid reserved
- 5 ounces baby spinach

In a medium shallow dish, lightly beat the egg whites. In a separate medium shallow dish, stir together the bread crumbs, pine nuts, salt, and pepper. Set the dishes and a large plate in a row, assembly-line fashion. Dip one piece of chicken in the egg whites, turning to coat and letting the excess drip off. Dip in the bread-crumb mixture, gently shaking off any excess. Using your fingertips, gently press so the coating adheres to the chicken. Transfer to the plate. Repeat with the remaining chicken.

In a large skillet, heat the oil over medium-high heat, swirling to coat the bottom. Cook the chicken for 3 to 5 minutes, or until lightly browned. Turn the chicken over.

Add the apricots. Cook for 3 to 5 minutes, or until the chicken is lightly browned on the outside and no longer pink in the center.

Pour in ¼ to ½ cup reserved apricot syrup, depending on how much sauce you want. Cook until the liquid is reduced to about half and reaches the desired consistency. Set aside.

In a separate large skillet, cook the spinach over medium-high heat for 2 to 3 minutes, or just until wilted, stirring constantly. Transfer to plates. Top with the chicken, apricots, and syrup.

····· **PER SERVING** ···

calories 315

total fat 7.5 g
  saturated fat 1.5 g
  trans fat 0.0 g
  polyunsaturated fat 2.0 g
  monounsaturated fat 3.5 g

cholesterol 66 mg
sodium 466 mg
carbohydrates 28 g
  fiber 4 g
  sugars 9 g
protein 34 g

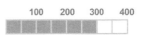

DIETARY EXCHANGES
1 starch, ½ fruit,
1 vegetable, 3½ lean meat

chicken breasts stuffed with goat cheese, dates, and spinach

serves 4; 3 ounces chicken per serving

Although many soft cheeses, such as goat and feta, are high in calories and saturated fat, you can still enjoy them in reasonable amounts. Thanks to their unmistakable flavors, a little goes a long way.

- 4 boneless, skinless chicken breast halves (about 4 ounces each), all visible fat discarded, flattened to ¼-inch thickness
- 2 ounces soft goat cheese
- ⅛ teaspoon cayenne
- 4 dried dates, chopped
- 2 ounces baby spinach
- ½ teaspoon paprika

Preheat the oven to 425°F. Line a rimmed baking sheet with cooking parchment.

Put the chicken with the smooth side down on the baking sheet. Spread each breast with 1 tablespoon goat cheese, leaving a ½-inch border uncovered. Sprinkle with the cayenne and dates. Top with the spinach, still leaving the border uncovered. Starting at the narrowest end, roll up the chicken jelly-roll style. Place with the seam side down on the baking sheet. Sprinkle with the paprika.

Bake for 20 minutes, or until the chicken is no longer pink in the center. Remove from the oven and let stand on the baking sheet for 5 minutes. Cut the rolls crosswise into ½-inch slices. (The slices will look like pinwheels.) Arrange the slices in a fanlike pattern on plates.

chicken breasts stuffed with fresh basil and red bell pepper

Omit the goat cheese, cayenne, dates, and spinach. Substitute 2 ounces fat-free brick cream cheese, softened; 2 teaspoons minced garlic; ¼ cup chopped red bell pepper; and 8 to 12 fresh basil leaves. Prepare as directed. If you prefer, you may omit the cream cheese.

COOK'S TIP ON COOKING PARCHMENT Cooking parchment keeps food from sticking to baking sheets without the need for added oil. It also keeps the bottom of the meat, vegetables, or baked goods from browning too quickly. Remember, however, that it cannot be used for broiling because it could ignite and cause a fire.

WITH GOAT CHEESE

PER SERVING

calories 193	cholesterol 72 mg
total fat 4.5 g	sodium 149 mg
saturated fat 2.5 g	carbohydrates 8 g
trans fat 0.0 g	fiber 1 g
polyunsaturated fat 0.5 g	sugars 5 g
monounsaturated fat 1.0 g	protein 29 g

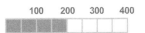

DIETARY EXCHANGES
½ fruit, 3½ lean meat

WITH CREAM CHEESE

PER SERVING

calories 146	cholesterol 68 mg
total fat 1.5 g	sodium 176 mg
saturated fat 0.5 g	carbohydrates 2 g
trans fat 0.0 g	fiber 0 g
polyunsaturated fat 0.5 g	sugars 1 g
monounsaturated fat 0.5 g	protein 29 g

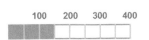

DIETARY EXCHANGES
3½ very lean meat

stuffed chicken breasts in lemon-oregano tomato sauce

serves 4; 3 ounces chicken per serving

A touch of lemon juice serves as a one-ingredient marinade for the chicken, which is stuffed with a combination of fresh tomatoes, parsley, kalamata olives, and feta cheese. The tomato sauce, enhanced with lemon zest and oregano, helps keep the chicken moist.

1 tablespoon fresh lemon juice

4 boneless, skinless chicken breast halves (about 4 ounces each), all visible fat discarded, flattened to ½-inch thickness

½ cup no-salt-added tomato sauce

1 teaspoon grated lemon zest

1 teaspoon dried oregano, crumbled

½ teaspoon crushed red pepper flakes

¼ teaspoon salt

2 medium Italian plum (Roma) tomatoes, diced

¼ cup crumbled low-fat feta cheese

2 tablespoons snipped fresh parsley or 1 teaspoon dried, crumbled

2 tablespoons chopped kalamata olives

1 medium green onion (green part only), chopped

Put the lemon juice in a large glass dish. Add the chicken, turning to coat. Let stand at room temperature for 10 minutes, or cover and refrigerate for up to 4 hours.

Preheat the oven to 350°F.

In a small bowl, stir together the tomato sauce, lemon zest, oregano, red pepper flakes, and salt. Set aside.

In another small bowl, stir together the remaining ingredients.

Drain the chicken, discarding the lemon juice. Put the chicken with the smooth side down on a flat work surface. Spoon the feta mixture down the center of each breast, leaving a ½-inch border uncovered. Starting at the narrowest end, roll up the chicken jelly-roll style. Place with the seam side down in a nonstick 8-inch square baking pan. Top with the tomato sauce mixture.

Bake, covered, for 40 to 45 minutes, or until the chicken is no longer pink in the center.

····· **PER SERVING** ·······

calories 177
total fat 3.5 g
  saturated fat 1.0 g
  trans fat 0.0 g
  polyunsaturated fat 0.5 g
  monounsaturated fat 1.5 g

cholesterol 69 mg
sodium 412 mg
carbohydrates 6 g
  fiber 1 g
  sugars 3 g
protein 29 g

100 200 300 400

DIETARY EXCHANGES
1 vegetable, 3 lean meat

chicken and snow pea stir-fry

serves 4; 1 cup per serving

When your schedule is packed and you have to get dinner on the table in a hurry, you may be tempted to stop for Chinese takeout. Instead, turn to this super-quick, healthier stir-fry, with far fewer calories. Try it with a side dish of soba noodles, rice noodles, or brown rice.

1 teaspoon canola or corn oil and 2 teaspoons canola or corn oil, divided use

1 pound boneless, skinless chicken breasts, all visible fat discarded, cut into very thin strips

½ medium onion, diced

4 medium garlic cloves, minced

6 ounces snow peas, trimmed if fresh, thawed if frozen

¼ cup slivered or sliced almonds, dry-roasted

½ teaspoon salt

In a large nonstick skillet, heat 1 teaspoon oil over medium-high heat, swirling to coat the bottom. Cook the chicken for 3 to 4 minutes, or until no longer pink in the center, stirring frequently. Transfer to a large plate.

In the same skillet, heat the remaining 2 teaspoons oil over medium-high heat, swirling to coat the bottom. Cook the onion for about 3 minutes, or until soft, stirring frequently.

Stir in the garlic. Cook for 10 seconds, stirring constantly.

Stir in the snow peas. Cook for 2 minutes, or until tender-crisp, stirring constantly.

Stir in the chicken and any accumulated juices. Remove from the heat. Stir in the almonds and salt.

PER SERVING

calories 222	cholesterol 66 mg
total fat 8.5 g	sodium 367 mg
saturated fat 1.0 g	carbohydrates 7 g
trans fat 0.0 g	fiber 2 g
polyunsaturated fat 2.0 g	sugars 3 g
monounsaturated fat 4.5 g	protein 29 g

100 200 300 400

DIETARY EXCHANGES
1 vegetable, 3 lean meat

chicken and bow-ties
with green beans

serves 4; 1½ cups per serving

Mild and creamy gorgonzola melts slightly to create a wonderfully aromatic dish that only tastes like it is high calorie.

3 quarts water

4 ounces dried whole-grain bow-tie pasta

6 ounces whole green beans, trimmed

1 teaspoon canola or corn oil

12 ounces boneless, skinless chicken breasts, all visible fat discarded, cut into thin strips

½ cup finely chopped red onion

1 medium garlic clove, minced

2 ounces Gorgonzola cheese, crumbled

2 tablespoons chopped fresh basil or 2 teaspoons dried, crumbled

2 teaspoons grated lemon zest

2 tablespoons lemon juice

2 teaspoons olive oil (extra-virgin preferred)

In a large saucepan, bring the water to a boil over high heat. Stir in the pasta. Boil for 6 minutes. Stir in the green beans. Boil for 5 minutes, or until the beans are tender-crisp. Drain well in a colander.

Meanwhile, in a large nonstick skillet, heat the oil over medium-high heat, swirling to coat the bottom. Cook the chicken for 2 minutes, stirring constantly.

Stir in the onion and garlic. Cook for 1 to 2 minutes, or until the chicken is no longer pink in the center, stirring constantly. Remove from the heat. Cover to keep warm. Set aside.

Pour the pasta mixture into a large bowl. Stir in the chicken mixture and remaining ingredients.

PER SERVING

calories 301	cholesterol 62 mg
total fat 9.5 g	sodium 251 mg
saturated fat 3.5 g	carbohydrates 27 g
trans fat 0.0 g	fiber 6 g
polyunsaturated fat 1.0 g	sugars 3 g
monounsaturated fat 3.0 g	protein 27 g

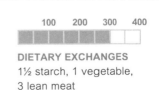

DIETARY EXCHANGES
1½ starch, 1 vegetable,
3 lean meat

cheesy chicken and quinoa stir-fry

serves 4; 1½ cups per serving

A typical Asian stir-fry in most respects, this dish has two twists—quinoa, a whole-grain replacement for the traditional white rice, and Parmesan cheese.

1 cup fat-free, low-sodium chicken broth

½ cup uncooked quinoa, rinsed and drained

1 teaspoon canola or corn oil

1 pound boneless, skinless chicken breasts, all visible fat discarded, cut into bite-size pieces

1 medium shallot, chopped

8 ounces button mushrooms, sliced

1 cup broccoli florets

1 large red bell pepper, cut into 1-inch strips

½ cup shredded carrot

1 tablespoon grated peeled gingerroot

2 teaspoons toasted sesame oil

3 medium garlic cloves, minced

¼ teaspoon pepper

⅛ teaspoon salt

⅓ cup chopped fresh basil

¼ cup shredded or grated Parmesan cheese

In a small saucepan, bring the broth to a boil over high heat. Stir in the quinoa. Return to a boil. Reduce the heat and simmer, covered, for 12 minutes, or until all the broth is absorbed. Remove from the heat. Fluff with a fork. Let stand, covered, for 15 minutes.

While the quinoa stands, in a large nonstick skillet, heat the canola oil over medium-high heat, swirling to coat the bottom. Cook the chicken and shallot for 4 to 5 minutes, or until the chicken is no longer pink in the center, stirring constantly.

Stir in the mushrooms, broccoli, bell pepper, and carrot. Cook for 5 minutes, or until the broccoli and bell pepper are tender-crisp, stirring frequently.

Stir in the gingerroot, sesame oil, garlic, pepper, and salt. Cook for 1 minute, stirring frequently. Remove from the heat. Stir in the quinoa, basil, and Parmesan.

····· **PER SERVING** ·········

calories 303	cholesterol 69 mg	
total fat 8.0 g	sodium 270 mg	
saturated fat 2.0 g	carbohydrates 23 g	
trans fat 0.0 g	fiber 4 g	
polyunsaturated fat 2.5 g	sugars 4 g	
monounsaturated fat 3.0 g	protein 35 g	

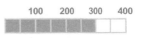

100   200   300   400

DIETARY EXCHANGES
1 starch, 2 vegetable,
3 lean meat

chicken fajitas

Don't think you can't still enjoy Mexican food just because you are watching your calories. Cilantro, jalapeño, and cumin spice up the sour cream and yogurt sauce that tops the fajitas in this diet-friendly dish.

- 8 ounces boneless, skinless chicken breasts, all visible fat discarded, cut into thin strips
- 2 tablespoons fresh lime juice
- ¾ cup fat-free sour cream
- ¼ cup fat-free plain yogurt
- 2 tablespoons finely snipped fresh cilantro
- 1 teaspoon finely chopped fresh jalapeño
- ⅛ teaspoon ground cumin
- 1 large green bell pepper, thinly sliced lengthwise
- 1 small red bell pepper, thinly sliced lengthwise
- 1 large onion, thinly sliced crosswise
- ½ cup fat-free, low-sodium chicken broth
- 8 6-inch fat-free flour tortillas (lowest sodium available)
- 2 cups shredded lettuce
- 2 medium tomatoes, chopped and drained

Put the chicken in a large shallow dish. Sprinkle with the lime juice. Cover and refrigerate for 15 to 30 minutes.

Meanwhile, in a small bowl, stir together the sour cream, yogurt, cilantro, jalapeño, and cumin. Set aside.

Heat a large nonstick skillet over medium heat. Cook the bell peppers, onion, and broth for 1 minute.

Stir the chicken into the bell pepper mixture. Cook for 2 to 4 minutes, or until the chicken is no longer pink in the center and the liquid has evaporated.

Meanwhile, warm the tortillas using the package directions. Keep covered until ready to serve.

Spoon the chicken mixture down the center of each tortilla. Top with the sour cream mixture, lettuce, and tomatoes. Roll up jelly-roll style. Serve immediately.

COOK'S TIP For a different meal for another day, double the chicken-vegetable filling. When you're ready to serve the additional half, heat it in a microwave oven and spoon it over cooked brown rice instead of in tortillas. While the chicken marinates in lime juice, you'll have plenty of time to make Quick Mexican-Style Soup (page 143).

COOK'S TIP ON BELL PEPPERS To safely slice a bell pepper, cut it in half lengthwise first. Discard the seeds and ribs. Slice the pepper from the inside, not the skin side. This will help prevent the knife from sliding on the slippery curved outer surface.

····· PER SERVING ·····

calories 315
total fat 1.5 g
  saturated fat 0.5 g
  trans fat 0.0 g
  polyunsaturated fat 0.5 g
  monounsaturated fat 0.0 g

cholesterol 41 mg
sodium 512 mg
carbohydrates 50 g
  fiber 6 g
  sugars 12 g
protein 24 g

100 200 300 400

DIETARY EXCHANGES
2½ starch, 2 vegetable,
2½ very lean meat

risotto with porcini mushrooms and chicken

serves 6; 1 cup per serving

The key to a creamy risotto is the slow absorption of the liquid, at least 20 minutes for this recipe. If you take the time to make it right, you will be rewarded with a rich-tasting result. Serve it with your favorite green vegetable and sliced tomatoes.

- 4 cups fat-free, low-sodium chicken broth or mushroom stock
- 1½ cups dry white wine (regular or nonalcoholic)
- ½ cup dried porcini mushrooms
- 8 ounces boneless, skinless chicken breasts, all visible fat discarded, cut into ½-inch cubes
- 2 teaspoons olive oil
- 1 large onion, chopped
- 2 cups uncooked arborio rice
- ½ teaspoon salt
- ½ teaspoon pepper
- ½ cup shredded or grated Parmesan cheese
- 2 tablespoons finely snipped Italian (flat-leaf) parsley

In a medium saucepan, bring the broth and wine to a boil over high heat. Stir in the dried mushrooms. Reduce the heat and simmer for 5 minutes. Drain the mushrooms through a coffee filter to remove any dirt, reserving the broth. Chop the mushrooms into bite-size pieces. Set aside. Return the broth to the saucepan. Bring to a simmer over low heat. Keep the broth at a simmer while preparing the risotto.

Meanwhile, heat a medium nonstick skillet over medium-high heat. Cook the chicken for 6 to 8 minutes, or until golden brown, stirring occasionally. Set aside.

In a large saucepan (heavy preferred), heat the oil over medium-high heat, swirling to coat the bottom. Cook the onion for about 3 minutes, or until soft, stirring frequently.

Add the rice, salt, and pepper to the onion, stirring to coat the rice grains.

Pour the simmering broth mixture 1 cup at a time into the rice mixture, stirring constantly until each addition of liquid is absorbed. After the last addition of broth is absorbed, stir in the chicken, Parmesan, and parsley.

COOK'S TIP If you prefer a moister risotto, you can add a bit more broth or wine before serving. It is important to keep the liquid hot while adding it to risotto so the finished dish will be creamy.

····· PER SERVING ·····

calories 413
total fat 5.0 g
  saturated fat 1.5 g
  trans fat 0.0 g
  polyunsaturated fat 0.5 g
  monounsaturated fat 2.0 g

cholesterol 27 mg
sodium 381 mg
carbohydrates 61 g
  fiber 5 g
  sugars 2 g
  protein 22 g

100 200 300 400

DIETARY EXCHANGES
3½ starch, 2 vegetable,
2 very lean meat

chicken and veggies with noodles

serves 4; 1½ cups per serving

Noodles topped with chicken strips and vegetables in a calorie-conscious creamy sauce is a family-pleasing combination.

Cooking spray

1 pound boneless, skinless chicken breasts, all visible fat discarded, cut into thin strips

1 large onion, thinly sliced crosswise

1 large green bell pepper, thinly sliced lengthwise

1 large rib of celery, thinly sliced crosswise

½ cup water

¾ teaspoon dried thyme, crumbled

⅛ teaspoon cayenne

4 ounces dried no-yolk noodles

1 10.75-ounce can low-fat condensed cream of chicken soup (lowest sodium available)

⅛ teaspoon salt

Lightly spray a Dutch oven with cooking spray. Heat over medium-high heat. Cook the chicken for 2 minutes, stirring constantly. Remove the pot from the heat. Transfer the chicken to a large plate.

Lightly spray the browned bits remaining in the pot with cooking spray. Put the onion, bell pepper, and celery in the pot. Lightly spray with cooking spray. Cook over medium-high heat for 4 minutes, or until the vegetables begin to brown, stirring frequently.

Stir in the chicken and any accumulated juices, water, thyme, and cayenne. Reduce the heat and simmer, covered, for 10 minutes, or until the celery is tender, stirring occasionally.

Meanwhile, prepare the pasta using the package directions, omitting the salt.

When the celery is tender, stir in the soup and salt. Cook for 1 minute, or until heated through. Serve over the pasta.

COOK'S TIP Adding the soup at the very end preserves the creaminess of the dish.

····· **PER SERVING** ·····

calories 311
total fat 3.5 g
  saturated fat 1.0 g
  trans fat 0.0 g
  polyunsaturated fat 0.5 g
  monounsaturated fat 0.5 g

cholesterol 69 mg
sodium 460 mg
carbohydrates 36 g
  fiber 4 g
  sugars 7 g
protein 32 g

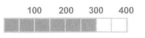

DIETARY EXCHANGES
2 starch, 1 vegetable,
3 very lean meat

chicken enchiladas

serves 6; 2 enchiladas per serving

With their fresh, wholesome vegetables and aromatic herbs and spices, these home-cooked enchiladas are sure to beat out any restaurant's version in overall good nutrition.

Cooking spray

filling

   1   large onion, diced
  ¾   cup diced green bell pepper
  ¾   cup diced carrot
  ¾   cup diced zucchini
   3   medium garlic cloves, minced
   8   ounces ground skinless chicken breast
   1   medium fresh jalapeño, seeds and ribs discarded, minced
   1   tablespoon chili powder
   2   teaspoons dried oregano, crumbled
   1   teaspoon ground cumin
   1   15.5-ounce can no-salt-added black beans, rinsed and drained
   1   cup fresh, frozen, or canned no-salt-added whole-kernel corn, cooked if fresh, thawed if frozen, drained if canned
   2   tablespoons fresh lime juice
   2   tablespoons snipped fresh cilantro

....

  12   6-inch corn tortillas
  ¼   cup low-fat Cheddar cheese and ½ cup low-fat Cheddar cheese, divided use
  2½   cups salsa (lowest sodium available)
  ¾   cup fat-free sour cream

Preheat the oven to 350°F. Lightly spray a 15 x 11 x 2-inch glass baking dish with cooking spray. Lightly spray a large skillet with cooking spray.

In the skillet, cook the onion, bell pepper, carrot, zucchini, and garlic over medium heat for 5 minutes, or until tender, stirring occasionally.

Stir in the chicken. Cook for 1 minute, or until no longer pink, stirring constantly.

Stir in the jalapeño, chili powder, oregano, and cumin. Cook for 1 minute, stirring constantly. Remove from the heat.

Stir in the remaining filling ingredients.

Spoon a heaping ¼ cup filling down the center of each tortilla. Sprinkle ¼ cup Cheddar over the filling, about 1 teaspoon for each tortilla. Roll up jelly-roll style. Place with the seam down in the baking dish. Pour the salsa over the enchiladas, covering each one.

Bake, covered, for 30 minutes. Sprinkle with the remaining ½ cup Cheddar. Bake, uncovered, for 5 minutes. Serve with a dollop of sour cream on each enchilada.

COOK'S TIP If you want to challenge your heat barometer when eating this festive Mexican dish, increase the amount of jalapeño or leave in the seeds and ribs.

···· PER SERVING ··

calories 312	cholesterol 30 mg	
total fat 3.0 g	sodium 584 mg	
saturated fat 1.0 g	carbohydrates 49 g	
trans fat 0.0 g	fiber 7 g	**DIETARY EXCHANGES**
polyunsaturated fat 0.5 g	sugars 13 g	3 starch, 1 vegetable,
monounsaturated fat 0.5 g	protein 22 g	2 very lean meat

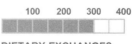

chicken pot pie
with mashed potato crust

This mashed-potato-topped version of chicken pot pie lets you turn leftovers into the epitome of comfort food. You'll save a whopping number of calories and add many other nutritional benefits by making your own pot pie instead of buying one from the freezer section of the grocery store.

Cooking spray

1 tablespoon olive oil and 2 tablespoons olive oil, divided use

½ cup chopped onion

1 medium garlic clove, minced

2 medium ribs of celery, cut crosswise into ¼-inch pieces

2 medium carrots, cut crosswise into ¼-inch pieces

¼ cup all-purpose flour

1 cup fat-free, low-sodium chicken broth and 1 cup fat-free, low-sodium chicken broth, divided use

3 cups chopped cooked skinless chicken or turkey breast, cooked without salt, all visible fat discarded

1 cup frozen baby green peas or leftover cooked or frozen vegetables

2 tablespoons chopped fresh Italian (flat-leaf) parsley

¼ teaspoon salt

Pepper to taste

Mashed Potatoes (recipe on next page) or about 4 cups leftover mashed potatoes, cooked without salt and margarine

Preheat the oven to 375°F. Lightly spray a 9-inch deep-dish pie pan or baking pan with cooking spray. Set aside.

In a Dutch oven, heat 1 tablespoon oil over medium-high heat, swirling to coat the bottom. Cook the onion and garlic for about 3 minutes, or until the onion is soft, stirring frequently.

Stir in the celery and carrots. Cook for 5 minutes, or until the celery begins to soften. Transfer to a medium plate.

Reduce the heat to medium. In the same pan, heat the remaining 2 tablespoons oil, swirling to coat the bottom. Whisk in the flour, thoroughly incorporating the oil. (The mixture will be dry.)

Gradually pour in 1 cup broth, whisking constantly. Cook for 2 to 3 minutes, or until the mixture begins to thicken and turn golden.

Stir in the onion mixture, chicken, peas, parsley, and enough of the remaining 1 cup broth for the desired consistency. Stir in the salt and pepper. Pour the mixture into the pie pan.

Spread the mashed potatoes over the chicken mixture.

Bake for 25 minutes, or until the potato crust is golden and the filling is bubbly.

mashed potatoes

    1 pound Yukon Gold potatoes, peeled and cut into 2-inch cubes
    4 cups fat-free, low-sodium chicken broth
    1 medium garlic clove

Put the potatoes in a large saucepan and add enough broth to cover. Add the garlic. Bring to a boil over high heat. Reduce the heat and cook at a low boil for 10 to 15 minutes, or until the potatoes are just tender. Drain immediately, reserving the broth.

In a large mixing bowl, using a potato masher or an electric mixer on low speed, mash or beat the potatoes and garlic until no large chunks remain. Gradually pour in the broth, mashing or beating after each addition, until the desired consistency.

···· PER SERVING ···

calories 219
total fat 7.0 g
　saturated fat 1.5 g
　trans fat 0.0 g
　polyunsaturated fat 1.0 g
　monounsaturated fat 4.5 g

cholesterol 45 mg
sodium 180 mg
carbohydrates 19 g
　fiber 3 g
　sugars 3 g
　protein 20 g

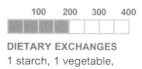

DIETARY EXCHANGES
1 starch, 1 vegetable,
2 lean meat

meats

Beef Tenderloin with Horseradish Cream

Filet Mignon with Balsamic Berry Sauce

Honey-Lime Flank Steak

Broiled Flank Steak in Barbecue-Style Marinade

Orange Beef Stir-Fry

Grilled Sirloin Kebabs with Creamy Herb Dipping Sauce

Satay-Style Sirloin with Peanut Dipping Sauce

Greek-Style Sirloin Cubes and Olive-Feta Rice

Beef Stroganoff with Baby Bella Mushrooms

Slow-Cooker Steak-and-Bean Chili

Slow-Cooker Barbecue Beef in Pitas

Meat Loaf with a Twist

Ground Beef Goulash with Red Wine

Moussaka-Style Eggplant Casserole

Chicken-Fried Steak with Creamy Gravy

Saucy Cube Steaks

Cube Steaks with Avocado Salsa

Chopped Beef Hash

Pork Tenderloin with Cranberry Salsa

Pork Tenderloin with Orange-Ginger Sweet Potatoes

Thai Coconut Curry with Pork and Vegetables

Pork Chops Parmesan

Ham and Broccoli with Rotini

Sausage and White Beans with Spinach

beef tenderloin with horseradish cream

serves 4; 3 ounces beef and 2 tablespoons sauce per serving

No need to splurge on calories for your next special-occasion entrée. Serve this beef tenderloin with a heavenly horseradish cream sauce for a meal to remember.

Cooking spray

sauce

3 tablespoons fat-free plain yogurt

3 tablespoons fat-free sour cream

2 tablespoons chopped green onions

2 teaspoons bottled white horseradish, or to taste, drained

½ teaspoon Worcestershire sauce (lowest sodium available)

beef

1 1-pound center-cut beef tenderloin, all visible fat and silver skin discarded

1 medium garlic clove, cut into 6 slices

1½ teaspoons spicy brown mustard

½ teaspoon garlic powder

¼ teaspoon pepper

Preheat the oven to 450°F. Lightly spray a shallow roasting pan with cooking spray. Set aside.

In a small bowl, whisk together the sauce ingredients. Cover and refrigerate until serving time.

Meanwhile, cut 6 small, evenly spaced slits into the top of the beef. Insert a garlic slice into each slit. Thinly spread the mustard all over the beef. Sprinkle with the garlic powder and pepper. Put the beef in the roasting pan.

Roast for 20 minutes. Reduce the temperature to 350°F. Roast for 20 to 25 minutes, or until the beef registers 140°F on an instant-read thermometer for medium-rare doneness or 155°F for medium doneness. Remove from the oven. Cover with aluminum foil. Let stand for at least 10 minutes before slicing. The temperature will rise about 5 degrees. Serve with the horseradish cream sauce.

COOK'S TIP Be sure to make the sauce before roasting the beef so the flavors in the sauce have time to blend.

COOK'S TIP ON BOTTLED HORSERADISH Freshly opened bottled horseradish is much hotter than horseradish that has been open for a while. Therefore, the amount you use, such as in this recipe, may be governed by how long it has been since the horseradish was first opened.

···· **PER SERVING** ··

calories 174
total fat 5.0 g
  saturated fat 2.5 g
  trans fat 0.0 g
  polyunsaturated fat 0.5 g
  monounsaturated fat 2.5 g

cholesterol 55 mg
sodium 97 mg
carbohydrates 4 g
  fiber 0 g
  sugars 2 g
protein 25 g

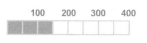

DIETARY EXCHANGES
3 lean meat

filet mignon with balsamic berry sauce

serves 4; 3 ounces beef and 2 tablespoons sauce per serving

Holiday time doesn't have to derail a healthy eating goal. Plan your menu around this beautiful cut of meat, served with a sweet, mellow, sophisticated sauce that is perfect for a special family celebration or an intimate dinner party. It pairs perfectly with Roasted Green Beans and Walnuts (page 363) and Smashed Potatoes with Aromatic Herbs (page 369) or Cream of Triple-Mushroom Soup (page 144).

sauce

½ cup water

¼ cup all-fruit blackberry spread

2 tablespoons balsamic vinegar

2 tablespoons soy sauce (lowest sodium available)

2 tablespoons Worcestershire sauce (lowest sodium available)

steaks

1 teaspoon canola or corn oil

4 filets mignons (about 4 ounces each), any bacon and all visible fat discarded

¼ teaspoon salt

¼ teaspoon pepper

In a small bowl, whisk together the sauce ingredients. Set aside.

In a large nonstick skillet, heat the oil over medium-high heat, swirling to coat the bottom. Add the beef. Sprinkle the top side with the salt and pepper. Using your fingertips, gently press so the salt and pepper adhere to the beef. Cook for 2 to 3 minutes, or until richly browned. Reduce the heat to medium. Turn the beef over. Cook for 2 minutes on each side, or to the desired doneness. Transfer with the browner side up to a large plate. Cover to keep warm.

Increase the heat to medium high. Pour the sauce into the skillet. Bring to a boil, scraping to dislodge any browned bits. Cook for 1 to 2 minutes, or until the liquid is reduced to ½ cup. Spoon over the beef.

····· PER SERVING ·····

calories 215
total fat 6.0 g
  saturated fat 2.5 g
  trans fat 0.0 g
  polyunsaturated fat 0.5 g
  monounsaturated fat 3.5 g

cholesterol 57 mg
sodium 403 mg
carbohydrates 13 g
  fiber 0 g
  sugars 10 g
protein 24 g

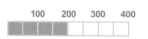

DIETARY EXCHANGES
1 fruit, 3 lean meat

honey-lime flank steak

serves 4; 3 ounces beef per serving (plus 8 ounces reserved)

This one easy-to-prepare dish actually is the base for two meals. Serve part of the grilled flank steak for a delicious dinner with your choice of vegetables, and refrigerate the rest of the cooked steak to use in Flank Steak Salad with Sesame-Lime Dressing (page 184) later in the week.

marinade

1½ to 2 tablespoons fresh lime juice

3 tablespoons honey

2 tablespoons plain rice vinegar

1 tablespoon soy sauce (lowest sodium available)

2 teaspoons toasted sesame oil

1 teaspoon grated peeled gingerroot

2 medium garlic cloves, minced

1½ pounds flank steak, all visible fat and silver skin discarded

Cooking spray (optional)

In a large shallow glass dish, whisk together the marinade ingredients. Add the beef, turning to coat. Cover and refrigerate for 2 to 12 hours, turning occasionally.

If using an outdoor grill, preheat on medium high. If using a ridged stovetop grill pan, lightly spray with cooking spray.

Drain the beef, discarding the marinade.

Grill the beef for 7 to 8 minutes on each side for medium-rare, or to the desired doneness (the stovetop grill also uses medium-high heat). Transfer to a cutting board. Let stand for 5 minutes. Cut diagonally across the grain into thin slices. Cover and refrigerate 8 ounces beef for use within three days in Flank Steak Salad with Sesame-Lime Dressing. Transfer the remaining beef to plates.

PER SERVING

calories 188	cholesterol 53 mg	
total fat 9.0 g	sodium 137 mg	
saturated fat 4.0 g	carbohydrates 0 g	
trans fat 0.5 g	fiber 0 g	
polyunsaturated fat 0.5 g	sugars 0 g	
monounsaturated fat 4.5 g	protein 25 g	

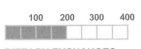

DIETARY EXCHANGES
3 lean meat

broiled flank steak in barbecue-style marinade

serves 4; 3 ounces beef per serving

With its spectacular aroma and taste, this steak out"flanks" the others. Serve it with Vegetable Salad Vinaigrette (page 167) and corn on the cob.

marinade

- ¼ cup no-salt-added ketchup
- ¼ cup red wine vinegar
- 1 tablespoon honey
- 1 tablespoon Worcestershire sauce (lowest sodium available)
- 2 medium garlic cloves, minced
- ½ teaspoon smoked paprika
- ⅛ teaspoon salt

- 1 pound flank steak, all visible fat and silver skin discarded
  Cooking spray

In a large shallow glass dish, whisk together the marinade ingredients. Add the steak, turning to coat. Cover and refrigerate for 2 to 12 hours, turning occasionally.

Preheat the broiler. Lightly spray a broiler pan and rack with cooking spray.

Drain the steak, discarding the marinade. Transfer the steak to the broiler rack.

Broil 2 to 3 inches from the heat for 4 to 5 minutes on each side for medium rare, or to the desired doneness. Transfer to a cutting board. Let stand for 5 minutes. Cut diagonally across the grain into very thin slices.

PER SERVING

calories 161	cholesterol 37 mg
total fat 6.0 g	sodium 140 mg
saturated fat 2.5 g	carbohydrates 0 g
trans fat 0.0 g	fiber 0 g
polyunsaturated fat 0.0 g	sugars 0 g
monounsaturated fat 2.0 g	protein 25 g

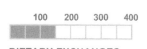

DIETARY EXCHANGES
3 lean meat

orange beef stir-fry

serves 4; 3 ounces beef per serving

You might want to make a double batch of this lower-calorie, healthier version of traditional takeout. It's every bit as tasty a day or two after it is prepared. Try the stir-fry over whole-grain or soba noodles instead of the usual white rice and add a side dish of steamed snow peas to round out the meal.

Cooking spray

1 pound flank steak, all visible fat and silver skin discarded, thinly sliced on the diagonal, then cut into bite-size pieces

1 teaspoon canola or corn oil

4 medium green onions, sliced

2 teaspoons grated peeled gingerroot

2 teaspoons grated orange zest

2 medium garlic cloves, minced

¼ cup fresh orange juice

2 tablespoons plain rice vinegar or white wine vinegar

1 tablespoon teriyaki sauce (lowest sodium available)

1½ tablespoons honey

1 teaspoon toasted sesame oil

2 teaspoons cornstarch

¼ cup cold water

Lightly spray a wok or large skillet with cooking spray. Cook the beef over high heat for 2 minutes, or until browned, stirring frequently. Transfer to a medium bowl. Set aside. Wipe the wok with paper towels.

Reduce the heat to medium. Pour the canola oil into the wok, swirling to coat the bottom. Cook the green onions, gingerroot, orange zest, and garlic for 3 minutes, or until the green onions are soft, stirring frequently.

Stir in the beef with any accumulated juices. Increase the heat to medium high. Stir in the orange juice, vinegar, teriyaki sauce, honey, and sesame oil. Cook for 1 to 2 minutes, or until the beef is the desired doneness and the mixture is hot, stirring occasionally.

Put the cornstarch in a cup. Add the water, whisking to dissolve. Stir into the beef mixture. Cook for 1 minute, or until thickened, stirring frequently.

COOK'S TIP If you make a double recipe, use two woks or skillets so the beef isn't crowded and doesn't steam instead of stir-fry.

COOK'S TIP ON SLICING RAW MEAT Freezing meat for about 30 minutes before slicing it makes the task much easier.

···· **PER SERVING** ··

calories 235	cholesterol 48 mg
total fat 9.0 g	sodium 158 mg
saturated fat 3.0 g	carbohydrates 13 g
trans fat 0.0 g	fiber 1 g
polyunsaturated fat 1.0 g	sugars 10 g
monounsaturated fat 4.5 g	protein 24 g

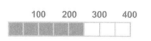

DIETARY EXCHANGES
1 carbohydrate, 3 lean meat

grilled sirloin kebabs with creamy herb dipping sauce

serves 4; 2 kebabs and 2 tablespoons sauce per serving

The sirloin in this dish can marinate for up to two days—the flavor just gets better and better the longer the beef cubes marinate—and the sauce can be made at the same time. Then when you come home from work, grill the kebabs and have dinner on the table within minutes.

1 pound boneless sirloin steak, all visible fat discarded, cut into 16 cubes

2 tablespoons soy sauce and 1 tablespoon soy sauce (lowest sodium available), divided use

1 teaspoon pepper (coarsely ground preferred)

½ cup fat-free sour cream

2 teaspoons Dijon mustard

1 teaspoon dried oregano, crumbled

1 medium garlic clove, minced

Cooking spray

1 medium onion

16 medium button mushrooms

1 medium zucchini, halved lengthwise, each half cut crosswise into 8 pieces

Place the beef cubes in a shallow glass dish. Pour 2 tablespoons soy sauce over the beef. Sprinkle with the pepper, turning to coat. Cover and refrigerate for 2 to 48 hours, turning occasionally.

In a small bowl, whisk together the sour cream, mustard, oregano, and garlic. Cover and refrigerate until serving time. (This sauce will keep even if you use the full two days of marinating time.)

At least 10 minutes before the grilling time, soak eight 12-inch wooden skewers in cold water to keep them from charring, or use metal skewers.

Lightly spray the grill rack with cooking spray. Preheat the grill on medium high.

Cut the onion into 4 wedges. Separate the layers, keeping 16 of the larger pieces for the kebabs and saving the remaining pieces for another use.

Drain the beef, discarding the marinade. Thread each skewer as follows: beef, mushroom, onion, zucchini, beef, mushroom, onion, zucchini.

Grill the kebabs for 3 to 4 minutes on each side, or until the beef is cooked to the desired doneness. Serve drizzled with the remaining 1 tablespoon soy sauce and with the dipping sauce on the side.

COOK'S TIP You can freeze the uncooked beef cubes in the marinade for up to one month, then thaw them in the refrigerator.

PER SERVING

calories 222	cholesterol 61 mg
total fat 5.0 g	sodium 426 mg
saturated fat 2.0 g	carbohydrates 14 g
trans fat 0.0 g	fiber 2 g
polyunsaturated fat 0.5 g	sugars 7 g
monounsaturated fat 2.0 g	protein 30 g

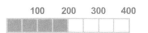

DIETARY EXCHANGES
1 vegetable, ½ carbohydrate, 3 lean meat

satay-style sirloin with peanut dipping sauce

serves 4; 3 ounces beef and 2 tablespoons sauce per serving

By grilling individual marinated steaks instead of assembling traditional satay meat skewers, you'll save a bit of prep time. Serve the steaks with Mixed Vegetable Grill (page 376) and quinoa.

marinade

- 4 medium green onions, thinly sliced
- 2 tablespoons fresh lime juice
- 2 teaspoons soy sauce (lowest sodium available)
- 1 teaspoon light brown sugar
- 1 teaspoon grated peeled gingerroot
- 1 teaspoon toasted sesame oil
- 2 medium garlic cloves, minced

- 1 pound boneless top sirloin steak, all visible fat discarded, cut into 4 equal pieces

sauce

- ⅓ cup fat-free half-and-half
- 2 tablespoons creamy peanut butter
- 2 teaspoons soy sauce (lowest sodium available)
- ½ teaspoon coconut extract
- ½ teaspoon chili paste (optional)

    Cooking spray (optional)

In a medium shallow glass dish, stir together the marinade ingredients. Add the beef, turning to coat. Cover and refrigerate for 15 minutes to 8 hours, turning occasionally if marinating more than 30 minutes.

Meanwhile, in a small bowl, whisk together the sauce ingredients. Cover and refrigerate until ready to use. (The sauce will keep for up to two days.)

Preheat the grill on medium high or preheat the broiler. If using a broiler, lightly spray the pan and rack with cooking spray.

Drain the beef, discarding the marinade.

Grill or broil about 6 inches from the heat for 8 to 10 minutes on each side for medium rare to medium, or to the desired doneness. Serve with the dipping sauce.

PER SERVING

calories 206
total fat 8.5 g
  saturated fat 2.5 g
  trans fat 0.0 g
  polyunsaturated fat 1.5 g
  monounsaturated fat 4.0 g

cholesterol 56 mg
sodium 235 mg
carbohydrates 5 g
  fiber 1 g
  sugars 2 g
protein 27 g

100   200   300   400

DIETARY EXCHANGES
½ carbohydrate,
3½ lean meat

greek-style sirloin cubes and olive-feta rice

serves 4; 1½ cups per serving

This dish of tender beef offers just the right combination of flavor, texture, and color. Serve with a salad of mixed greens, red and yellow tomatoes, and red onions.

2   teaspoons olive oil
1   cup frozen pearl onions
1   14.5-ounce can no-salt-added diced tomatoes, undrained
¼   cup water
1   teaspoon grated lemon zest
1   teaspoon fresh lemon juice
1   teaspoon dried oregano, crumbled
¼   teaspoon salt
⅛   teaspoon pepper
1¼ cups fat-free, low-sodium chicken broth
2   tablespoons chopped kalamata olives
2   tablespoons slivered almonds, dry-roasted
1   cup uncooked instant brown rice
2   tablespoons crumbled low-fat feta cheese
1   pound boneless top sirloin steak, all visible fat discarded, cut into ¾-inch cubes

In a medium saucepan, heat the oil over medium-high heat, swirling to coat the bottom. Cook the onions for 4 to 5 minutes, or until almost thawed and slightly golden brown, stirring occasionally.

Stir in the tomatoes with liquid, water, lemon zest, lemon juice, oregano, salt, and pepper. Bring to a simmer, stirring occasionally. Reduce the heat and simmer, covered, for 15 minutes, stirring occasionally.

Meanwhile, in a separate medium saucepan, stir together the broth, olives, and almonds. Bring to a simmer over medium-high heat. Stir in the rice. Reduce the heat and simmer, covered, for 10 minutes, or until the rice is tender. Stir in the feta. Remove from the heat and cover to keep warm.

In a large nonstick skillet, cook the beef over medium-high heat for 5 to 6 minutes, or until browned on the outside and slightly pink in the center, stirring occasionally.

Stir the beef into the tomato mixture. Reduce the heat to low and cook for 1 minute, or until the mixture is heated through, stirring occasionally. Serve over the rice.

COOK'S TIP ON DRY-ROASTING NUTS Place the nuts in a single layer in a small skillet. Dry-roast over medium heat for about 4 minutes, or just until fragrant, stirring frequently. Watch carefully so they don't burn. Remove the nuts from the skillet so they don't continue to cook.

PER SERVING

calories 356	cholesterol 62 mg
total fat 11.0 g	sodium 377 mg
saturated fat 2.5 g	carbohydrates 31 g
trans fat 0.0 g	fiber 3 g
polyunsaturated fat 2.0 g	sugars 5 g
monounsaturated fat 6.0 g	protein 31 g

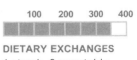

DIETARY EXCHANGES
1 starch, 3 vegetable,
3 lean meat

beef stroganoff with baby bella mushrooms

serves 4; 1 cup beef mixture and ½ cup noodles per serving

By watching portion size and making judicious ingredient choices, you can still enjoy many of your favorite classic dishes, such as beef stroganoff, while losing or managing your weight. In this version, delicate pearl onions and baby bella mushrooms are cooked until they are so tender they seem to melt into the sauce. Serve with a salad of crisp romaine, shredded carrots, and juicy red tomatoes.

- 3 ounces dried no-yolk noodles
- 2 tablespoons all-purpose flour
- ½ teaspoon salt-free all-purpose seasoning blend
- 1 pound boneless top round steak, all visible fat discarded, cut into thin slices
- Cooking spray
- 1 teaspoon olive oil
- 1 pound baby bella mushrooms, sliced
- 1 cup frozen pearl onions
- 1 cup fat-free, no-salt-added beef broth
- ¼ cup dry white wine (regular or nonalcoholic)
- 2 tablespoons steak sauce (lowest sodium available)
- ¼ teaspoon salt
- ¼ teaspoon pepper
- ⅓ cup fat-free sour cream

Prepare the noodles using the package directions, omitting the salt. Drain well in a colander. Cover to keep warm.

Meanwhile, in a medium shallow glass dish, stir together the flour and seasoning blend. Add the beef, turning to coat.

Lightly spray a large skillet with cooking spray. Add the oil and heat over medium-high heat, swirling to coat the bottom. Cook the beef mixture, including any flour remaining in the dish, for 6 to 8 minutes, or until the beef is browned on the outside and slightly pink in the center. Transfer to a medium plate.

In the same skillet, cook the mushrooms and onions for 3 to 4 minutes, or until the mushrooms are soft and the onions are almost thawed, stirring occasionally.

Stir in the remaining ingredients except the sour cream. Bring to a simmer, stirring occasionally. Reduce the heat and simmer, covered, for 20 to 25 minutes, or until the beef is tender and the sauce is thickened (no stirring needed).

Put the sour cream in a small bowl. Stir in a small amount of the beef mixture (to reduce the risk of curdling). Stir the sour cream mixture into the remaining beef mixture. Cook over low heat for 1 to 2 minutes, or until heated through, stirring occasionally. Serve over the noodles.

····· PER SERVING ···

calories 340
total fat 5.0 g
  saturated fat 1.5 g
  trans fat 0.0 g
  polyunsaturated fat 0.5 g
  monounsaturated fat 2.5 g

cholesterol 60 mg
sodium 290 mg
carbohydrates 37 g
  fiber 3 g
  sugars 7 g
  protein 33 g

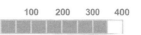

DIETARY EXCHANGES
1½ starch, 3 very lean meat

slow-cooker steak-and-bean chili

serves 6; 1½ cups per serving

This chili is hearty, spicy, and savory. Round up your gang for a mouth-watering bowl tonight!

Cooking spray

chili

1 28-ounce can no-salt-added crushed tomatoes, undrained

1 14.5-ounce can no-salt-added diced tomatoes, undrained

1 pound boneless top round steak, all visible fat discarded, cut into ½-inch cubes

1 cup frozen whole-kernel corn

1 cup chopped red onion

1 medium green bell pepper, chopped

1 tablespoon chili powder

1 tablespoon ground cumin

½ to 1 teaspoon sugar

½ teaspoon dried oregano, crumbled

½ teaspoon pepper

½ teaspoon cayenne

¼ teaspoon salt

1 15.5-ounce can no-salt-added red kidney beans, rinsed and drained

toppings

¾ cup fat-free sour cream

¾ cup shredded low-fat 4-cheese Mexican blend or Cheddar cheese

2 tablespoons chopped red onion

Lightly spray a 3½- or 4-quart slow cooker with cooking spray. Put the chili ingredients except the beans in the slow cooker, stirring to combine. Cook, covered, on low for 6 to 7 hours, or until the beef is tender.

Stir in the beans. Cook, covered, for 15 minutes, or until heated through.

Serve topped with the sour cream, cheese, and onion.

COOK'S TIP If you're pressed for time, you can cook the chili using your slow cooker's high setting for 3 to 3½ hours, but the beef will not be quite so tender.

····· **PER SERVING** ···

calories 313	cholesterol 46 mg
total fat 3.5 g	sodium 267 mg
saturated fat 1.5 g	carbohydrates 39 g
trans fat 0.0 g	fiber 7 g
polyunsaturated fat 0.5 g	sugars 13 g
monounsaturated fat 1.5 g	protein 31 g

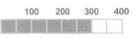

DIETARY EXCHANGES
1½ starch, 3 vegetable,
3 very lean meat

slow-cooker barbecue beef in pitas

serves 6; ½ cup beef mixture and 1 pita half per serving

There's nothing like coming home to a kitchen filled with the aroma of barbecue that's been simmering all day in a slow cooker. Be sure you have plenty of napkins on hand when you serve this saucy dish! Add a side of Carrot-Pineapple Slaw (page 170) or Multicolored Marinated Slaw (page 171) and some pinto beans to make the meal complete.

1 tablespoon canola or corn oil

Cooking spray

1 pound boneless round steak, all visible fat discarded, cut into 1-inch cubes

½ cup water

1 medium onion, chopped

1 8-ounce can no-salt-added tomato sauce

¼ cup firmly packed dark brown sugar

2 tablespoons balsamic vinegar

1 teaspoon Worcestershire sauce (lowest sodium available)

½ teaspoon ground cumin

¼ teaspoon ground allspice

1 tablespoon liquid smoke

½ teaspoon salt

3 6-inch whole-grain pita pockets, halved

In a large nonstick skillet, heat the oil over medium-high heat, swirling to coat the bottom. Cook the beef for 1 to 2 minutes, or until browned, stirring frequently.

Lightly spray a 3½- or 4-quart slow-cooker with cooking spray. Transfer the beef to the slow cooker.

In the same skillet, bring the water to a boil over medium-high heat, scraping to dislodge any browned bits. Pour over the beef.

Stir in the onion, tomato sauce, brown sugar, vinegar, Worcestershire sauce, cumin, and allspice. Cook, covered, for 5½ hours on high or 11 hours on low, or until the beef is very tender.

About 15 minutes before serving, stir in the liquid smoke and salt. Leaving the heat on and the beef in the slow cooker, use a fork to shred the larger pieces of beef. Stir. Re-cover the slow cooker and finish the cooking time.

Warm the pita pockets using the package directions. Fill with the beef mixture.

···· **PER SERVING** ···

calories 255
total fat 5.0 g
  saturated fat 1.0 g
  trans fat 0.0 g
  polyunsaturated fat 1.0 g
  monounsaturated fat 2.5 g

cholesterol 38 mg
sodium 390 mg
carbohydrates 32 g
  fiber 3 g
  sugars 14 g
  protein 21 g

100 200 300 400

DIETARY EXCHANGES
1½ starch, 1 vegetable,
2½ lean meat

meat loaf with a twist

serves 6; 1 slice per serving

Grated zucchini provides extra moisture for this traditional meat loaf, and horseradish gives a bit of bite to the glaze.

Cooking spray

meat loaf

1 medium zucchini

1 pound extra-lean ground beef

½ cup uncooked rolled oats

1 small onion, chopped

2 large egg whites, lightly beaten

2 tablespoons shredded or grated Parmesan cheese

2 tablespoons fat-free milk

1 tablespoon snipped fresh parsley

2 medium garlic cloves, minced

½ teaspoon dried basil, crumbled

½ teaspoon dried oregano, crumbled

¼ teaspoon salt

glaze

¼ cup no-salt-added ketchup

1 tablespoon light brown sugar

1 teaspoon Dijon honey mustard

1 teaspoon bottled white horseradish, drained

⅛ teaspoon salt

....

½ teaspoon paprika (optional)

Preheat the oven to 350°F. Lightly spray a broiler pan and rack with cooking spray. Set aside.

Shred enough zucchini to measure 1 cup. Squeeze dry between paper towels. Pat dry with more paper towels. Cut the remaining zucchini crosswise into thin slices. Set the slices aside.

In a large bowl, using your hands or a spoon, combine the shredded zucchini with the remaining meat loaf ingredients. Place the mixture on the broiler rack. Shape into an 8 x 3½ x 2-inch loaf.

Bake for 1 hour.

Meanwhile, in a small bowl, whisk together the glaze ingredients.

Remove the meat loaf from the oven. Spoon the glaze over the top and sides of the loaf. Arrange the reserved zucchini slices on top. Sprinkle the paprika over the zucchini slices.

Bake for 10 to 15 minutes, or until the meat loaf registers 160°F on an instant-read thermometer and is no longer pink in the center. Let stand for 5 minutes before slicing.

···· PER SERVING ···

calories 175

total fat 5.0 g

  saturated fat 2.0 g

  trans fat 0.0 g

  polyunsaturated fat 0.5 g

  monounsaturated fat 2.0 g

cholesterol 43 mg

sodium 262 mg

carbohydrates 14 g

  fiber 2 g

  sugars 7 g

protein 20 g

100　200　300　400

DIETARY EXCHANGES

1 carbohydrate,

2½ lean meat

ground beef goulash with red wine

serves 4; 1 cup beef mixture and ½ cup pasta per serving

Here's a home-style dish that's ready in short order—simply brown the beef, stir in the other ingredients, and let the mixture simmer while you boil some whole-grain pasta.

   Cooking spray
1 teaspoon olive oil and 1 tablespoon olive oil, divided use
1 pound extra-lean ground beef
1 14.5-ounce can no-salt-added stewed tomatoes, undrained
1 medium onion, diced
4 ounces button mushrooms, sliced
¼ cup dry red wine (regular or nonalcoholic)
2 tablespoons balsamic vinegar
2 tablespoons soy sauce (lowest sodium available)
2 teaspoons dried oregano, crumbled
1 teaspoon Worcestershire sauce (lowest sodium available)
4 ounces dried whole-grain rotini
¼ teaspoon salt

Lightly spray a Dutch oven with cooking spray. Heat 1 teaspoon oil over medium-high heat, swirling to coat the bottom. Cook the beef for 1 to 2 minutes, or until browned on the outside and no longer pink in the center, stirring frequently to turn and break up the beef.

Stir in the tomatoes with liquid, onion, mushrooms, wine, vinegar, soy sauce, oregano, and Worcestershire sauce. Increase the heat to high and bring to a boil. Reduce the heat and simmer, covered, for 25 minutes, or until the onion is very soft, stirring occasionally.

Meanwhile, prepare the pasta using the package directions, omitting the salt. Drain well in a colander.

Stir the salt and remaining 1 tablespoon oil into the beef mixture. Simmer, uncovered, for 3 to 5 minutes, or until slightly thickened, stirring occasionally. Spoon over the pasta.

····· PER SERVING ···

calories 364
total fat 11.0 g
  saturated fat 3.0 g
  trans fat 0.5 g
  polyunsaturated fat 1.5 g
  monounsaturated fat 6.0 g

cholesterol 62 mg
sodium 445 mg
carbohydrates 34 g
  fiber 6 g
  sugars 10 g
protein 30 g

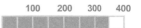

DIETARY EXCHANGES
1½ starch, 2 vegetable,
3 lean meat

moussaka-style eggplant casserole

serves 4; 1½ cups per serving

You don't need to peel the eggplant or chop the tomatoes for this easier version of moussaka.

Cooking spray

filling

8 ounces extra-lean ground beef

1 teaspoon canola or corn oil

1 small eggplant (about 12 ounces), cut into ½-inch cubes

1 large onion, finely chopped

1 14.5-ounce can no-salt-added stewed tomatoes, undrained

1 tablespoon sugar

1½ teaspoons ground cumin

1 teaspoon ground cinnamon

¼ teaspoon ground allspice

2 ounces dried whole-grain elbow macaroni

sauce

3 tablespoons light tub margarine

2 tablespoons all-purpose flour

½ teaspoon salt

1 cup fat-free milk

Preheat the oven to 350°F. Lightly spray an 11 x 7 x 2-inch glass baking dish with cooking spray. Set aside.

In a large nonstick skillet, cook the beef over medium-high heat for 3 to 4 minutes, or until browned on the outside and no longer pink in the center, stirring occasionally to turn and break up the beef. Spoon into a small bowl, discarding any liquid. Set aside.

Reduce the heat to medium. In the same skillet, heat the oil, swirling to coat the bottom. Cook the eggplant and onion for 4 to 5 minutes, or until the onion is soft, stirring frequently.

Stir in the tomatoes with liquid, sugar, cumin, cinnamon, allspice, and beef. Increase the heat to medium high and bring to a simmer. Simmer for 10 minutes, or until the eggplant is tender, stirring occasionally. Remove from the heat. Stir in the pasta.

Meanwhile, in a small saucepan, melt the margarine over medium-high heat, swirling to coat the bottom. Whisk in the flour and remaining ½ teaspoon salt. Gradually whisk in the milk. Cook for 3 to 4 minutes, or until thickened, scraping the bottom of the pan constantly (a heat-resistant rubber scraper works well).

Spread the beef mixture in the baking dish. Spoon the sauce over all.

Bake for 25 minutes, or until bubbly. Remove from the oven. Let stand for 10 minutes before serving so the flavors blend.

PER SERVING

calories 287	cholesterol 32 mg
total fat 8.0 g	sodium 444 mg
saturated fat 1.5 g	carbohydrates 36 g
trans fat 0.0 g	fiber 8 g
polyunsaturated fat 1.5 g	sugars 16 g
monounsaturated fat 4.0 g	protein 19 g

100   200   300   400

DIETARY EXCHANGES
1½ starch, 3 vegetable, 2 lean meat

chicken-fried steak with creamy gravy

serves 4; 3 ounces beef and 2 tablespoons gravy per serving

Whole-grain cracker crumbs provide the crunchy crust you expect with chicken-fried steak, and chicken broth and fat-free half-and-half combine in a wonderful creamy gravy. All this southern classic lacks are the calories, saturated fats, and cholesterol you don't want anyway!

¼ cup all-purpose flour

1 teaspoon salt-free all-purpose seasoning blend

½ cup low-fat buttermilk

¾ cup finely crushed whole-grain crackers (about 30)

4 cube steaks (about 4 ounces each), all visible fat discarded

2 teaspoons olive oil

Cooking spray

¼ cup fat-free, low-sodium chicken broth

¼ cup fat-free half-and-half

¼ teaspoon salt

In a large shallow dish, stir together the flour and seasoning blend. In a small bowl, set aside 2 teaspoons of this mixture. Put the buttermilk and cracker crumbs in two separate large shallow dishes. Set the dishes with the flour mixture, the buttermilk, and the cracker crumbs in a row, assembly-line fashion. Dip the beef in the flour mixture, turning to coat and gently shaking off any excess. Dip in the buttermilk, turning to coat and letting the excess drip off. Dip in the cracker crumbs, turning to coat. Using your fingertips, gently press so the coating adheres to the beef. Transfer the beef to a large plate. Cover and refrigerate for 30 minutes to 4 hours. (This will further help the coating adhere to the beef during cooking.)

In a large nonstick skillet, heat the oil over medium-high heat, swirling to coat the bottom. Cook the beef on one side for 4 to 5 minutes, or until golden brown. Remove the skillet from the heat. Lightly spray the uncooked side of the beef twice with cooking spray. Turn over. Cook for 4 to 5 minutes, or until browned on the outside and no longer pink in the center. Transfer to a platter. Cover to keep warm. Remove the skillet from the heat to cool slightly. (A pan that is too hot at this point will evaporate the gravy liquid.)

In a small bowl, whisk together the broth, half-and-half, salt, and reserved 2 teaspoons flour mixture. Pour into the skillet. Cook over medium heat for 2 to 3 minutes, or until the mixture comes to a simmer and thickens, stirring occasionally. Spoon over the steaks.

COOK'S TIP Cube steaks are usually easy to find, but if you don't spot them in the counter, ask the butcher to tenderize, or "cube," eye-of-round, top round, or bottom round steaks. You can also tenderize your own steaks at home with a meat-tenderizing mallet. Just pound both sides firmly with the mallet without tearing the meat.

···· PER SERVING ··

calories 285
total fat 8.5 g
  saturated fat 2.5 g
  trans fat 0.0 g
  polyunsaturated fat 1.5 g
  monounsaturated fat 4.0 g

cholesterol 58 mg
sodium 344 mg
carbohydrates 22 g
  fiber 2 g
  sugars 3 g
protein 30 g

100 200 300 400

DIETARY EXCHANGES
1½ starch, 3 lean meat

saucy cube steaks

serves 4; 1 cube steak per serving

Pop sweet potatoes in the microwave and steam some broccoli on the stovetop while you prepare this simple skillet dish.

¾ cup water

2 tablespoons dry sherry

2 teaspoons cornstarch

2 teaspoons very low sodium beef bouillon granules

1 teaspoon Worcestershire sauce (lowest sodium available)

½ teaspoon dried oregano, crumbled, and ½ teaspoon dried oregano, crumbled, divided use

¼ teaspoon sugar

⅛ teaspoon garlic powder

4 cube steaks (about 4 ounces each), all visible fat discarded

¼ teaspoon salt

⅛ teaspoon pepper

1 teaspoon canola or corn oil

2 teaspoons light tub margarine

2 tablespoons finely snipped fresh parsley

In a small bowl, whisk together the water, sherry, cornstarch, bouillon granules, Worcestershire sauce, ½ teaspoon oregano, sugar, and garlic powder until the cornstarch is dissolved. Set aside.

Sprinkle the beef with the salt, pepper, and remaining ½ teaspoon oregano. Using your fingertips, gently press so the seasonings adhere to the beef.

In a large nonstick skillet, heat the oil over medium-high heat, swirling to coat the bottom. Cook the beef for 4 to 5 minutes on each side, or until brown on the outside and no longer pink in the center. Transfer to a large plate.

Reduce the heat to medium high. Pour the water mixture into the skillet. Bring to a boil, scraping to dislodge any browned bits. Cook for 1 minute, or until thickened slightly, stirring constantly. Remove from the heat. Stir in the margarine and parsley. Spoon over the beef.

··· **PER SERVING** ··

calories 172

total fat 4.9 g

  saturated fat 1.3 g

  trans fat 0.1 g

  polyunsaturated fat 0.7 g

  monounsaturated fat 2.6 g

cholesterol 57 mg

sodium 197 mg

carbohydrates 3 g

  fiber 0 g

  sugars 1 g

protein 25 g

100   200   300   400

DIETARY EXCHANGES

3 lean meat

cube steaks
with avocado salsa

serves 4; 1 cube steak and 3 tablespoons salsa per serving

Cube steak goes Tex-Mexican when served with an avocado-based salsa that can double as a snack with veggie dippers.

salsa

1	medium Italian plum (Roma) tomato, diced
½	medium avocado, diced
¼	cup chopped red onion
2	tablespoons snipped fresh cilantro
1	tablespoon diced fresh jalapeño, seeds and ribs discarded
1	tablespoon fresh lime juice
1	medium garlic clove, minced
⅛	teaspoon salt

steaks

1	teaspoon smoked paprika
½	teaspoon garlic powder
½	teaspoon pepper
4	cube steaks (about 4 ounces each)
1	teaspoon olive oil

In a small bowl, gently stir together the salsa ingredients. Set aside.

Sprinkle the paprika, garlic powder, and pepper over both sides of the beef. Using your fingertips, gently press so the seasonings adhere to the beef.

In a large nonstick skillet, heat the oil over medium-high heat, swirling to coat the bottom. Cook the beef for 4 to 5 minutes on each side, or until no longer pink in the center. Serve topped with the salsa.

PER SERVING

calories 199
total fat 7.5 g
  saturated fat 2.0 g
  trans fat 0.0 g
  polyunsaturated fat 1.0 g
  monounsaturated fat 4.5 g

cholesterol 58 mg
sodium 146 mg
carbohydrates 6 g
  fiber 2 g
  sugars 1 g
protein 27 g

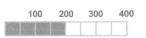

DIETARY EXCHANGES
1 vegetable, 3 lean meat

chopped beef hash

serves 4; 1½ cups per serving

Using frozen hash browns and leftover roast beef, you can serve this one-skillet dinner in just minutes.

1 teaspoon olive oil

1 medium red bell pepper, diced

1 medium green bell pepper, diced

1 medium onion, diced

1 2-ounce jar diced pimientos, drained

3 cups frozen diced hash browns, thawed

2 cups chopped cooked lean roast beef, cooked without salt (about 8 ounces), all visible fat discarded

1 teaspoon dried marjoram, crumbled

1 teaspoon Worcestershire sauce (lowest sodium available)

½ teaspoon dried thyme, crumbled

¼ teaspoon salt

¼ teaspoon pepper

In a large nonstick skillet, heat the oil over medium-high heat, swirling to coat the bottom. Cook the bell peppers, onion, and pimientos for 3 to 4 minutes, or until tender, stirring occasionally.

Stir in the hash browns. Cook for 4 to 5 minutes, or until the potatoes are golden brown and heated through, stirring occasionally.

Stir in the remaining ingredients. Cook for 3 to 4 minutes, or until the mixture is heated through.

PER SERVING

calories 256
total fat 3.0 g
  saturated fat 1.0 g
  trans fat 0.0 g
  polyunsaturated fat 0.5 g
  monounsaturated fat 1.5 g

cholesterol 40 mg
sodium 223 mg
carbohydrates 35 g
  fiber 5 g
  sugars 5 g
  protein 23 g

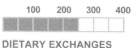

DIETARY EXCHANGES
2 starch, 1 vegetable,
2½ very lean meat

pork tenderloin with cranberry salsa

serves 4; 3 ounces pork and ½ cup salsa per serving

Pineapple, cranberries, and cinnamon combine in a tangy salsa that's great for the winter holidays and refreshing enough for a hot summer's day.

salsa

1 cup chopped fresh pineapple or canned pineapple chunks packed in their own juice, drained

½ cup sweetened dried cranberries

¼ cup finely chopped red onion

1 medium poblano pepper, seeds and ribs discarded, finely chopped

1 teaspoon grated peeled gingerroot

½ teaspoon ground cinnamon

pork

1 1-pound pork tenderloin, all visible fat discarded

¼ teaspoon paprika

¼ teaspoon salt

¼ teaspoon pepper

⅛ teaspoon garlic powder

Preheat the oven to 425°F.

In a medium bowl, gently stir together the salsa ingredients. Set aside.

Place the pork on a baking sheet, tucking the narrow end under so the pork is an even thickness.

In a small bowl, stir together the remaining ingredients. Sprinkle over the pork. Using your fingertips, gently press the mixture so it adheres to the pork.

Bake for 20 to 25 minutes, or until the pork registers 150°F on an instant-read thermometer. Transfer to a cutting board. Let stand for about 5 minutes before slicing. The pork will continue to cook during the standing time, reaching about 160°F. It should be a little pink in the center. Serve with the salsa on the side.

COOK'S TIP For a milder dish or if poblanos are not available, use a medium green bell pepper instead. If you'd still like a little heat, add ⅛ teaspoon crushed red pepper flakes to the salsa.

PER SERVING

calories 206
total fat 2.5 g
  saturated fat 1.0 g
  trans fat 0.0 g
  polyunsaturated fat 0.5 g
  monounsaturated fat 1.0 g

cholesterol 74 mg
sodium 207 mg
carbohydrates 21 g
  fiber 2 g
  sugars 17 g
  protein 24 g

100   200   300   400

DIETARY EXCHANGES
1½ fruit, 3 very lean meat

pork tenderloin with orange-ginger sweet potatoes

serves 6; 3 ounces pork and ¾ cup sweet potato mixture per serving

You've probably eaten applesauce and pork together, but you may not have tried them quite like they're prepared in this dish. The applesauce makes a terrific coating that adds flavor and moistness to the pork. Complete your meal with steamed spinach or Sesame Kale (page 364).

pork

1 teaspoon ground coriander

½ teaspoon ground cumin

½ teaspoon ground cinnamon

½ teaspoon salt

Pepper to taste

1 1-pound pork tenderloin, all visible fat discarded

½ cup unsweetened applesauce

sweet potatoes

2 medium sweet potatoes, pierced in several places with a fork

1 teaspoon olive oil

1 10-ounce can mandarin oranges, canned in juice, well drained

¼ cup snipped fresh parsley

¼ teaspoon ground ginger

Preheat the oven to 450°F.

Line a baking sheet with cooking parchment. On the baking sheet, stir together the coriander, cumin, cinnamon, salt, and pepper.

Tuck the narrow end of the pork under so the pork is an even thickness. Tie with kitchen twine about every 2 inches. Spread the applesauce all over the pork. Sprinkle the coriander mixture all over the pork.

Bake for 20 minutes, or until the pork registers 150°F on an instant-read thermometer. Transfer to a cutting board. Let stand for about 5 minutes before slicing. The pork will continue to cook during the standing time, reaching about 160°F. It should be a little pink in the center.

Meanwhile, put the sweet potatoes on a large microwaveable plate or on the microwave turntable. Microwave on 100 percent power (high) for 3 to 4 minutes, or until tender enough to be pierced easily with a fork. Peel the potatoes and cut into large chunks, about 2 inches.

In a large skillet, heat the oil over medium-high heat, swirling to coat the bottom. Cook the sweet potatoes, mandarin oranges, parsley, and ginger for 3 to 5 minutes, or until the sweet potatoes are soft and the mixture is well blended, stirring frequently. Serve with the pork.

···· **PER SERVING** ···

calories 159
total fat 2.5 g
  saturated fat 0.5 g
  trans fat 0.0 g
  polyunsaturated fat 0.5 g
  monounsaturated fat 1.0 g

cholesterol 49 mg
sodium 269 mg
carbohydrates 17 g
  fiber 3 g
  sugars 8 g
protein 17 g

100   200   300   400

DIETARY EXCHANGES
½ starch, ½ fruit,
2½ very lean meat

thai coconut curry with pork and vegetables

serves 4; 1½ cups per serving

Tempt your palate with the exciting flavors of Thai cuisine, including light coconut milk, lemongrass, and red curry paste. Serve this dish with chilled slices of cantaloupe and honeydew melon.

Cooking spray

4 boneless center-cut pork chops (about 4 ounces each), all visible fat discarded, cut into ½-inch cubes

1 cup baby carrots

½ medium onion, cut into 1-inch pieces

1 stalk lemongrass or 1 teaspoon grated lemon zest

1½ cups fat-free, low-sodium chicken broth

1 teaspoon Thai red curry paste

1 cup uncooked instant brown rice

4 medium green onions, chopped

2 tablespoons cornstarch

½ cup light coconut milk

4 ounces broccoli florets

Lightly spray a large skillet with cooking spray. Cook the pork over medium-high heat for 3 to 4 minutes, or until browned, stirring occasionally.

Stir in the carrots and onion. Cook for 3 to 4 minutes, or until the carrots are tender-crisp and the onion is soft, stirring frequently.

Meanwhile, trim and discard about 6 inches from the slender tip of the lemongrass stalk. Remove the outer layer of leaves from the bottom part of the stalk. Cut the stalk in half lengthwise.

Stir the lemongrass, broth, and red curry paste into the pork mixture. Bring to a simmer. Reduce the heat and simmer, covered, for 15 to 20 minutes, or until the pork is a little pink in the center and the carrots are tender, stirring occasionally.

Meanwhile, prepare the rice using the package directions, omitting the salt and margarine and adding the green onions. Cover to keep warm.

Put the cornstarch in a small bowl. Add the coconut milk, whisking until smooth. Stir into the pork mixture. Stir in the broccoli. Increase the heat to medium high and return to a simmer. Reduce the heat and simmer, covered, for 3 to 4 minutes, or until the mixture is thickened and the broccoli is tender, stirring occasionally. Discard the lemongrass. Serve the pork mixture over the rice.

····· **PER SERVING** ·····

calories 320
total fat 9.0 g
  saturated fat 3.5 g
  trans fat 0.0 g
  polyunsaturated fat 1.0 g
  monounsaturated fat 3.5 g

cholesterol 67 mg
sodium 137 mg
carbohydrates 30 g
  fiber 4 g
  sugars 5 g
protein 27 g

100   200   300   400

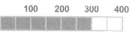

DIETARY EXCHANGES
1½ starch, 2 vegetable,
3 lean meat

pork chops parmesan

serves 4; 1 pork chop per serving

A coating of soft whole-grain bread crumbs and chopped fresh herbs adds flavor to these baked pork chops.

Cooking spray

2 tablespoons all-purpose flour

¼ cup egg substitute

2 slices whole-grain bread (lowest sodium available)

¼ cup snipped fresh parsley or 1 tablespoon dried, crumbled

¼ cup shredded or grated Parmesan cheese

10 medium to large fresh basil leaves or 1 teaspoon dried, crumbled

2 teaspoons fresh thyme or ½ teaspoon dried, crumbled

2 teaspoons fresh oregano or ½ teaspoon dried, crumbled

1 teaspoon garlic powder

1 teaspoon olive oil

¼ teaspoon pepper

4 boneless center-cut pork chops (about 4 ounces each), all visible fat discarded

Preheat the oven to 375°F. Lightly spray an 8-inch square baking pan with cooking spray. Set aside.

Put the flour and egg substitute in separate medium shallow dishes.

In a food processor or blender, process the remaining ingredients except the pork chops until the bread is chopped into crumbs and the herbs are coarsely chopped. Transfer the mixture to a third medium shallow dish. Set the dishes and the baking pan in a row, assembly-line fashion.

Dip one pork chop in the flour, turning to coat and gently shaking off any excess. Dip in the egg substitute, turning to coat and letting the excess drip off. Dip in the bread crumb mixture, turning to coat and gently shaking off any excess. Using your fingertips, gently press the coating so it adheres to the pork chops. Transfer to the baking pan. Repeat with the remaining pork chops.

Bake for 45 minutes, or until the pork chops are a little pink in the center.

···· PER SERVING ···

calories 237	cholesterol 82 mg	
total fat 7.5 g	sodium 251 mg	100 200 300 400
saturated fat 2.5 g	carbohydrates 10 g	
trans fat 0.0 g	fiber 1 g	DIETARY EXCHANGES
polyunsaturated fat 0.5 g	sugars 1 g	½ starch, 3½ lean meat
monounsaturated fat 3.0 g	protein 31 g	

ham and broccoli with rotini

serves 4; 1½ cups per serving

This really quick and easy one-dish meal is like mac and cheese, only better. The "mac" is whole-grain pasta, the cheese is low-fat, the corn provides more whole grain, and the broccoli and red bell pepper add veggies.

4 quarts water

6 ounces dried whole-grain rotini

3 ounces small broccoli florets

1 large red bell pepper, cut lengthwise into thin strips

1 cup frozen whole-kernel corn, thawed

4 ¾-ounce slices low-fat American cheese, quartered

3 ounces lower-sodium, low-fat ham, all visible fat discarded, thinly sliced and chopped

2 tablespoons fat-free milk

¼ to ½ teaspoon dried thyme, crumbled

⅛ teaspoon cayenne

In a stockpot, bring the water to a boil over high heat. Boil the pasta for 7 minutes.

Stir in the broccoli and bell pepper. Cook for 2 to 3 minutes, or until the broccoli is tender-crisp. Drain well in a colander. Return to the pot.

Stir in the remaining ingredients until the cheese is melted.

PER SERVING

calories 270	cholesterol 17 mg
total fat 4.0 g	sodium 493 mg
saturated fat 1.5 g	carbohydrates 45 g
trans fat 0.0 g	fiber 7 g
polyunsaturated fat 0.5 g	sugars 5 g
monounsaturated fat 1.5 g	protein 17 g

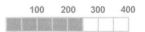

100   200   300   400

DIETARY EXCHANGES
2½ starch, 1 vegetable, 1 very lean meat

sausage and white beans with spinach

serves 4; 1½ cups per serving

The flavors of sausage and basil explode in this warm comfort dish—Mediterranean style. The beans are a good source of fiber, which helps give you that full feeling at the end of a meal.

Cooking spray

6 ounces low-fat bulk ground sausage

1 tablespoon dried basil, crumbled

2 medium garlic cloves, minced

1 15.5-ounce can no-salt-added navy or cannellini beans, rinsed and drained

¼ cup water and 1¾ cups water, divided use

1½ cups uncooked quick-cooking brown rice

2 ounces spinach, coarsely chopped

¼ teaspoon salt

Lightly spray a large skillet with cooking spray. Cook the sausage over medium-high heat for 3 to 4 minutes, or until no longer pink in the center, stirring constantly and breaking up any large pieces.

Stir in the basil and garlic. Cook for 15 seconds, stirring constantly.

Stir in the beans and ¼ cup water. Bring to a boil. Remove from the heat. Cover and set aside.

Meanwhile, in a medium saucepan, bring the remaining 1¾ cups water to a boil. Stir in the rice. Cook using the package directions, omitting the salt and margarine. Stir the rice into the bean mixture. Gently stir in the spinach and salt.

COOK'S TIP The heat of the other ingredients gently warms and wilts the spinach without leaching out its brilliant color and rich vitamins.

PER SERVING

calories 286
total fat 2.5 g
  saturated fat 0.5 g
  trans fat 0.0 g
  polyunsaturated fat 0.5 g
  monounsaturated fat 0.5 g

cholesterol 21 mg
sodium 419 mg
carbohydrates 45 g
  fiber 6 g
  sugars 4 g
protein 16 g

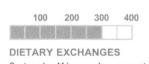

DIETARY EXCHANGES
3 starch, 1½ very lean meat

vegetarian entrées

Fresh Veggie Marinara with Feta

Italian Veggie Burgers

Pesto Florentine Pasta

Pasta e Fagioli Stew

Stuffed Shells with Arugula and Four Cheeses

Make-Ahead Manicotti

Soba Noodles in Peanut Sauce

Lentils with Basil and Feta

Spinach and Bean Quesadillas with Homemade Salsa

Slow-Cooker Black Bean Chili

Braised Edamame with Bok Choy

Mediterranean Wraps

Miami Pita Sandwiches

Mediterranean Vegetable Stew

Broccoli Bake with Three Cheeses

Spinach and Ricotta Frittata

One-Pot Vegetable and Grain Medley

Cajun Red Beans and Brown Rice

Fried Rice with Snow Peas, Bell Pepper,
and Water Chestnuts

Almond-Topped Bok Choy, Sugar Snap Pea,
and Tofu Stir-Fry

Speed-Dial Stuffed Peppers

Creole Ratatouille

Vegetable and Bulgur Curry

fresh veggie marinara with feta

serves 4; 1 cup vegetable mixture and ½ cup pasta per serving

Here's a great opportunity to experience the joys of soy.

- 6 ounces dried whole-grain penne
- 1 teaspoon canola or corn oil
- 1 large zucchini, chopped
- 1 large green bell pepper, chopped
- 1 medium onion, chopped
- 1 tablespoon dried basil, crumbled
- 2 medium garlic cloves, minced
- ⅛ teaspoon crushed red pepper flakes
- ½ medium eggplant (about 8 ounces), diced, or 8 ounces button mushrooms, sliced
- 1½ cups spaghetti sauce (lowest sodium available)
- 6 ounces frozen soy crumbles
- 2 ounces fat-free tomato and basil feta cheese, crumbled

Prepare the pasta using the package directions, omitting the salt. Drain well in a colander.

Meanwhile, in a Dutch oven, heat the oil over medium-high heat, swirling to coat the bottom. Cook the zucchini, bell pepper, onion, basil, garlic, and red pepper flakes for 4 minutes, or until the onion is soft, stirring frequently.

Stir in the eggplant. Reduce the heat to medium low. Cook, covered, for 4 minutes, or until the eggplant is soft, stirring occasionally.

Stir in the spaghetti sauce. Cook, covered, for 5 minutes.

Stir in the soy crumbles. Cook, covered, for 2 minutes, or until heated through. Serve over the pasta. Sprinkle with the feta.

COOK'S TIP Frozen soy crumbles are precooked. You should heat them, not cook them, so they retain their "ground beef" texture and don't begin to break apart.

····· **PER SERVING** ···

calories 373
total fat 8.0 g
  saturated fat 2.5 g
  trans fat 0.0 g
  polyunsaturated fat 1.5 g
  monounsaturated fat 1.5 g

cholesterol 10 mg
sodium 596 mg
carbohydrates 57 g
  fiber 14 g
  sugars 16 g
  protein 21 g

100   200   300   400

DIETARY EXCHANGES
2½ starch, 4 vegetable,
1½ lean meat

italian veggie burgers

Give classic cheeseburgers a healthy makeover with veggie patties topped with mozzarella and hot cooked vegetables.

- 4 frozen low-fat vegetarian burgers, such as grilled soy protein burgers
- 1 large zucchini, thinly sliced crosswise
- 1 medium onion, thinly sliced crosswise
- 1 medium green bell pepper, cut lengthwise into thin strips
- 1 tablespoon chopped fresh basil or 1 teaspoon dried, crumbled
- ⅛ teaspoon crushed red pepper flakes
  Cooking spray
- ⅛ teaspoon salt
- 2 ounces shredded low-fat mozzarella cheese

Cook the burgers using the package directions for the stovetop. Transfer to a platter. Do not cover.

Add the zucchini, onion, bell pepper, basil, and red pepper flakes to the pan. Lightly spray with cooking spray. Increase the heat to medium high and cook for 5 minutes, or until the edges of the onion begin to lightly brown, stirring frequently. Remove from the heat. Stir in the salt.

Sprinkle the burgers with the mozzarella. Top with the zucchini mixture.

COOK'S TIP Covering the cooked burgers to keep them warm might change the texture of the product. The heat from the cooked vegetables will reheat the patties while melting the cheese.

PER SERVING

calories 177	cholesterol 6 mg
total fat 5.5 g	sodium 447 mg
saturated fat 1.0 g	carbohydrates 18 g
trans fat 0.0 g	fiber 4 g
polyunsaturated fat 1.5 g	sugars 6 g
monounsaturated fat 2.5 g	protein 16 g

100 200 300 400

DIETARY EXCHANGES
½ starch, 2 vegetable,
2 lean meat

pesto florentine pasta

serves 6; 1 cup per serving

Fresh baby spinach sneaks a nutrition boost into traditional pesto in this quick-to-prepare entrée.

12 ounces dried whole-grain linguine or other flat pasta

pesto

3 cups baby spinach

3 tablespoons shredded or grated Parmesan cheese

2 tablespoons chopped fresh basil

1 tablespoon plus 1 teaspoon fresh lemon juice

1 large garlic clove

½ teaspoon salt

¼ teaspoon pepper

1½ tablespoons olive oil (extra-virgin preferred)

Prepare the pasta using the package directions, omitting the salt. Drain well in a colander. Transfer to a large serving bowl.

Meanwhile, in a food processor or blender, process the pesto ingredients except the oil for 25 seconds, or until smooth. With the processor running, slowly pour the oil through the food tube. Process for 10 seconds, or until blended. Stir into the pasta to coat completely.

COOK'S TIP You can easily double the amount of pesto you make from this recipe. The extra pesto is a wonderful topping for chicken, fish, and roasted vegetables.

PER SERVING

calories 250
total fat 5.5 g
  saturated fat 1.0 g
  trans fat 0.0 g
  polyunsaturated fat 1.0 g
  monounsaturated fat 3.0 g

cholesterol 2 mg
sodium 256 mg
carbohydrates 43 g
  fiber 7 g
  sugars 2 g
  protein 8 g

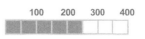

DIETARY EXCHANGES
3 starch, 1 fat

pasta e fagioli stew

serves 5; 1½ cups per serving

There are at least as many variations of pasta e fagioli (*fah-JYOH-lee*)—pasta and beans—as there are types of pasta. Unlike traditional recipes for pasta e fagioli, which are for soup, this hearty version is more stewlike, making it an ideal vegetarian meal.

1 teaspoon olive oil

2 cups chopped sweet onion, such as Vidalia, Maui, or Oso Sweet

3 medium garlic cloves, minced

2 15.5-ounce cans no-salt-added cannellini or white kidney beans, rinsed and drained

1 28-ounce can no-salt-added diced tomatoes, undrained

2 cups low-sodium vegetable broth

1 tablespoon dried oregano, crumbled

1 teaspoon dried basil, crumbled

½ teaspoon dried thyme, crumbled

⅛ teaspoon salt

1 cup dried whole-grain elbow macaroni

2 cups coarsely chopped Swiss chard leaves or spinach

2 tablespoons Worcestershire sauce (lowest sodium available)

¼ cup shredded or grated Parmesan cheese

In a large, heavy saucepan or Dutch oven, heat the oil over medium-high heat, swirling to coat the bottom. Cook the onion for about 3 minutes, or until soft, stirring frequently.

Stir in the garlic. Cook for 30 seconds, stirring frequently.

Stir in the beans, tomatoes with liquid, broth, oregano, basil, thyme, and salt. Increase the heat to high and bring to a boil, stirring occasionally.

Stir in the pasta. Reduce the heat and simmer for 10 minutes, or until the pasta is tender, stirring frequently. Stir in the Swiss chard and Worcestershire sauce. (The chard will wilt quickly from the heat.) Serve sprinkled with the Parmesan.

COOK'S TIP ON SWISS CHARD Related to the beet family, Swiss chard is colorful, delicious, and packed with nutrients. The leaves are green, and the stalks can be yellow, red, or white. You can use younger, smaller leaves in salads, but chop and cook larger leaves and stalks. If Swiss chard is not available, you can substitute spinach in many recipes, including this one.

····· **PER SERVING** ··

calories 312	cholesterol 3 mg	
total fat 4.0 g	sodium 250 mg	100 200 300 400
saturated fat 1.0 g	carbohydrates 55 g	
trans fat 0.0 g	fiber 12 g	**DIETARY EXCHANGES**
polyunsaturated fat 1.5 g	sugars 10 g	2½ starch, 3 vegetable,
monounsaturated fat 1.0 g	protein 15 g	1 very lean meat

stuffed shells with arugula and four cheeses

serves 12; 3 shells per serving

Even classic Italian dishes with lots of cheese, such as these stuffed shells, can be part of a healthful diet. Using fat-free and low-fat cheese keeps the calories—and the saturated fat—in line. These delicious shells are excellent for a big gathering, or use part for dinner and freeze individual portions for quick meals at a later time.

16 ounces dried jumbo pasta shells (about 36)

sauce

1 tablespoon olive oil

2 large garlic cloves, minced

¼ cup chopped fresh basil

2 tablespoons chopped fresh marjoram

3 pints cherry tomatoes, halved (about 6 cups)

½ teaspoon pepper

⅛ teaspoon salt

2 tablespoons snipped fresh Italian (flat-leaf) parsley

filling

16 ounces fat-free cottage cheese

15 ounces fat-free ricotta cheese

2 cups shredded low-fat mozzarella cheese

¼ cup shredded or grated Parmesan cheese

¼ teaspoon salt

¼ teaspoon pepper

4 ounces arugula, chopped

½ cup chopped dry-packed sun-dried tomatoes

2 tablespoons snipped fresh Italian (flat-leaf) parsley

Prepare the pasta using the package directions, omitting the salt and boiling for 10 minutes. Do not overcook the shells; they should remain very firm so they hold up during baking. Drain well in a colander. Arrange with the smooth side up on a dish towel to cool.

Preheat the oven to 375°F.

In a large skillet, heat the oil over high heat, swirling to coat the bottom. Cook the garlic for 1 to 2 minutes, or until fragrant, stirring frequently.

Stir in the basil and marjoram. Cook for 1 minute, stirring frequently.

Stir in the cherry tomatoes, ½ teaspoon pepper, and ⅛ teaspoon salt. Reduce the heat and simmer for 10 minutes. Stir in 2 tablespoons parsley.

Meanwhile, in a food processor or blender, process the cottage cheese and ricotta until smooth. Transfer to a large bowl. Stir in the mozzarella, Parmesan, remaining ¼ teaspoon salt, and remaining ¼ teaspoon pepper. Stir in the arugula and sun-dried tomatoes. Gently fill the shells with the mixture.

Ladle enough sauce into a 13 x 9 x 2-inch casserole dish to cover the bottom (1½ to 2 cups). Place the shells with the seam side down on the sauce. Ladle the remaining sauce over the shells.

Bake, covered, for 30 minutes. Sprinkle with the remaining 2 tablespoons parsley.

····· PER SERVING ····································

calories 280
total fat 4.5 g
  saturated fat 1.5 g
  trans fat 0.0 g
  polyunsaturated fat 0.5 g
  monounsaturated fat 2.0 g

cholesterol 12 mg
sodium 453 mg
carbohydrates 40 g
  fiber 3 g
  sugars 8 g
protein 20 g

100   200   300   400

DIETARY EXCHANGES
2 starch, 2 vegetable,
2 very lean meat

make-ahead manicotti

serves 7; 2 shells per serving

This dish is a "convenience food" because you don't precook the pasta. Best of all, you can assemble the casserole the night before you need it, then just sprinkle with cheese and bake while you prepare a salad to complete the meal.

Cooking spray

sauce

2 8-ounce cans no-salt-added tomato sauce

1 14.5-ounce can no-salt-added stewed tomatoes, undrained

1 cup spaghetti sauce (tomato-basil preferred) (lowest sodium available)

1 cup water

filling

15 ounces fat-free ricotta cheese

10 ounces frozen chopped spinach, thawed and squeezed dry

2 large egg whites

¼ cup shredded or grated Romano cheese

2 tablespoons chopped fresh basil

1 tablespoon sugar

2 medium garlic cloves, minced

⅛ teaspoon pepper

14 dried manicotti shells

2 tablespoons shredded or grated Romano cheese

Lightly spray a 13 x 9 x 2-inch baking pan with cooking spray. Set aside.

In a medium bowl, stir together the sauce ingredients, breaking up the large tomato pieces with a spoon.

In a large bowl, stir together the filling ingredients. Stuff the uncooked pasta shells with the mixture.

Spread 1 cup sauce in the baking pan. Arrange the shells in a single layer on the sauce. Pour the remaining sauce on top. Cover and refrigerate for 8 to 24 hours. (The refrigeration time is needed so the uncooked shells will soften when they are baked.)

About 30 minutes before baking, remove the casserole from the refrigerator. Sprinkle with the remaining 2 tablespoons Romano.

Preheat the oven to 350°F.

Bake, uncovered, for 40 to 45 minutes, or until heated through.

COOK'S TIP ON STUFFING MANICOTTI You can use a small spoon, iced tea spoon, or butter knife to stuff manicotti. Another technique is to use a pastry bag. If you don't have one, you can easily turn a resealable plastic bag into a disposable pastry bag. Spoon the ricotta mixture into the bag, pushing the mixture toward a bottom corner. Twist the bag closed, pushing out any air. Using scissors, make a diagonal cut in the corner of the bag about ¾ inch from the bottom. Squeeze the filling through the hole into the shells.

···· **PER SERVING** ···

calories 284	cholesterol 10 mg	
total fat 2.5 g	sodium 379 mg	100 200 300 400
saturated fat 1.0 g	carbohydrates 45 g	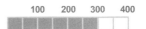
trans fat 0.0 g	fiber 5 g	**DIETARY EXCHANGES**
polyunsaturated fat 0.5 g	sugars 14 g	2 starch, 3 vegetable,
monounsaturated fat 0.5 g	protein 19 g	1½ very lean meat

soba noodles
in peanut sauce

serves 4; 1½ cups per serving

A dead ringer for the noodles in peanut sauce that you'll find on the menus of many Asian restaurants, this version is a much better fit in a healthy diet.

10   ounces soba (buckwheat) or whole-grain noodles

sauce

¼   cup plus 2 tablespoons hot water

2½   tablespoons plain rice vinegar

2   tablespoons soy sauce (lowest sodium available) or teriyaki sauce (lowest sodium available)

2   tablespoons creamy peanut butter

1   tablespoon honey

2   teaspoons minced peeled gingerroot

2   medium garlic cloves, minced

¼   teaspoon pepper

¼   teaspoon crushed red pepper flakes

2   small ribs of celery, chopped

½   large green bell pepper, chopped

½   medium carrot, grated

4   medium green onions, thinly sliced

1½   teaspoons toasted sesame oil

2   tablespoons sesame seeds

Prepare the noodles using the package directions, omitting the salt. Drain well in a colander. Return the noodles to the pot.

Meanwhile, in a medium bowl, whisk together the sauce ingredients.

Stir the remaining ingredients except the sesame seeds into the noodles. Stir in the sauce. Stir in the sesame seeds.

PER SERVING

calories 373	cholesterol 0 mg
total fat 9.0 g	sodium 345 mg
saturated fat 1.5 g	carbohydrates 65 g
trans fat 0.0 g	fiber 6 g
polyunsaturated fat 3.0 g	sugars 12 g
monounsaturated fat 4.0 g	protein 14 g

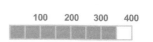

100   200   300   400

DIETARY EXCHANGES
4 starch, 1 vegetable, 1 fat

lentils with basil and feta

serves 4; 1¼ cups per serving

Lentils simmered with green and orange vegetables top whole-grain penne, then get a hefty sprinkling of feta. The result is a hearty, fiber-filled one-dish meal.

  4 ounces dried whole-grain penne
  1 teaspoon olive oil
  1 medium green bell pepper, diced
  1 medium carrot, thinly sliced crosswise
  1 medium zucchini, diced
1¼ cups water
  1 cup grape tomatoes, quartered
  ½ cup dried lentils, sorted for stones and shriveled lentils and rinsed
1½ tablespoons dried basil, crumbled
  ½ teaspoon salt
  2 ounces fat-free feta cheese, crumbled

Prepare the pasta using the package directions, omitting the salt. Drain well in a colander. Set aside.

Meanwhile, in a large nonstick skillet, heat the oil over medium-high heat, swirling to coat the bottom. Cook the bell pepper, carrot, and zucchini for 5 minutes, or until tender, stirring frequently.

Stir in the water, tomatoes, lentils, and basil. Bring to a simmer. Reduce the heat and simmer, covered, for about 25 minutes, or until the lentils are very tender, stirring occasionally. Stir in the salt. Serve over the pasta. Sprinkle with the feta.

COOK'S TIP The lentil mixture is also very good when served over 2 cups of cooked bulgur instead of pasta.

···· PER SERVING ·······

calories 251
total fat 2.5 g
  saturated fat 0.0 g
  trans fat 0.0 g
  polyunsaturated fat 0.5 g
  monounsaturated fat 1.0 g

cholesterol 0 mg
sodium 537 mg
carbohydrates 46 g
  fiber 9 g
  sugars 8 g
  protein 15 g

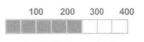

DIETARY EXCHANGES
2½ starch, 2 vegetable,
1 very lean meat

spinach and bean quesadillas with homemade salsa

serves 4; 2 quesadilla halves and 2 tablespoons salsa per serving (plus 1 cup salsa reserved)

A healthy alternative to most restaurant varieties, these quesadillas get pizzazz from the cilantro-flavored salsa. As a bonus, you'll have leftover salsa—perfect to use later in the week as a snack with raw vegetables or baked tortilla chips (just watch the sodium).

salsa

3 medium garlic cloves
½ cup snipped fresh cilantro
1 14.5-ounce can no-salt-added stewed tomatoes, undrained
2 to 3 teaspoons fresh lime juice
¼ teaspoon dried ground chipotle pepper (optional)
⅛ teaspoon salt

quesadillas

1 15.5-ounce can no-salt-added pinto beans, rinsed and drained
1 teaspoon salt-free onion-and-herb seasoning blend
2 tablespoons snipped fresh cilantro
4 medium garlic cloves, minced
⅛ teaspoon salt
4 8-inch fat-free flour tortillas (lowest sodium available)
10 ounces frozen leaf spinach, thawed and squeezed dry
1 medium red bell pepper, chopped
1½ ounces crumbled soft goat cheese
½ cup fat-free sour cream (optional)

Turn on a food processor or blender. With the motor running, drop in 3 garlic cloves. Process for 5 seconds, or until finely minced. Add ½ cup cilantro and pulse until finely chopped. Add the remaining salsa ingredients. Pulse several times, until the tomatoes are the desired size. Pour the salsa into a small bowl. Set aside.

In the food processor or blender (no need to clean it first), process the beans for 15 to 20 seconds, or until almost smooth. Transfer to a separate small bowl. Stir in the seasoning blend and remaining 2 tablespoons cilantro, 4 garlic cloves, and ⅛ teaspoon salt.

Place the tortillas on a flat work surface. Spread the bean mixture on half of each tortilla. Top the bean mixture with the spinach, bell pepper, and goat cheese. Fold the tortillas over to enclose the filling.

Heat a large nonstick skillet over medium-high heat. Cook 2 quesadillas, covered, for 2 minutes on each side, or until golden brown and heated through. Repeat with the remaining quesadillas. Cut each quesadilla in half. Top each half with 1 tablespoon salsa and 1 tablespoon sour cream. Cover and refrigerate the remaining salsa for another use within three days.

COOK'S TIP ON BEANS Beans are an excellent source of fiber, with about 6 grams of fiber per ½ cup serving. Look for canned beans with no added salt because regular canned beans are typically extremely high in sodium.

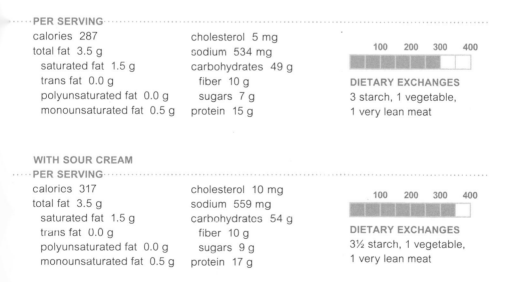

PER SERVING

calories 287	cholesterol 5 mg	100 200 300 400
total fat 3.5 g	sodium 534 mg	
saturated fat 1.5 g	carbohydrates 49 g	
trans fat 0.0 g	fiber 10 g	**DIETARY EXCHANGES**
polyunsaturated fat 0.0 g	sugars 7 g	3 starch, 1 vegetable,
monounsaturated fat 0.5 g	protein 15 g	1 very lean meat

WITH SOUR CREAM
PER SERVING

calories 317	cholesterol 10 mg	100 200 300 400
total fat 3.5 g	sodium 559 mg	
saturated fat 1.5 g	carbohydrates 54 g	
trans fat 0.0 g	fiber 10 g	**DIETARY EXCHANGES**
polyunsaturated fat 0.0 g	sugars 9 g	3½ starch, 1 vegetable,
monounsaturated fat 0.5 g	protein 17 g	1 very lean meat

slow-cooker black bean chili

serves 4; 1 cup chili and ½ cup pasta per serving

This satisfying chili-and-pasta dish should keep you full for hours. You certainly won't miss the meat or the extra calories. Make extra and freeze it (see the Cook's Tip) to use when you don't have time to cook or to take to work for lunch so you won't be tempted to grab fast food.

- 1 teaspoon olive oil
- 1 medium onion, chopped
- 1 15.5-ounce can no-salt-added black beans, rinsed and drained
- 1 14.5-ounce can no-salt-added stewed tomatoes, undrained
- 1 cup frozen whole-kernel corn, thawed
- 1 4-ounce can green chiles, undrained
- ½ cup water
- 2 tablespoons chili powder
- 1 teaspoon ground cumin
- ½ teaspoon salt
- 4 ounces dried whole-grain rotini
- ½ cup fat-free sour cream
- ½ cup shredded fat-free Cheddar cheese
- ¼ cup snipped fresh cilantro

In a medium nonstick skillet, heat the oil over medium-high heat, swirling to coat the bottom. Cook the onion for about 2 minutes, or until tender-crisp, stirring frequently.

Put the onion, beans, tomatoes with liquid, corn, green chiles with liquid, water, chili powder, cumin, and salt in a 3½- or 4-quart slow cooker, stirring to combine. Cook, covered, on high for 3 hours or on low for 6 hours, or until the onion is very soft.

About 15 minutes before serving time, prepare the pasta using the package directions, omitting the salt. Drain well in a colander.

Serve the chili over the pasta. Top with the sour cream. Sprinkle with the Cheddar and cilantro.

COOK'S TIP If you want enough chili for another meal, double the chili part of this recipe. (You don't need to increase the cooking time.) Refrigerate the extra cooked chili until it is thoroughly chilled, then freeze it in an airtight freezer container. The chili will keep for up to one month in the freezer. Let it thaw in the refrigerator for about 24 hours. While you heat the chili, prepare some pasta and get the toppings ready.

··· PER SERVING ·····

calories 356
total fat 3.0 g
  saturated fat 0.5 g
  trans fat 0.0 g
  polyunsaturated fat 1.0 g
  monounsaturated fat 1.5 g

cholesterol 8 mg
sodium 617 mg
carbohydrates 65 g
  fiber 13 g
  sugars 15 g
  protein 19 g

100 200 300 400

DIETARY EXCHANGES
3½ starch, 2 vegetable,
1 very lean meat

braised edamame with bok choy

serves 4; 1½ cups per serving

Convenient frozen shelled edamame cooks so quickly that you'll make this interesting Asian-style dish in no time. It is braised in toasted sesame oil and hoisin sauce and served over fluffy brown rice.

1   cup uncooked instant brown rice

1   teaspoon canola or corn oil

1   medium red bell pepper, diced

1   medium onion, diced

2   cups frozen shelled edamame (green soybeans)

1   cup low-sodium vegetable broth

½   cup canned baby corn, rinsed and drained

3   tablespoons hoisin sauce

1   tablespoon light brown sugar

1   tablespoon plain rice vinegar

1   teaspoon toasted sesame oil

2   large stalks of bok choy (green and white parts), cut crosswise into ½-inch pieces (about 2 cups)

Prepare the rice using the package directions, omitting the salt. Cover to keep warm.

Meanwhile, in a large saucepan, heat the oil over medium-high heat, swirling to coat the bottom. Cook the bell pepper and onion for about 3 minutes, or until tender, stirring frequently.

Stir in the remaining ingredients except the bok choy. Bring to a simmer. Reduce the heat and simmer, covered, for 6 to 8 minutes, or until the edamame is tender.

Stir in the bok choy. Simmer, covered, for 2 to 3 minutes, or until the bok choy is tender-crisp, stirring occasionally. Spoon over the rice.

PER SERVING

calories 288	cholesterol 0 mg
total fat 8.0 g	sodium 167 mg
saturated fat 1.5 g	carbohydrates 39 g
trans fat 0.0 g	fiber 9 g
polyunsaturated fat 3.5 g	sugars 11 g
monounsaturated fat 2.5 g	protein 14 g

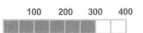

DIETARY EXCHANGES
2 starch, 2 vegetable,
1 very lean meat, 1 fat

mediterranean wraps

serves 4; 1 wrap per serving

With its many layers of color, this wrap is almost too pretty to eat.

1 cup canned no-salt-added chickpeas, rinsed and drained

1 medium cucumber, peeled, seeded, and chopped

1 small tomato, chopped

¼ cup snipped fresh parsley

¼ cup chopped red onion

2 tablespoons unsweetened dried cranberries

2 tablespoons crumbled soft goat cheese

2 tablespoons fresh lemon juice

1 tablespoon capers, drained

Dash of pepper

4 10-inch fat-free flour tortillas (lowest sodium available)

4 cups spinach

2 cups shredded carrots

In a medium bowl, stir together the chickpeas, cucumber, tomato, parsley, onion, cranberries, goat cheese, lemon juice, capers, and pepper. Set aside.

In a large skillet, lightly heat 1 tortilla on medium-high heat for about 30 seconds on each side to make the tortilla easier to wrap. Transfer to a medium plate.

Place 1 cup spinach on the tortilla, leaving a 1-inch border. Spread ½ cup carrots over the spinach. Top with ½ cup chickpea mixture. Roll up about 1 inch from the bottom of the tortilla. Fold over 1 inch from both sides. Starting back at the bottom, roll up the tortilla jelly-roll style, pushing in any filling before reaching the top. Turn over. Place a toothpick about one-third from each end, securing the loose end. Cut the wrap in half. Repeat with the remaining ingredients.

PER SERVING

calories 311	cholesterol 3 mg
total fat 3.0 g	sodium 643 mg
saturated fat 1.0 g	carbohydrates 60 g
trans fat 0.0 g	fiber 9 g
polyunsaturated fat 0.5 g	sugars 10 g
monounsaturated fat 0.5 g	protein 13 g

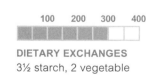

100 200 300 400

DIETARY EXCHANGES
3½ starch, 2 vegetable

miami pita sandwiches

serves 4; 1 sandwich per serving

These Miami-influenced sandwiches include some traditional Cuban ingredients, such as black beans and papaya. They provide good-for-you food that has interesting taste and texture without a lot of calories.

2 cups frozen whole-kernel corn, thawed

1 cup canned no-salt-added black beans, rinsed and drained

½ cup seeded and diced papaya, honeydew melon, Crenshaw melon, or cantaloupe

½ cup snipped fresh cilantro

1 small red onion, or to taste, cut into rings

¼ medium red bell pepper, diced

1 tablespoon fresh lime juice

1 tablespoon balsamic vinegar

⅛ teaspoon cayenne

⅛ teaspoon salt

Dash of pepper

4 cups chopped romaine

4 6-inch whole-grain pita pockets, halved

In a medium bowl, stir together the corn, beans, papaya, cilantro, onion, bell pepper, lime juice, vinegar, cayenne, salt, and pepper.

Spoon ½ cup romaine and ¼ cup corn mixture into each pita half.

PER SERVING

calories 326
total fat 2.5 g
  saturated fat 0.5 g
  trans fat 0.0 g
  polyunsaturated fat 1.0 g
  monounsaturated fat 0.5 g

cholesterol 0 mg
sodium 403 mg
carbohydrates 69 g
  fiber 11 g
  sugars 12 g
  protein 13 g

100   200   300   400

DIETARY EXCHANGES
4 starch, ½ fruit,
½ very lean meat

mediterranean vegetable stew

serves 6; 1⅔ cups per serving

Eggplant, zucchini, and chickpeas team up for a hearty vegetarian stew with Mediterranean overtones.

1 medium eggplant, cut into bite-size cubes
½ teaspoon salt and ½ teaspoon salt, divided use
1½ tablespoons olive oil
3 medium garlic cloves, minced
2 teaspoons dried Italian seasoning, crumbled
1 28-ounce can no-salt-added diced tomatoes, undrained
2 10-ounce cans no-salt-added chickpeas, rinsed and drained
1 medium to large zucchini, thinly sliced crosswise
3 medium dried bay leaves
 Pepper to taste

Put the eggplant in a medium bowl. Sprinkle with ½ teaspoon salt. (This will help keep the eggplant from absorbing too much oil.) After about 10 minutes, pat the eggplant dry with paper towels.

In a large skillet, heat the oil over medium-high heat, swirling to coat the bottom. Cook the eggplant and garlic for 3 to 5 minutes, or until they begin to soften, stirring occasionally. Push to the side.

Put the Italian seasoning in the center of the skillet. Cook for 1 minute, or until fragrant.

Stir in the tomatoes with liquid, chickpeas, zucchini, bay leaves, pepper, and remaining ½ teaspoon salt. Cook for 10 minutes, stirring occasionally. Discard the bay leaves before serving the stew.

PER SERVING

calories 184
total fat 4.5 g
 saturated fat 0.5 g
 trans fat 0.0 g
 polyunsaturated fat 1.0 g
 monounsaturated fat 3.0 g

cholesterol 0 mg
sodium 430 mg
carbohydrates 30 g
 fiber 8 g
 sugars 8 g
 protein 8 g

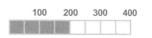

100   200   300   400

DIETARY EXCHANGES
1 starch, 3 vegetable, ½ fat

broccoli bake
with three cheeses

serves 4; 1 cup per serving

Even with three cheeses—ricotta, Cheddar, and Parmesan—this vegetarian entrée can fit into anyone's healthy meal plan.

Cooking spray

1½ pounds broccoli (about 3 bunches), stalks trimmed and separated, keeping the florets attached

1¼ cups fat-free ricotta cheese

¾ cup shredded low-fat sharp Cheddar cheese

2 or 3 medium green onions, chopped

3 tablespoons egg substitute

1½ teaspoons Worcestershire sauce (lowest sodium available)

¾ teaspoon salt-free onion-and-herb seasoning blend

⅓ cup plain dry bread crumbs (lowest sodium available)

1 tablespoon shredded or grated Parmesan cheese

½ teaspoon garlic powder

½ teaspoon dried parsley, crumbled

Preheat the oven to 350°F. Lightly spray a shallow 1½-quart glass casserole dish with cooking spray. Set aside.

In a large saucepan, steam the broccoli for 6 to 8 minutes, or until tender-crisp. Drain well.

Meanwhile, in a medium bowl, stir together the ricotta, Cheddar, green onions, egg substitute, Worcestershire sauce, and seasoning blend. Set aside.

In a small bowl, stir together the remaining ingredients.

Put the broccoli in the casserole dish. Spread the ricotta mixture over the broccoli. Sprinkle with the bread crumb mixture. Lightly spray with cooking spray.

Bake for 15 to 20 minutes, or until the broccoli is heated through and a knife inserted into the topping comes out clean.

···· PER SERVING ··········

calories 206	cholesterol 12 mg	
total fat 3.0 g	sodium 454 mg	
saturated fat 1.5 g	carbohydrates 23 g	
trans fat 0.0 g	fiber 6 g	
polyunsaturated fat 0.5 g	sugars 7 g	
monounsaturated fat 0.5 g	protein 23 g	

100 200 300 400

DIETARY EXCHANGES
½ starch, 3 vegetable,
2 very lean meat

spinach and ricotta frittata

serves 4; 1 wedge per serving

This dish is great for *any* meal—breakfast, brunch, lunch, or dinner. Serve it with fresh fruit or a tossed salad, or better yet, for a combination of the two, try Fruit and Spinach Salad with Fresh Mint (page 165).

Cooking spray
½ medium onion, sliced
1 cup egg substitute
1 cup fat-free ricotta cheese
4 cups baby spinach

Preheat the oven to 400°F.

Lightly spray an 8-inch ovenproof skillet with cooking spray. Cook the onion over medium-low heat for about 12 minutes, or until it begins to caramelize and turn brown on the edges, stirring occasionally.

Meanwhile, in a medium bowl, whisk together the egg substitute and ricotta until thoroughly combined. Set aside.

Stir the spinach into the cooked onion. Cook for about 1 minute, or until the spinach is lightly wilted, stirring constantly. Spread the mixture in the skillet.

Pour in the egg substitute mixture, covering the spinach mixture.

Bake for 20 minutes, or until a knife inserted in the center comes out clean. Cut into wedges.

COOK'S TIP You can make this frittata using leftover green beans, carrots, corn, chicken, turkey, black beans, or whatever else you have on hand that sounds good and is healthy. You can substitute roasted garlic for the onions, too. Be sure to use the ricotta, however; it adds the body needed for this dish.

PER SERVING

calories 91
total fat 0.0 g
  saturated fat 0.0 g
  trans fat 0.0 g
  polyunsaturated fat 0.0 g
  monounsaturated fat 0.0 g

cholesterol 5 mg
sodium 284 mg
carbohydrates 7 g
  fiber 2 g
  sugars 4 g
protein 15 g

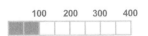

DIETARY EXCHANGES
½ carbohydrate,
2 very lean meat

one-pot vegetable and grain medley

serves 4; 1½ cups per serving

As tasty as it is colorful, this recipe requires almost no effort to prepare. All you need to complete the meal is fresh berries or sliced peaches. Both the barley (an excellent source of fiber) and the corn (a moderate source) count toward your daily servings of grains. If there are any leftovers of the medley, you'll find that they taste even better the next day, so plan to take the extra to work for lunch.

1 teaspoon olive oil
2 medium bell peppers (orange and green preferred)
2 medium shallots, coarsely chopped
2 cups frozen whole-kernel corn
2 cups low-sodium vegetable broth
1 14.5-ounce can no-salt-added diced tomatoes, undrained
½ cup uncooked pearl barley
1 teaspoon dried oregano, crumbled
1 teaspoon dried rosemary, crushed
¼ teaspoon salt
¼ teaspoon pepper
¼ cup shredded or grated Parmesan cheese

In a Dutch oven or large saucepan, heat the oil over medium-high heat, swirling to coat the bottom. Cook the bell peppers and shallots for 2 to 3 minutes, or until tender-crisp, stirring occasionally.

Stir in the remaining ingredients except the Parmesan. Bring to a simmer. Reduce the heat and simmer, covered, for 40 to 45 minutes, or until the barley is tender. Just before serving, stir in the Parmesan.

PER SERVING

calories 226
total fat 3.5 g
  saturated fat 1.0 g
  trans fat 0.0 g
  polyunsaturated fat 0.5 g
  monounsaturated fat 1.5 g

cholesterol 4 mg
sodium 261 mg
carbohydrates 43 g
  fiber 8 g
  sugars 7 g
protein 9 g

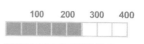

DIETARY EXCHANGES
2½ starch, 2 vegetable

cajun red beans and brown rice

serves 6; 1 cup beans and ½ cup rice per serving

In times past, cooks would simmer dried red beans all day while attending to the family's laundry. "Monday's Beans" provided a substantial, nutritious meal that required little attention while the cook labored at the washboard. Our updated version combines canned beans with a variety of seasonings, and dinner is ready in just about an hour.

Cooking spray

beans

2   15.5-ounce cans no-salt-added red beans, such as kidney beans, undrained

3   large ribs of celery, chopped

1   large onion, chopped

1   medium green bell pepper, chopped

1   8-ounce can no-salt-added tomato sauce

2   tablespoons snipped fresh parsley

2   tablespoons no-salt-added ketchup

6   medium garlic cloves, minced

2   teaspoons salt-free all-purpose seasoning blend

2   teaspoons Worcestershire sauce (lowest sodium available)

2   medium dried bay leaves

1   teaspoon chili powder or cayenne

¼   teaspoon salt

1   cup uncooked brown rice

Ground dried chipotle chiles to taste (optional)

Lightly spray a Dutch oven with cooking spray. Put all the beans ingredients in the Dutch oven, stirring to combine. Bring to a boil over medium-high heat. Reduce the heat and simmer, covered, for 1 hour. Thin the mixture with water if needed. Discard the bay leaves.

Meanwhile, prepare the rice using the package directions, omitting the salt and margarine. Top with the bean mixture. Sprinkle with the ground chipotles.

COOK'S TIP ON CHIPOTLE CHILES Chipotle chiles, which are dried smoked jalapeños, are available in several forms at the supermarket. The whole dried chiles are usually in the produce area, jars of ground dried chiles are in the international or spice section, and cans of chipotles in adobo sauce also are in the international area. Add your choice when you want a bit of heat and smoky flavor.

COOK'S TIP ON RICE COOKERS A rice cooker is the perfect appliance for cooking rice—it's quick and simple to use, and it's almost foolproof. As soon as the rice absorbs all the water and gets to the right temperature, the cooker changes from cooking mode to warming mode. It will keep the rice warm for hours. If your rice cooker has a brown rice setting, by all means use that when preparing brown rice. If it has no such setting, try using two parts uncooked brown rice to three parts water.

····· **PER SERVING** ···

calories 277	cholesterol 0 mg
total fat 1.5 g	sodium 168 mg
saturated fat 0.0 g	carbohydrates 54 g
trans fat 0.0 g	fiber 9 g
polyunsaturated fat 0.5 g	sugars 8 g
monounsaturated fat 0.5 g	protein 11 g

100   200   300   400

DIETARY EXCHANGES
3 starch, 2 vegetable,
½ very lean meat

fried rice with snow peas, bell pepper, and water chestnuts

serves 4; 1½ cups per serving

Fresh gingerroot imparts its distinctive flavor to this satisfying rice-and-vegetable mixture, and red hot-pepper sauce kicks up the heat.

½ cup uncooked brown rice

½ cup egg substitute or 3 large egg whites

1 tablespoon canola or corn oil

1 medium red bell pepper, coarsely chopped

4 medium green onions, sliced

2 medium ribs of celery, sliced on the diagonal

2 to 3 teaspoons minced peeled gingerroot

2 medium garlic cloves, minced

6 ounces fresh or frozen snow peas or sugar snap peas, trimmed if fresh or thawed if frozen, halved if large

1 8-ounce can sliced water chestnuts, drained

¾ cup low-sodium vegetable broth or fat-free, low-sodium chicken broth

1½ tablespoons soy sauce (lowest sodium available) or teriyaki sauce (lowest sodium available)

¼ teaspoon red hot-pepper sauce

Prepare the rice using the package directions, omitting the salt and margarine.

About 10 minutes before the rice is ready, pour the egg substitute into a large nonstick skillet. Cook over medium-high heat for about 1 minute, or until set. Using a spoon or whisk, break the egg "pancake" into small pieces. Transfer the pieces to a small plate. Wipe the skillet with paper towels.

Add the oil to the skillet, swirling to coat the bottom. Cook the bell pepper, green onions, celery, gingerroot, and garlic over medium-high heat for 3 to 4 minutes, or until the bell pepper and celery are tender-crisp, stirring frequently.

Stir in the peas. Cook for 2 to 3 minutes, or until tender-crisp, stirring occasionally.

Stir in the water chestnuts, rice, and egg pieces. Cook for 2 minutes, or until heated through, stirring occasionally.

Stir in the broth, soy sauce, and hot-pepper sauce. Cook for 2 to 3 minutes, or until the mixture is hot, stirring occasionally.

···· PER SERVING ···

calories 199	cholesterol 0 mg	
total fat 4.5 g	sodium 265 mg	
saturated fat 0.5 g	carbohydrates 32 g	
trans fat 0.0 g	fiber 6 g	
polyunsaturated fat 1.5 g	sugars 6 g	
monounsaturated fat 2.5 g	protein 8 g	

100 200 300 400

DIETARY EXCHANGES
1 starch, 3 vegetable, 1 fat

almond-topped bok choy, sugar snap pea, and tofu stir-fry

serves 4; 1 cup vegetable mixture and ½ cup rice per serving

Splash a sweetly spicy soy sauce mixture over stir-fried vegetables, tofu, and brown rice just before serving for a very enjoyable dinner.

2   tablespoons soy sauce (lowest sodium available)
1   tablespoon sugar
1   tablespoon cider vinegar
⅛   teaspoon crushed red pepper flakes
1¼ cups water and ¼ cup water, divided use
¾   cup uncooked quick-cooking brown rice
1   teaspoon canola or corn oil
1   large onion, cut crosswise, then halved
2   medium carrots, thinly sliced crosswise
2   medium garlic cloves, minced
3   medium stalks bok choy (green and white parts), cut crosswise (about 2 cups)
3   ounces fresh or frozen sugar snap peas or snow peas, trimmed if fresh and thawed if frozen, halved if large
2   ounces light firm tofu, drained, patted dry, and cut into ½-inch cubes
2   ounces slivered almonds, dry-roasted

In a small bowl, whisk together the soy sauce, sugar, vinegar, and red pepper flakes until the sugar is dissolved. Set aside.

In a medium saucepan, bring 1¼ cups water to a simmer over high heat. Stir in the rice. Cook using the package directions, omitting the salt and margarine. Set aside.

Meanwhile, in a large nonstick skillet, heat the oil over medium-high heat, swirling to coat the bottom. Cook the onion and carrots for 4 to 5 minutes, or until the onion is soft, stirring frequently.

Stir the garlic into the onion mixture. Cook for 10 seconds, stirring constantly.

Stir in the bok choy, peas, tofu, and remaining ¼ cup water. Cook for 2 minutes, or until the water has evaporated and the vegetables are tender-crisp, stirring constantly. Remove from the heat.

Spoon the rice onto plates. Top with the onion mixture. Drizzle with the soy sauce mixture. (Don't stir.) Sprinkle with the almonds.

PER SERVING

calories 229	cholesterol 0 mg
total fat 9.0 g	sodium 241 mg
saturated fat 0.5 g	carbohydrates 30 g
trans fat 0.0 g	fiber 5 g
polyunsaturated fat 2.5 g	sugars 10 g
monounsaturated fat 5.5 g	protein 8 g

100 200 300 400

DIETARY EXCHANGES
1½ starch, 2 vegetable, ½ lean meat, 1 fat

speed-dial stuffed peppers

serves 4; 1 bell pepper half per serving

In this quick one-skillet vegetarian dish, bell pepper halves are cooked right on top of their rice and pine nut stuffing.

¾ cup pine nuts (about 3 ounces)

1½ teaspoons ground cumin

1 teaspoon curry powder

½ teaspoon ground cinnamon

1 teaspoon canola or corn oil

1 large onion, finely chopped

1 cup uncooked quick-cooking brown rice

2 ounces light firm tofu, drained, patted dry, and cut into ½-inch cubes

2 cups water

2 large green or red bell peppers, or a combination, halved lengthwise

1 teaspoon sugar

½ teaspoon salt

In a large nonstick skillet, dry-roast the pine nuts for 2 minutes over medium-high heat, or until beginning to lightly brown, stirring constantly. Watch carefully so they don't burn. Transfer to a medium plate. Set aside.

In the same skillet, stir together the cumin, curry powder, and cinnamon. Cook for 30 seconds, or until fragrant, stirring constantly. Watch carefully so the spices don't burn. Add to the pine nuts.

Add the oil to the skillet, swirling to coat the bottom. Cook the onion, still over medium high, for 5 minutes, or until beginning to brown, stirring frequently.

Stir in the rice and tofu. Cook for 2 minutes, or until the tofu is beginning to lightly brown, stirring occasionally. Stir in the water.

Place the bell peppers with the cut side down on the rice mixture. Bring to a simmer. Reduce the heat and simmer, covered, for 12 to 15 minutes, or until the bell peppers are tender. Transfer the bell peppers with the cut side up to plates.

Stir the pine nut mixture, sugar, and salt into the rice mixture. Spoon into the bell peppers.

COOK'S TIP Dry-roasting the pine nuts and spices intensifies their flavor. Adding them to the food right before serving intensifies its flavor as well.

······ PER SERVING ··

calories 258
total fat 13.5 g
 saturated fat 2.0 g
 trans fat 0.0 g
 polyunsaturated fat 5.0 g
 monounsaturated fat 5.0 g

cholesterol 0 mg
sodium 311 mg
carbohydrates 31 g
 fiber 5 g
 sugars 8 g
 protein 10 g

100   200   300   400

DIETARY EXCHANGES
1½ starch, 2 vegetable,
1 lean meat, 2 fat

creole ratatouille

serves 4; 1 cup vegetable mixture and ½ cup rice per serving

French ratatouille *(ra-tuh-TOO-ee)* gets a Creole twist with celery, okra, and–of course–a dash of red hot-pepper sauce!

Cooking spray

1 medium green bell pepper, cut into 1-inch pieces

1 medium onion, cut into ½-inch wedges

2 medium ribs of celery, chopped

2 cups fresh or frozen cut okra, cut crosswise into ½-inch pieces if fresh

1 14.5-ounce can no-salt-added tomatoes, undrained, or 1 pound fresh tomatoes, chopped

¾ cup water

2 teaspoons Worcestershire sauce (lowest sodium available)

½ teaspoon dried thyme, crumbled

½ teaspoon sugar

1 cup uncooked quick-cooking brown rice

½ cup snipped fresh parsley

1 teaspoon olive oil (extra-virgin preferred)

½ teaspoon salt

⅛ teaspoon red hot-pepper sauce, or to taste (optional)

3 ounces shredded low-fat mozzarella cheese

Lightly spray a Dutch oven with cooking spray. Cook the bell pepper, onion, and celery over medium heat for 6 minutes, or until beginning to brown on the edges, stirring frequently.

Stir in the okra, tomatoes with liquid, water, Worcestershire sauce, thyme, and sugar. Increase the heat to high and bring to a boil. Reduce the heat and simmer, covered, for 20 minutes, or until the bell pepper is tender, stirring occasionally. Remove from the heat.

Meanwhile, prepare the rice using the package directions, omitting the salt and margarine.

Stir the remaining ingredients except the mozzarella into the okra mixture. Let stand, covered, for 10 minutes so the flavors blend. Serve over the rice. Top with the mozzarella.

COOK'S TIP The flavors of this dish will improve if it is refrigerated overnight and reheated over medium heat. If you prefer a thinner consistency, pour in ¼ cup water before reheating.

····· **PER SERVING** ···

calories 196	cholesterol 8 mg
total fat 4.0 g	sodium 567 mg
saturated fat 1.0 g	carbohydrates 31 g
trans fat 0.0 g	fiber 6 g
polyunsaturated fat 0.5 g	sugars 8 g
monounsaturated fat 2.0 g	protein 11 g

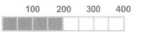

100 200 300 400

DIETARY EXCHANGES
1 starch, 3 vegetable,
1 lean meat

vegetable and bulgur curry

serves 4; 1½ cups per serving

Raisins, coconut, peanuts, fresh orange zest, and, of course, curry powder liven up the bulgur, carrots, and green peas in this delicious one-dish meal. The bulgur, a whole grain, is an excellent source of fiber.

1   cup uncooked bulgur

1   teaspoon curry powder

3   ounces unsalted peanuts or pecans, finely chopped

¼   cup sweetened flaked coconut

1   teaspoon canola or corn oil

1   large onion, chopped

2   medium carrots, chopped

¼   cup raisins

¼   cup water

¼   teaspoon salt and ¼ teaspoon salt, divided use

1   cup frozen green peas, thawed

1   to 2 teaspoons grated orange zest

1   teaspoon ground cumin

½   teaspoon ground cinnamon

¼   teaspoon cayenne

In a medium saucepan, prepare the bulgur using the package directions, omitting the salt and adding the curry powder. Remove from the heat. Fluff with a fork. Set aside.

Meanwhile, in a large nonstick skillet, dry-roast the peanuts for 2 minutes over medium-high heat, or until just beginning to lightly brown, stirring frequently.

Stir the coconut into the peanuts. Cook for 1 minute, or until the coconut is golden, stirring constantly. Pour onto a small plate.

In the same skillet, heat the oil, still on medium high, swirling to coat the bottom. Cook the onion and carrots for 8 to 10 minutes, or until richly browned, stirring occasionally. Stir in the raisins, water, and ¼ teaspoon salt. Remove from the heat.

Stir the peas, orange zest, cumin, cinnamon, cayenne, and remaining ¼ teaspoon salt into the bulgur. Serve topped with the onion mixture and sprinkled with the peanut mixture.

····· PER SERVING ··

calories 375	cholesterol 0 mg	
total fat 14.0 g	sodium 379 mg	
saturated fat 3.0 g	carbohydrates 55 g	
trans fat 0.0 g	fiber 13 g	
polyunsaturated fat 4.0 g	sugars 16 g	
monounsaturated fat 6.0 g	protein 13 g	

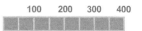

DIETARY EXCHANGES
2 starch, 1 fruit,
2 vegetable, 1 lean meat,
2 fat

vegetables and side dishes

Asparagus with Gremolata

Asparagus and Two Red Peppers with Orzo

Italian Barley and Mushrooms

French Brussels Sprouts

Bulgur and Black Beans with Lime

Red Cabbage Braised with Balsamic Vinegar

Orange-Glazed Carrots

Roasted Green Beans and Walnuts

Sesame Kale

Creole Lentils

Orzo with Tomato and Capers

Stir-Fried Sugar Snap Peas with Shallots and Walnuts

Smashed Potatoes with Aromatic Herbs

Quinoa Pilaf

Lemon-Herb Brown Rice

Pesto and Pecan Rice

Spinach with Almonds and Lemon Zest

Butternut Squash with Apple and Pecans

Stewed Zucchini and Cherry Tomatoes

Mixed Vegetable Grill

Vibrant-Veggie Roast

asparagus with gremolata

serves 4; about 6 spears per serving

Gremolata (or gremolada), an aromatic mixture of parsley, lemon zest, and garlic, livens up steamed asparagus. We added dillweed and pepper to the gremolata for even more flavor.

1 pound medium asparagus spears (about 24), trimmed

1 tablespoon salt-free all-purpose seasoning blend

gremolata

¼ cup finely snipped fresh parsley

1 tablespoon snipped fresh dillweed

1 teaspoon grated lemon zest

1 medium garlic clove, minced

⅛ teaspoon pepper

Sprinkle the asparagus with the seasoning blend. Steam in a large saucepan for 2 to 3 minutes, or until tender-crisp. Drain well. Transfer to a serving bowl.

Meanwhile, in a small bowl, stir together the gremolata ingredients. Sprinkle over the asparagus. Stir gently to coat.

COOK'S TIP ON TRIMMING ASPARAGUS When using fresh asparagus, discard about the bottom 1 inch of the stalk ends (breaking where the stalk bends).

PER SERVING

calories 27
total fat 0.0 g
  saturated fat 0.0 g
  trans fat 0.0 g
  polyunsaturated fat 0.0 g
  monounsaturated fat 0.0 g

cholesterol 0 mg
sodium 2 mg
carbohydrates 6 g
  fiber 3 g
  sugars 3 g
protein 3 g

100 200 300 400

DIETARY EXCHANGES
1 vegetable

asparagus and two red peppers with orzo

serves 8; ½ cup per serving

Orzo, the rice-shaped pasta, and asparagus make an enticing side dish. Combined with colorful red bell pepper, they provide an attractive addition for any table.

- 6 cups water and ¼ cup water, divided use
- ¾ cup dried orzo
- 1 pound medium asparagus, trimmed, cut into 1-inch pieces, or 9 ounces frozen cut asparagus, thawed for about 2 minutes
- ½ medium red bell pepper, cut lengthwise into thin strips
- 1 medium shallot, thinly sliced
- 1½ teaspoons honey or maple syrup
- 1 teaspoon dried oregano, crumbled
- 1 teaspoon white wine vinegar
- ¼ teaspoon crushed red pepper flakes
- 1 teaspoon olive oil (extra-virgin preferred)
- ¼ teaspoon salt
  Dash of pepper

In a medium saucepan, bring 6 cups water to a boil. Stir in the orzo. Cook for 8 minutes, or until tender. Drain well in a colander.

Meanwhile, in a large skillet, stir together the asparagus, bell pepper, shallot, honey, oregano, vinegar, red pepper flakes, and remaining ¼ cup water. Bring to a simmer over medium-low heat. Simmer for 5 minutes, or until the asparagus is cooked but still crisp to the bite. (If cooked longer, the asparagus will lose its bright green color.)

In a medium bowl, stir together the orzo, asparagus mixture, oil, salt, and pepper.

PER SERVING

calories 84
total fat 1.0 g
  saturated fat 0.0 g
  trans fat 0.0 g
  polyunsaturated fat 0.0 g
  monounsaturated fat 0.5 g

cholesterol 0 mg
sodium 74 mg
carbohydrates 16 g
  fiber 2 g
  sugars 3 g
protein 3 g

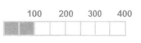

DIETARY EXCHANGES
1 starch

italian barley
and mushrooms

serves 4; ½ cup per serving

This pilaf-like dish features quick-cooking barley, a high-fiber whole grain. Try barley as a replacement for rice in other dishes when you want a change of pace.

1 cup water
½ cup uncooked quick-cooking barley
1 teaspoon very low sodium beef bouillon granules
  Olive oil spray
8 ounces button mushrooms, sliced
2 medium green onions, minced
1 medium garlic clove, minced
½ teaspoon dried oregano, crumbled
½ cup snipped fresh Italian (flat-leaf) parsley
2 teaspoons olive oil (extra-virgin preferred)
¼ teaspoon salt
⅛ teaspoon pepper

In a small saucepan, bring the water to a boil over high heat. Stir in the barley and bouillon granules. Reduce the heat and simmer, covered, for 12 minutes, or until the barley is tender.

Meanwhile, lightly spray a large skillet with olive oil spray. Add the mushrooms and lightly spray with olive oil spray. Cook over medium-high heat for 4 minutes, or until beginning to lightly brown, stirring frequently.

Stir in the green onions, garlic, and oregano. Cook for 15 seconds, stirring constantly. Remove from the heat.

Stir in the barley and remaining ingredients.

PER SERVING

calories 107
total fat 3.0 g
  saturated fat 0.5 g
  trans fat 0.0 g
  polyunsaturated fat 0.5 g
  monounsaturated fat 1.5 g

cholesterol 0 mg
sodium 159 mg
carbohydrates 18 g
  fiber 3 g
  sugars 2 g
protein 4 g

100 200 300 400

DIETARY EXCHANGES
1 starch, ½ fat

french brussels sprouts

serves 8; ½ cup per serving

This one-pan side dish blends brussels sprouts with the classic French flavoring combination known as mirepoix (*mihr-PWAH*)—onions, celery, and carrots—as well as with a bit of turkey bacon.

10 ounces small brussels sprouts (about 20), trimmed, damaged or yellow outer leaves discarded

1 slice turkey bacon, chopped

⅓ cup sliced green onions (white part only)

⅓ cup diced celery

⅓ cup diced or shredded carrots

1 tablespoon water (as needed)

Put the brussels sprouts in a medium saucepan. Add cold water to cover. Bring to a boil over medium-high heat. Cook for 15 minutes, or until tender when tested with the tip of a sharp knife or fork. Transfer the sprouts to a colander. Run under cold water to stop the cooking process and maintain the bright color of the sprouts. Drain well. Transfer to a serving bowl and cover.

In the same saucepan, cook the bacon over medium-low heat for about 8 minutes, or until it begins to brown. Stir in the green onions, celery, and carrots. Cook, covered, for 3 minutes.

Stir in the brussels sprouts. Reduce the heat to low and cook, covered, for 5 minutes, or until heated through, stirring occasionally. If the vegetables begin to stick to the pan, add 1 tablespoon water. Drain if needed. Transfer to the serving bowl.

PER SERVING

calories 24	cholesterol 2 mg
total fat 0.5 g	sodium 39 mg
saturated fat 0.0 g	carbohydrates 4 g
trans fat 0.0 g	fiber 2 g
polyunsaturated fat 0.0 g	sugars 1 g
monounsaturated fat 0.0 g	protein 2 g

100   200   300   400

DIETARY EXCHANGES

1 vegetable

bulgur and black beans with lime

serves 4; ½ cup per serving

Bulgur wheat, a whole grain, is traditionally used in Middle Eastern dishes such as tabbouleh. Here it is combined with black beans to make a fiber-packed side dish. Try bulgur as an alternative to white rice in a variety of dishes.

1¼ cups water
⅓ cup uncooked bulgur
½ 15.5-ounce can no-salt-added black beans, rinsed and drained
½ cup diced tomatoes (optional)
2 tablespoons snipped fresh cilantro
1 medium fresh jalapeño, seeds and ribs discarded, finely chopped
1 to 1½ tablespoons fresh lime juice
¼ teaspoon salt
1 tablespoon olive oil (extra-virgin preferred)

In a medium saucepan, bring the water to a rolling boil over high heat. Stir in the bulgur. Reduce the heat and simmer, covered, for 10 to 12 minutes, or until most of the water has evaporated. Remove from the heat.

Stir in the remaining ingredients except the oil. Drizzle with the oil. (Don't stir.)

WITH TOMATOES
PER SERVING

calories 123
total fat 3.5 g
  saturated fat 0.5 g
  trans fat 0.0 g
  polyunsaturated fat 0.5 g
  monounsaturated fat 2.5 g

cholesterol 0 mg
sodium 151 mg
carbohydrates 19 g
  fiber 5 g
  sugars 3 g
  protein 5 g

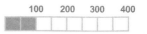

DIETARY EXCHANGES
1½ starch, ½ very lean meat, ½ fat

red cabbage braised with balsamic vinegar

serves 4; ½ cup per serving

Eye-catching red cabbage with a touch of blackberry spread, balsamic vinegar, and lemon zest teams well with baked pork chops, such as Pork Chops Parmesan (page 312) or poached salmon.

1   teaspoon olive oil
2   medium leeks (white part only), thinly sliced
½   medium red cabbage (about 1 pound), thinly sliced
¼   cup unsweetened apple juice
2   tablespoons all-fruit seedless blackberry spread
1   tablespoon balsamic vinegar
1   teaspoon grated lemon zest
¼   teaspoon pepper

In a medium saucepan, heat the oil over medium heat, swirling to coat the bottom. Cook the leeks for 2 to 3 minutes, or until tender-crisp, stirring occasionally.

Stir in the cabbage. Cook for 2 to 3 minutes, or until tender-crisp, stirring occasionally.

Stir in the remaining ingredients. Reduce the heat and simmer, covered, for 20 to 25 minutes, or until the cabbage is tender, stirring occasionally.

PER SERVING

calories 112
total fat 1.5 g
  saturated fat 0.0 g
  trans fat 0.0 g
  polyunsaturated fat 0.5 g
  monounsaturated fat 1.0 g

cholesterol 0 mg
sodium 49 mg
carbohydrates 25 g
  fiber 4 g
  sugars 14 g
  protein 3 g

100   200   300   400

DIETARY EXCHANGES
½ fruit, 3 vegetable, ½ fat

orange-glazed carrots

serves 4; ½ cup per serving

Try these sweet carrots with grilled or broiled beef or poultry.

1 medium orange
4 medium carrots, cut crosswise into ⅛-inch pieces
¼ teaspoon ground cinnamon
2 tablespoons firmly packed dark brown sugar
⅛ teaspoon salt
1 tablespoon light tub margarine

Grate 1 teaspoon zest from the orange. Set the zest aside. Squeeze the juice from the orange. Pour the juice into a large nonstick skillet. Bring to a boil over medium-high heat.

Stir in the carrots and cinnamon. Return to a boil. Reduce the heat and simmer, covered, for 8 to 9 minutes, or until the carrots are tender.

Increase the heat to medium-high. Stir in the brown sugar and salt. Bring to a boil. Cook for 1 to 2 minutes, or until the carrots are richly glazed, stirring constantly. Remove from the heat.

Stir in the margarine and reserved orange zest until the margarine has melted.

PER SERVING

calories 76
total fat 1.5 g
  saturated fat 0.0 g
  trans fat 0.0 g
  polyunsaturated fat 0.5 g
  monounsaturated fat 0.5 g

cholesterol 0 mg
sodium 147 mg
carbohydrates 16 g
  fiber 2 g
  sugars 12 g
  protein 1 g

100   200   300   400

DIETARY EXCHANGES
2 vegetable,
½ carbohydrate

roasted green beans and walnuts

serves 4; ½ cup per serving

While the green beans are roasting, the walnuts are toasting, bringing out the full flavors of each.

Cooking spray
12 ounces fresh green beans, trimmed
2 tablespoons finely chopped walnuts
2 tablespoons finely snipped fresh parsley
¼ teaspoon salt
⅛ teaspoon cayenne

Preheat the oven to 425°F. Lightly spray a large baking sheet with cooking spray.

Arrange the beans in a single layer on the baking sheet. Sprinkle with the walnuts. Lightly spray the tops with cooking spray.

Bake for 10 minutes, stirring once halfway through. Serve sprinkled with the parsley, salt, and cayenne.

COOK'S TIP ON WALNUTS Walnuts are an excellent source of omega-3 fatty acids, an important nutrient in a healthy diet. Use them for snacks, on high-fiber cereal, or in fat-free yogurt. Enjoy the nuts but be mindful of the portion—about seven halves equal 100 calories.

PER SERVING

calories 51
total fat 2.5 g
  saturated fat 0.5 g
  trans fat 0.0 g
  polyunsaturated fat 2.0 g
  monounsaturated fat 0.5 g

cholesterol 0 mg
sodium 152 mg
carbohydrates 7 g
  fiber 3 g
  sugars 1 g
protein 2 g

100 200 300 400

DIETARY EXCHANGES
1 vegetable, ½ fat

sesame kale

serves 6; ½ cup per serving

If you are unfamiliar with kale, a leafy, high-fiber member of the cabbage family, this simple-to-prepare recipe will give you a good introduction. The red pepper flakes add just the right kick, and the sesame seeds provide a hint of crunch.

- 2 cups water
- 8 ounces kale, chopped
  Olive oil spray
- 1 teaspoon olive oil
- 1 cup chopped red onion
- ½ teaspoon crushed red pepper flakes
- 1 large garlic clove, minced
- 1 teaspoon toasted sesame oil
- ⅛ teaspoon salt
- 2 tablespoons sesame seeds, dry-roasted

In a large skillet, bring the water to a boil over high heat. Cook the kale for 5 minutes, or until tender and beginning to wilt, stirring occasionally. Drain well in a colander. Discard the liquid in the skillet.

Lightly spray the same skillet with olive oil spray. Add the oil, swirling to coat the bottom. Cook the onion and red pepper flakes over medium-high heat for about 3 minutes, or until the onion is soft, stirring frequently.

Stir in the garlic. Cook for 30 seconds, stirring frequently.

Stir the kale into the onion mixture. Cook for 1 to 2 minutes, or until heated through, stirring occasionally. Remove from the heat. Stir in the sesame oil and salt. Serve sprinkled with the sesame seeds.

COOK'S TIP ON DRY-ROASTED SESAME SEEDS Look in the spice aisle for bottled dry-roasted sesame seeds or prepare them yourself. Dry-roast them in a small skillet over medium-high heat for 1 to 2 minutes, or until lightly browned, stirring frequently. Watch carefully so they don't burn. Remove the seeds from the skillet so they don't continue to cook.

TIME-SAVER Check your supermarket for packages of prewashed, pre-chopped kale.

··· **PER SERVING** ··

calories 64

total fat 3.5 g

  saturated fat 0.5 g

  trans fat 0.0 g

  polyunsaturated fat 1.5 g

  monounsaturated fat 1.5 g

cholesterol 0 mg

sodium 70 mg

carbohydrates 7 g

  fiber 2 g

  sugars 1 g

protein 2 g

100   200   300   400

DIETARY EXCHANGES

1 vegetable, 1 fat

creole lentils

serves 4; ½ cup per serving

Simmer lentils to tenderness with tomatoes, bell peppers, celery, onion, and okra. A touch of hot sauce adds zip.

Cooking spray

1 medium green bell pepper, chopped

1 medium rib of celery, finely chopped

½ cup chopped onion

2 medium tomatoes, chopped

1 cup fresh or frozen cut okra, cut crosswise into ½-inch pieces if fresh

¾ cup water

½ cup dried lentils, sorted for stones and shriveled lentils and rinsed

½ teaspoon dried thyme, crumbled

2 medium dried bay leaves

¼ cup snipped fresh parsley

2 teaspoons olive oil (extra-virgin preferred)

¼ teaspoon salt

¼ teaspoon red hot-pepper sauce

Lightly spray a large saucepan with cooking spray. Cook the bell pepper, celery, and onion over medium-high heat for 3 minutes, or until the onion is soft, stirring frequently.

Increase the heat to high. Stir in the tomatoes, okra, water, lentils, thyme, and bay leaves. Bring to a boil. Reduce the heat and simmer, covered, for 30 minutes, or until the lentils are tender. Remove from the heat. Discard the bay leaves.

Stir in the remaining ingredients. Let stand, covered, for 5 minutes so the flavors blend.

PER SERVING

calories 144
total fat 2.5 g
  saturated fat 0.5 g
  trans fat 0.0 g
  polyunsaturated fat 0.5 g
  monounsaturated fat 1.5 g

cholesterol 0 mg
sodium 166 mg
carbohydrates 24 g
  fiber 6 g
  sugars 5 g
  protein 9 g

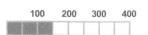

DIETARY EXCHANGES
1 starch, 2 vegetable,
½ lean meat

orzo with tomato and capers

serves 4; ½ cup per serving

This versatile Mediterranean combination is delectable both as a hot or room temperature side dish and as a cold pasta salad.

3 ounces dried orzo

1 small tomato, diced

¼ cup snipped fresh parsley

1 tablespoon capers, drained

2 teaspoons dried basil, crumbled

2 teaspoons olive oil (extra-virgin preferred)

½ to 1 teaspoon cider vinegar

½ medium garlic clove, minced

⅛ teaspoon salt

⅛ teaspoon crushed red pepper flakes

Prepare the orzo using the package directions, omitting the salt. Drain well in a colander.

Meanwhile, in a medium bowl, stir together the remaining ingredients.

Stir the orzo into the tomato mixture. Serve hot, at room temperature, or chilled.

PER SERVING

calories 107	cholesterol 0 mg
total fat 2.5 g	sodium 137 mg
saturated fat 0.5 g	carbohydrates 18 g
trans fat 0.0 g	fiber 1 g
polyunsaturated fat 0.5 g	sugars 2 g
monounsaturated fat 1.5 g	protein 3 g

100 200 300 400

DIETARY EXCHANGES
1 starch, ½ fat

stir-fried sugar snap peas with shallots and walnuts

serves 4; ½ cup per serving

Dress up any meal from grilled chicken to meat loaf with this super side dish of crisp, rather sweet sugar snaps enhanced with imitation bacon bits and fragrant five-spice powder.

1 teaspoon canola or corn oil

2 medium shallots, chopped

8 ounces fresh or frozen sugar snap peas, trimmed if fresh

2 tablespoons imitation bacon bits

1 teaspoon toasted sesame oil

¼ teaspoon five-spice powder (optional)

1 tablespoon crushed dry-roasted walnuts

In a large nonstick skillet, heat the canola oil over medium heat, swirling to coat the bottom. Cook the shallots for 1 to 2 minutes, or until tender-crisp, stirring constantly.

Stir in the remaining ingredients except the walnuts. Cook for 1 to 2 minutes, or until the sugar snap peas are tender-crisp. Serve sprinkled with the walnuts.

PER SERVING

calories 72
total fat 4.0 g
  saturated fat 0.5 g
  trans fat 0.0 g
  polyunsaturated fat 1.5 g
  monounsaturated fat 1.5 g

cholesterol 0 mg
sodium 43 mg
carbohydrates 7 g
  fiber 2 g
  sugars 3 g
  protein 3 g

100   200   300   400

DIETARY EXCHANGES
½ starch, 1 fat

smashed potatoes with aromatic herbs

serves 4; ½ cup per serving

Parsley, rosemary, and horseradish set these coarsely mashed potatoes apart from similar recipes. Leaving the skins on the potatoes provides more fiber, a nutrient that helps you battle the bulge.

- 1 pound red or yellow-skinned potatoes, such as Yukon Gold (about 4 medium)
- ½ cup fat-free half-and-half
- 1 tablespoon snipped fresh parsley or 1 teaspoon dried, crumbled
- 1 tablespoon finely chopped or minced fresh rosemary or 1 teaspoon dried, crushed
- 2 teaspoons bottled white horseradish, drained
- 1 medium garlic clove, minced
- ⅛ teaspoon salt
- ⅛ teaspoon pepper

Put the potatoes in a medium saucepan. Fill the pan with water to cover the potatoes by 1 inch. Bring to a boil over high heat. Reduce the heat and simmer, partially covered, for about 30 minutes, or until the potatoes are tender when pierced with the tip of a sharp knife or a fork. Drain well, leaving the potatoes in the pan.

Add the remaining ingredients. Using a potato masher or hand-held electric mixer, coarsely mash or beat the mixture.

COOK'S TIP Feel free to replace the rosemary with basil, oregano, dillweed, thyme, savory, or sliced green onions (green part only).

PER SERVING

calories 103	cholesterol 0 mg
total fat 0.0 g	sodium 118 mg
saturated fat 0.0 g	carbohydrates 23 g
trans fat 0.0 g	fiber 2 g
polyunsaturated fat 0.0 g	sugars 3 g
monounsaturated fat 0.0 g	protein 4 g

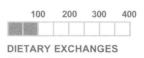

100 200 300 400

DIETARY EXCHANGES
1½ starch

quinoa pilaf

serves 4; ½ cup per serving

This pilaf stars quinoa, which is sometimes referred to as a supergrain because it is high in protein and many other key nutrients.

- 1 cup fat-free, low-sodium chicken broth
- 3 ounces button mushrooms, sliced
- ¼ cup chopped onion
- ½ cup quinoa, rinsed and drained
- ¼ cup frozen green peas, thawed
- ¼ cup shredded or grated Parmesan cheese

In a small saucepan, stir together the broth, mushrooms, and onion. Bring to a boil over high heat.

Stir in the quinoa. Return to a boil. Reduce the heat and simmer, covered, for 12 minutes, or until all the broth is absorbed. Remove the pan from the heat.

Stir in the peas. Let stand, covered, for 10 minutes. Stir in the Parmesan.

COOK'S TIP For a special presentation, spoon a serving of the pilaf into a ½-cup measuring cup, packing it lightly, and invert onto a large plate. Repeat with the remaining pilaf.

COOK'S TIP ON QUINOA Quinoa has a bitter coating called saponin, which should be rinsed off. Put the quinoa in a fine-mesh strainer and rinse under running water for 1 to 2 minutes. Shake off any excess water. Many cooks like to rinse even quinoa that is prerinsed before packaging, just to be sure no saponin remains.

PER SERVING

calories 116	cholesterol 4 mg
total fat 3.0 g	sodium 111 mg
saturated fat 1.0 g	carbohydrates 17 g
trans fat 0.0 g	fiber 2 g
polyunsaturated fat 1.0 g	sugars 1 g
monounsaturated fat 1.0 g	protein 7 g

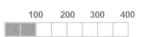

100   200   300   400

DIETARY EXCHANGES
1 starch, ½ lean meat

lemon-herb brown rice

serves 4; ½ cup per serving

Adding the margarine spray at the very end and not stirring it into the rice mixture lets the flavor stay on top so you can taste it with every bite.

- 1 cup uncooked quick-cooking brown rice
- ¼ cup finely snipped fresh parsley
- 1 teaspoon dried basil, crumbled
- ½ to 1 teaspoon grated lemon zest
- 1 tablespoon fresh lemon juice
- ¼ teaspoon salt
- 20 sprays fat-free liquid margarine spray

Prepare the rice using the package directions, omitting the salt and margarine. Transfer to a serving bowl.

Stir in the remaining ingredients except the margarine spray.

Spray the top of the rice mixture with margarine spray. Don't stir.

PER SERVING

calories 88
total fat 1.0 g
  saturated fat 0.0 g
  trans fat 0.0 g
  polyunsaturated fat 0.5 g
  monounsaturated fat 0.5 g

cholesterol 0 mg
sodium 157 mg
carbohydrates 18 g
  fiber 1 g
  sugars 0 g
  protein 2 g

100   200   300   400

DIETARY EXCHANGES
1 starch

pesto and pecan rice

serves 4; ½ cup per serving

Small amounts of pesto and pecans go a long way in turning brown rice into an attention-getting side dish.

Cooking spray

½ medium green bell pepper, chopped

½ cup onion, chopped

1 medium rib of celery, chopped

1 medium garlic clove, minced

½ cup uncooked brown rice

1½ cups fat-free, low-sodium chicken broth and 1½ teaspoons fat-free, low-sodium chicken broth, divided use

¼ teaspoon pepper

⅛ teaspoon salt

1½ teaspoons prepared pesto

2 teaspoons coarsely chopped pecans, dry-roasted

1 tablespoon chopped fresh basil (optional)

Lightly spray a medium saucepan with cooking spray. Cook the bell pepper, onion, celery, and garlic over medium-high heat for about 3 minutes, or until the onion is soft, stirring frequently. Remove the pan from the heat. Transfer the mixture to a medium plate.

Respray the pan. Cook the rice for 1 to 2 minutes, or until lightly toasted, stirring occasionally.

Stir in 1½ cups broth, the pepper, and salt. Increase the heat to high and bring to a boil. Reduce the heat and simmer, covered, for 40 to 45 minutes, or until the rice is tender.

Meanwhile, in a small bowl, whisk together the pesto and remaining 1½ teaspoons broth until smooth. Stir with the bell pepper mixture into the cooked rice. Sprinkle with the pecans and basil.

PER SERVING

calories 121	cholesterol 1 mg
total fat 2.5 g	sodium 124 mg
saturated fat 0.5 g	carbohydrates 21 g
trans fat 0.0 g	fiber 2 g
polyunsaturated fat 0.5 g	sugars 2 g
monounsaturated fat 1.5 g	protein 4 g

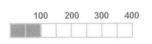

100 200 300 400

DIETARY EXCHANGES
1½ starch

spinach with almonds and lemon zest

serves 4; ½ cup per serving

....

When you need an easy side dish, you will love this combination of baby spinach, dry-roasted almonds, caramelized onions, lemon zest, and Parmesan— it takes less than 15 minutes of cooking time. Try it with pan-seared or grilled fish, such as Grilled Trout with Horseradish Sour Cream (page 214), or baked pork chops.

  1 teaspoon olive oil
  1 medium onion, thinly sliced crosswise
  1 teaspoon light brown sugar
  1 medium garlic clove, minced
  1 pound baby spinach
  1 tablespoon Worcestershire sauce (lowest sodium available)
  1 teaspoon grated lemon zest
1½ tablespoons shredded or grated Parmesan cheese
  1 tablespoon slivered almonds, dry-roasted

In a large nonstick skillet, heat the oil over medium-high heat, swirling to coat the bottom. Cook the onion for 7 to 8 minutes, or until golden brown, stirring occasionally. (Watch carefully so the onion doesn't burn.)

Stir in the brown sugar and garlic. Cook for 1 minute.

Stir in the spinach, Worcestershire sauce, and lemon zest. Cook for 3 to 4 minutes, or until the spinach is wilted, stirring occasionally. Serve sprinkled with the Parmesan and almonds.

····· PER SERVING ·····

calories 92
total fat 2.5 g
  saturated fat 0.5 g
  trans fat 0.0 g
  polyunsaturated fat 0.5 g
  monounsaturated fat 1.5 g

cholesterol 1 mg
sodium 219 mg
carbohydrates 17 g
  fiber 6 g
  sugars 4 g
protein 4 g

100 200 300 400

DIETARY EXCHANGES
3 vegetable, ½ fat

butternut squash with apple and pecans

serves 4; 1 squash wedge and ⅓ cup apple mixture per serving

A whole raw butternut squash can be difficult to cut and take quite a while to cook, but using the microwave lets you make quick work of getting this yummy side dish on the table. Although the combination of butternut squash and apple "feels" like fall, this dish is good any time of the year.

- 1 medium butternut squash (about 2 pounds), pierced in several places with a fork
- ¼ cup water
- 1 medium apple, such as Gala or Jonathan, chopped
- 2 tablespoons golden raisins
- 2 tablespoons maple syrup
- 2 tablespoons finely chopped pecans, dry-roasted
- 1 tablespoon light tub margarine
- ⅛ teaspoon ground nutmeg

Put the squash in a microwaveable pie pan or large rimmed plate. Microwave on 100 percent power (high) for 2 minutes, turning over once.

Cut the squash lengthwise into quarters, discarding the seeds and strings. Place the squash with one cut side down in the pie pan. Pour in the water. Microwave, covered, on 100 percent power (high) for 10 minutes, or until the squash is tender when pierced with a fork. Remove from the microwave. Let stand, covered, for 2 minutes.

Meanwhile, in a medium nonstick skillet, cook the apple, raisins, and maple syrup over medium-high heat for 4 minutes, or until the apple is beginning to lightly brown, stirring frequently.

Stir the pecans, margarine, and nutmeg into the apple mixture. Cook for 1 minute, or until the margarine is melted, stirring constantly. Spoon over the cut side of the squash.

PER SERVING

calories 167	cholesterol 0 mg
total fat 4.0 g	sodium 31 mg
saturated fat 0.5 g	carbohydrates 35 g
trans fat 0.0 g	fiber 7 g
polyunsaturated fat 1.0 g	sugars 17 g
monounsaturated fat 2.0 g	protein 2 g

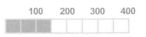

100 200 300 400

DIETARY EXCHANGES
1½ starch, 1 fruit, ½ fat

stewed zucchini and cherry tomatoes

serves 4; ½ cup per serving

Weighing in at only 51 calories per serving, this colorful vegetable combo is a delightful companion to grilled seafood, such as Grilled Fish with Cucumber Salsa (page 194), or grilled or baked chicken breasts.

1 teaspoon canola or corn oil

4 medium garlic cloves

2 medium zucchini, cut crosswise into ½-inch slices

2 tablespoons fat-free, low-sodium chicken broth

½ cup cherry tomatoes, halved

2 tablespoons chopped fresh basil or 1 teaspoon dried, crumbled

⅛ teaspoon pepper

2 tablespoons shredded or grated Romano cheese

In a medium saucepan, heat the oil over medium heat, swirling to coat the bottom. Cook the garlic for 2 to 3 minutes, or until light golden brown, stirring occasionally.

Stir in the zucchini. Cook for 1 to 2 minutes, or until tender-crisp, stirring occasionally.

Pour in the broth. Reduce the heat and simmer, covered, for 5 minutes, or until the zucchini is tender, stirring occasionally.

Stir in the tomatoes, basil, and pepper. Cook for 1 to 2 minutes, or until the tomatoes are warmed through. Serve sprinkled with the Romano.

COOK'S TIP ON CRINKLE-CUTTERS You can find crinkle-cutters at gourmet shops and some supermarkets. They are easy-to-use gadgets that make attractive wavy cuts on foods such as zucchini, yellow summer squash, cucumbers, carrots, and various melons. Try one on the zucchini for this recipe.

PER SERVING

calories 51
total fat 2.5 g
  saturated fat 1.0 g
  trans fat 0.0 g
  polyunsaturated fat 0.5 g
  monounsaturated fat 1.0 g

cholesterol 3 mg
sodium 69 mg
carbohydrates 6 g
  fiber 2 g
  sugars 3 g
  protein 3 g

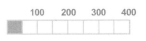

DIETARY EXCHANGES
1 vegetable, ½ fat

mixed vegetable grill

serves 4; ½ cup per serving

Here is a combination of just a few of the many very low calorie vegetables that are delicious when grilled. Cut the zucchini into long slices that go directly on the grill and skewer the tomatoes and mushrooms for an appealing side dish with different shapes and colors.

Olive oil spray

2 medium zucchini, cut lengthwise into ½-inch-thick slices

12 medium button mushrooms, trimmed so that the stems are even with the bottom of the caps

12 cherry tomatoes

10 fresh basil leaves (optional)

Fat-free liquid margarine spray

⅛ teaspoon salt

Pepper to taste

Balsamic vinegar, to taste

Soak four 8-inch wooden skewers for at least 10 minutes in cold water to keep them from charring, or use metal skewers.

Meanwhile, lightly spray the grill with olive oil spray. Preheat on medium high.

Put 6 mushrooms on each of two skewers. On the remaining two skewers, alternate the tomatoes and basil leaves, beginning and ending with a tomato. (The zucchini slices don't go on the skewers.) Lightly spray the surface of the zucchini, mushrooms, and tomatoes with the margarine spray. Sprinkle with the salt and pepper.

Grill the zucchini and the vegetables on the skewers for 8 to 12 minutes, or until lightly charred and the desired doneness, turning the zucchini occasionally, the tomatoes frequently, and the mushrooms once. Remove the zucchini and the skewers from the grill as they become done. Lightly brush with the vinegar before serving.

PER SERVING

calories 37
total fat 0.5 g
  saturated fat 0.0 g
  trans fat 0.0 g
  polyunsaturated fat 0.0 g
  monounsaturated fat 0.0 g

cholesterol 0 mg
sodium 95 mg
carbohydrates 7 g
  fiber 2 g
  sugars 3 g
  protein 3 g

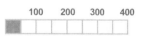

DIETARY EXCHANGES
1 vegetable

vibrant-veggie roast

serves 6; ½ cup per serving

Roast colorful root vegetables and bell pepper, then seal them in aluminum foil and let them stand for a short time so they can slowly release their delicious juices.

- 2 medium carrots, quartered lengthwise and cut crosswise into 3-inch pieces
- 1 medium red bell pepper, cut into 1-inch squares
- 1 medium beet, peeled and cut into ½-inch wedges
- 1 small sweet potato, peeled and cut into 1-inch cubes
- ½ medium red onion, cut into ½-inch wedges
- 12 medium garlic cloves, peeled and left whole
- 1 tablespoon canola or corn oil and 1 ½ teaspoons canola or corn oil, divided use
- ¼ teaspoon salt
- ¼ teaspoon pepper (coarsely ground preferred)

Preheat the oven to 425°F. Line a large baking sheet with aluminum foil.

Place the carrots, bell pepper, beet, sweet potato, onion, and garlic on the baking sheet. Drizzle 1 tablespoon oil over all. Stir together. Arrange in a single layer on the baking sheet.

Roast for 30 minutes, or until the vegetables are tender and beginning to brown on the edges. Remove from the oven.

Drizzle the remaining 1½ teaspoons oil over all. Sprinkle with the salt and pepper. Lift the edges of the foil and make a package to wrap the vegetables and garlic, sealing tightly. Leaving the package on the baking sheet, let stand for 10 to 12 minutes so the flavors blend and the vegetables release their juices. (This is a very important step. Don't skip it.)

COOK'S TIP To help prevent beet stains, peel the beets under running water, and wash your hands and the cutting board right after handling the beets.

PER SERVING

calories 85	cholesterol 0 mg	
total fat 3.5 g	sodium 139 mg	
saturated fat 0.5 g	carbohydrates 12 g	
trans fat 0.0 g	fiber 3 g	
polyunsaturated fat 1.0 g	sugars 4 g	
monounsaturated fat 2.0 g	protein 2 g	

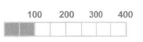

DIETARY EXCHANGES
½ starch, 1 vegetable, ½ fat

breads and breakfast dishes

apple and dried cherry quick bread

serves 18; 1 slice per serving

This fruity loaf is short in stature (only about 2 inches tall) but long in taste.

Cooking spray
2 cups whole-wheat pastry flour or all-purpose flour
⅓ cup firmly packed light or dark brown sugar
2 teaspoons baking powder
1 teaspoon ground cinnamon
1 teaspoon grated lemon zest
⅛ teaspoon salt
1 cup unsweetened applesauce
½ cup unsweetened apple juice
¼ cup egg substitute or 2 large egg whites
1 large apple, such as Granny Smith or Braeburn, peeled and diced
½ cup unsweetened dried cherries

Preheat the oven to 350°F. Lightly spray a 9 x 5 x 3-inch loaf pan with cooking spray. Set aside.

In a large bowl, stir together the flour, brown sugar, baking powder, cinnamon, lemon zest, and salt.

In a medium bowl, whisk together the applesauce, apple juice, and egg substitute. Add the applesauce mixture, apple, and cherries to the flour mixture. Stir until the flour mixture is just moistened but no flour is visible. Don't overmix; the batter should be slightly lumpy. Spoon into the loaf pan, gently smoothing the top.

Bake for 50 to 55 minutes, or until a wooden toothpick inserted in the center comes out clean. Let cool for 5 minutes. Using a metal spatula, loosen the bread from the pan. Turn out onto a cooling rack and let cool completely.

PER SERVING

calories 82	cholesterol 0 mg	
total fat 0.0 g	sodium 69 mg	
saturated fat 0.0 g	carbohydrates 19 g	
trans fat 0.0 g	fiber 2 g	
polyunsaturated fat 0.0 g	sugars 9 g	
monounsaturated fat 0.0 g	protein 2 g	

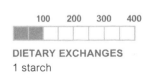

100 200 300 400

DIETARY EXCHANGES
1 starch

pan-style whole-wheat dinner rolls

serves 16; 1 roll per serving

Quick-rise yeast helps speed up the rising process for the fresh-baked goodness of these yeast dinner rolls.

1½ cups whole-wheat flour

1½ cups all-purpose flour

1 ¼-ounce package fast-rising yeast

½ cup fat-free milk

½ cup water

¼ cup egg substitute

2 tablespoons honey

1 tablespoon olive oil

¼ teaspoon salt

Cooking spray

2 tablespoons hulled unsalted sunflower seeds

In a large bowl, stir together the flours. Remove 1 cup flour mixture and set aside. Stir the yeast into the 2 cups flour mixture remaining in the bowl. Set aside.

If using the stove (rather than the microwave), in a small saucepan, cook the milk and water over medium-low heat for 2 to 3 minutes, or until the mixture registers 120°F to 130°F on an instant-read thermometer. (The yeast will not activate if the liquid gets too hot.) If using the microwave, heat the milk and water in a microwaveable container on 100 percent power (high) for 30 seconds, or until the mixture reaches the proper temperature.

Pour the milk mixture into the flour mixture. Stir in the egg substitute, honey, oil, and salt. Beat with a spoon for about 30 seconds, or until smooth.

Gradually add up to ¾ cup of the reserved flour, stirring after each addition, until the dough starts to pull away from the side of the bowl.

Sprinkle the remaining ¼ cup flour over a flat work surface. Put the dough on the floured surface. Knead for 5 to 6 minutes, or until smooth and elastic, adding more flour if needed. Leaving the dough on the flat surface, cover it with a dry dish towel. Let rest for 10 minutes.

Lightly spray a 13 x 9 x 2-inch baking pan with cooking spray.

Press the dough evenly into the pan. Using a dull knife, divide the dough into 16 squares without cutting all the way through. (This will slightly separate the rolls so they will rise and bake together but break apart easily after they are baked.) Sprinkle with the sunflower seeds. Cover with a dry dish towel. Let the dough rise for 30 to 45 minutes, or until doubled in bulk.

Meanwhile, preheat the oven to 400°F.

Bake for 20 to 22 minutes, or until the rolls are golden brown and sound hollow when tapped on the top. Transfer the pan to a cooling rack. Let cool for 5 minutes before separating and serving the rolls.

····· **PER SERVING** ···

calories 108

total fat 2.0 g

  saturated fat 0.0 g

  trans fat 0.0 g

  polyunsaturated fat 0.5 g

  monounsaturated fat 1.0 g

cholesterol 0 mg

sodium 49 mg

carbohydrates 20 g

  fiber 2 g

  sugars 3 g

protein 4 g

100   200   300   400

DIETARY EXCHANGES

1½ starch

blueberry pancakes

serves 5; 2 4-inch pancakes and heaping 1½ tablespoons blueberry topping per serving

Kick-start your day with a healthy dose of fiber and protein from these pancakes, bursting with a double dose of blueberry flavor. Complete your breakfast with a glass of fat-free milk.

¼ cup fat-free plain yogurt

¼ cup all-fruit blueberry spread

½ cup all-purpose flour

⅓ cup whole-wheat flour

¼ cup toasted wheat germ

3 tablespoons firmly packed light brown sugar

¾ teaspoon baking powder

½ teaspoon ground cinnamon

¼ teaspoon baking soda

¾ cup low-fat buttermilk

½ cup unsweetened applesauce

¼ cup egg substitute

1 tablespoon canola or corn oil

½ teaspoon vanilla extract

¾ cup blueberries

....

¼ cup chopped pecans

If your griddle is not large enough to hold 10 pancakes and you want to serve all the pancakes at once, preheat the oven to 200°F. Place a cooling rack on a baking sheet. Set aside.

In a small bowl, whisk together the yogurt and blueberry spread. Set aside.

In a medium bowl, stir together the flours, wheat germ, brown sugar, baking powder, cinnamon, and baking soda.

In a small bowl, whisk together the buttermilk, applesauce, egg substitute, oil, and vanilla. Stir into the flour mixture just until combined but no flour is visible. Don't overmix. Gently fold in the blueberries.

Heat a nonstick griddle over medium heat. Sprinkle a few drops of water on it. If the water evaporates quickly, the griddle is ready. Pour about ¼ cup batter for each pancake onto the griddle (you may need to make several batches). Cook for 2 to 3 minutes, or until bubbles appear all over the surface and the bottoms are golden brown. Turn the pancakes over. Cook for 1 to 2 minutes, or until cooked through and golden brown on the bottoms. Place the pancakes in a single layer on the cooling rack, leaving space between. Don't cover the pancakes. Put in the oven to keep warm. Repeat with the remaining batter (you should have a total of 10 pancakes).

Spoon the blueberry topping over the pancakes. Sprinkle with the pecans.

COOK'S TIP ON NUTS Enjoy about 10 pecan halves for a 100-calorie snack, crush them to add to smoothies, or chop them to top salads.

PER SERVING

calories 273	cholesterol 2 mg
total fat 8.0 g	sodium 200 mg
saturated fat 1.0 g	carbohydrates 44 g
trans fat 0.0 g	fiber 4 g
polyunsaturated fat 2.5 g	sugars 23 g
monounsaturated fat 4.0 g	protein 8 g

100 200 300 400

DIETARY EXCHANGES
2 starch, 1 fruit, 1 fat

peach cornmeal waffles

serves 8; 1 waffle per serving

These homey, peach-studded waffles are perfect for a weekend brunch.

1⅓ cups all-purpose flour

⅔ cup yellow cornmeal

¼ cup sugar

2 teaspoons baking powder

½ teaspoon baking soda

¼ teaspoon ground nutmeg

1½ cups low-fat buttermilk

1 cup diced peaches, fresh, unsweetened frozen, or canned in fruit juice, peeled if fresh, thawed if frozen, or drained if canned

½ cup egg substitute

1 tablespoon canola or corn oil

If you want to serve all the waffles at once, put a large baking sheet in the oven and preheat the oven to 200°F. Preheat a nonstick waffle iron (Belgian or regular) according to the manufacturer's directions.

Meanwhile, in a large bowl, stir together the flour, cornmeal, sugar, baking powder, baking soda, and nutmeg. Make a well in the center.

In a medium bowl, whisk together the remaining ingredients. Pour into the well. Stir just until moistened but no flour is visible. Don't overmix.

Spread a scant ½ cup batter onto the hot waffle iron. Cook for 5 to 7 minutes, or until the waffle is golden brown and cooked through.

As each waffle finishes cooking, transfer it to the baking sheet, making a single layer. Don't cover the waffles. Put in the oven to keep warm. Repeat with the remaining batter (you should have a total of 8 waffles).

PER SERVING

calories 192
total fat 2.5 g
  saturated fat 0.5 g
  trans fat 0.0 g
  polyunsaturated fat 0.5 g
  monounsaturated fat 1.5 g

cholesterol 2 mg
sodium 259 mg
carbohydrates 37 g
  fiber 2 g
  sugars 11 g
protein 6 g

100 200 300 400

DIETARY EXCHANGES
2½ starch

crisp french toast

serves 4; 1½ slices per serving

Thanks mostly to the egg substitute and whole-grain bread, this breakfast dish is protein packed. A coating of coarsely crushed cereal provides the crunchy texture.

1 cup egg substitute

1½ tablespoons fat-free half-and-half

½ teaspoon vanilla extract

1 cup toasted rice flakes cereal, coarsely crushed

1 teaspoon canola or corn oil and 1 teaspoon canola or corn oil, divided use

6 slices whole-grain bread (lowest sodium available), halved lengthwise

Preheat the oven to 200°F.

In a medium shallow dish, whisk together the egg substitute, half-and-half, and vanilla. Spread the cereal crumbs on a large plate. Set the plate next to the dish. Set aside.

In a large nonstick skillet, heat 1 teaspoon oil over medium heat, swirling to coat the bottom.

Quickly dip one piece of bread into the egg substitute mixture, turning to coat and letting any excess drip off. Immediately coat well with the cereal crumbs. Repeat with enough pieces of bread to make one layer in the skillet.

Cook the bread for 1 to 2 minutes on each side, or until the coating is golden brown and the egg is cooked through. Transfer to an oven-proof platter and keep warm, uncovered, in the oven.

Repeat with the remaining 1 teaspoon oil and remaining pieces of bread.

PER SERVING

calories 168	cholesterol 0 mg
total fat 2.0 g	sodium 350 mg
saturated fat 0.5 g	carbohydrates 24 g
trans fat 0.0 g	fiber 3 g
polyunsaturated fat 1.0 g	sugars 5 g
monounsaturated fat 0.5 g	protein 13 g

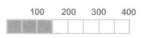

100   200   300   400

DIETARY EXCHANGES

1½ starch, 1 very lean meat

cheesy florentine egg cups

serves 6; 1 egg cup per serving

Portion control is a breeze when a mixture of egg substitute, vegetables, and cheeses is baked in individual muffin cups. The finished product tastes much like a crustless spinach quiche. Enjoy with a bowl of cut-up fresh fruit and half of a whole-grain English muffin.

      Cooking spray
1   teaspoon olive oil
3   ounces chopped button mushrooms
2   medium green onions, chopped
1½   ounces baby spinach
¾   cup egg substitute
½   cup grated low-fat 4-cheese Mexican blend or Cheddar cheese
3   tablespoons shredded or grated Parmesan cheese
1   tablespoon all-purpose flour
¼   teaspoon pepper
¼   teaspoon red hot-pepper sauce

Preheat the oven to 350°F. Lightly spray a 6-cup muffin pan with cooking spray.

In a small nonstick skillet, heat the oil over medium-high heat, swirling to coat the bottom. Cook the mushrooms and green onions for 3 minutes, or until soft, stirring frequently.

Stir in the spinach. Cook for about 1 minute, or until wilted, stirring frequently. Set aside.

In a medium bowl, whisk together the remaining ingredients.

Stir the mushroom mixture into the egg substitute mixture until well blended. Spoon into the muffin cups.

Bake for 25 to 30 minutes, or until the tip of a sharp knife inserted in the center comes out clean and the mixture is slightly golden. If needed for removal, run a flat knife around the inside of the muffin cups.

COOK'S TIP Are you always rushing out the door without breakfast because you have no time? These egg cups may be your solution. Make them ahead, then take one to work, put it on a small plate or a paper towel, place a paper towel on top, and reheat for 20 to 30 seconds on 100 percent (high) in the microwave.

···· PER SERVING ··

calories 73
total fat 3.5 g
  saturated fat 1.5 g
  trans fat 0.0 g
  polyunsaturated fat 0.0 g
  monounsaturated fat 1.0 g

cholesterol 8 mg
sodium 193 mg
carbohydrates 4 g
  fiber 1 g
  sugars 1 g
protein 7 g

100   200   300   400

DIETARY EXCHANGES
1 lean meat

fruit-and-cinnamon oatmeal

serves 4; 1 cup per serving

A steamy bowl of this oatmeal is packed with sweet and fruity flavors—plus a hint of cinnamon—and with protein and fiber to get you ready for your day.

3¾ cups water

2 cups uncooked quick-cooking oatmeal

½ cup raisins or chopped dried apricots

⅓ cup firmly packed dark brown sugar

1 teaspoon ground cinnamon

1 teaspoon light tub margarine (optional)

½ teaspoon vanilla extract or vanilla, butter, and nut flavoring

⅛ teaspoon salt

In a medium saucepan, bring the water to a boil over high heat. Stir in the oatmeal and raisins. Reduce the heat and simmer for 3 minutes, stirring occasionally. Remove from the heat.

Stir in the remaining ingredients.

PER SERVING

calories 292

total fat 2.5 g

  saturated fat 0.5 g

  trans fat 0.0 g

  polyunsaturated fat 1.0 g

  monounsaturated fat 1.0 g

cholesterol 0 mg

sodium 89 mg

carbohydrates 63 g

  fiber 5 g

  sugars 31 g

  protein 7 g

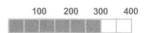

DIETARY EXCHANGES

2 starch, 2 fruit

fruit-and-yogurt breakfast parfaits

serves 4; 1 cup per serving

If you think you don't have time to fix a nourishing breakfast, give this parfait a try. It gives you a combo of dairy, whole grains, and fruit and is ready in minutes.

2 cups fat-free plain yogurt

⅓ cup sweet orange marmalade

1 cup whole-grain wheat-and-barley cereal flakes

1 large banana, sliced

1 cup hulled and sliced strawberries

2 tablespoons toasted wheat germ

In a small bowl, stir together the yogurt and orange marmalade.

In each parfait glass, wine glass, or mug, layer the ingredients as follows: ¼ cup yogurt mixture, ¼ cup cereal, ¼ of the banana slices, ¼ cup strawberries, and ¼ cup yogurt mixture. Top with the wheat germ. Serve soon after preparing so the cereal will remain crisp.

COOK'S TIP If you want to take your breakfast to work, slice a fourth of the banana and put it in a travel mug or insulated container. Add ½ cup of yogurt, 1 heaping tablespoon of marmalade, and ¼ cup of sliced strawberries. Put ¼ cup of cereal and 1½ teaspoons of wheat germ in a snack-size resealable plastic bag. When you get to the office, stir the cereal into the "parfait" and top with the wheat germ. It won't look as pretty, but it will taste just as good.

PER SERVING

calories 228	cholesterol 3 mg
total fat 1.0 g	sodium 157 mg
saturated fat 0.5 g	carbohydrates 48 g
trans fat 0.0 g	fiber 3 g
polyunsaturated fat 0.5 g	sugars 34 g
monounsaturated fat 0.0 g	protein 10 g

100 200 300 400

DIETARY EXCHANGES
1 starch, 1 fruit,
1 fat-free milk

desserts

Peach and Berry Crumble

Peach and Pineapple Upside-Down Cake

Orange and Almond Pudding Cake

Clafouti

Assorted Biscotti

    Cinnamon-Walnut Biscotti

    Dried Fruit and Marsala Biscotti

    Chocolate Chocolate Biscotti

Pumpkin Oatmeal Cookies

Apple and Pear Strudel

Lemon-Blueberry Cream

Mango-Berry Sweet Cream Tarts

Pumpkin Praline Mousse

Tapioca Pudding with Blueberries

Mocha Meringue Shells with Raspberries

Chocolate-Hazelnut Fondue

Fruit Sauce

Citrus Freeze Bars

peach and berry crumble

serves 4; ½ cup per serving

By using frozen fruits, you can whip up this crumble for a little cozy comfort regardless of the season.

Cooking spray
12 ounces frozen unsweetened peach slices, thawed and halved
4 ounces frozen unsweetened raspberries
⅓ cup sweetened dried cranberries
2 teaspoons cornstarch
2 teaspoons fresh orange juice or water
½ teaspoon vanilla extract
⅓ cup uncooked quick-cooking oatmeal
¼ cup sugar
1 tablespoon all-purpose flour
¼ teaspoon ground cinnamon
2 tablespoons light tub margarine

Preheat the oven to 350°F. Lightly spray an 8½ x 4½ x 2½-inch loaf pan with cooking spray.

In a medium bowl, stir together the peaches, raspberries, cranberries, cornstarch, orange juice, and vanilla until the cornstarch is dissolved. Pour into the pan.

In a small bowl, stir together the remaining ingredients except the margarine. Cut the margarine into the oatmeal mixture until the pieces are about the size of small peas. Sprinkle over the peach mixture.

Bake for 25 minutes, or until the peaches are tender. Set aside.

Preheat the broiler. Broil the crumble about 4 inches from the heat for 3 to 4 minutes, or until the topping begins to brown. Remove from the broiler. Let stand for about 30 minutes so the flavors blend.

···· PER SERVING ···

calories 193	cholesterol 0 mg	
total fat 3.5 g	sodium 46 mg	100 200 300 400
saturated fat 0.0 g	carbohydrates 39 g	
trans fat 0.0 g	fiber 4 g	**DIETARY EXCHANGES**
polyunsaturated fat 1.0 g	sugars 26 g	2½ carbohydrate, ½ fat
monounsaturated fat 1.5 g	protein 2 g	

peach and pineapple upside-down cake

serves 16; 2 x 2-inch piece per serving

This fruity delight is fat-free and fabulous! It's only about 100 calories, all of which definitely are the upside to this upside-down cake.

    Cooking spray

⅓ cup firmly packed light brown sugar

1 8-ounce can sliced peaches in fruit juice

1 8-ounce can pineapple tidbits in their own juice

1½ cups whole-wheat pastry flour or all-purpose flour

2 teaspoons baking powder

½ teaspoon ground cinnamon

½ cup sugar

½ cup unsweetened applesauce

¼ cup egg substitute

1 teaspoon vanilla extract

Preheat the oven to 350°F. Lightly spray an 8-inch square baking pan with cooking spray.

Sprinkle the brown sugar in the pan.

Drain the peaches and pineapple well, reserving a total of ¾ cup juice. Chop the peaches. Arrange the peaches and pineapple attractively on the brown sugar. Set aside.

In a large bowl, stir together the flour, baking powder, and cinnamon. Make a well in the center.

In a medium bowl, whisk together the ¾ cup reserved fruit juice and remaining ingredients. Pour into the well in the flour mixture. Stir just until the flour mixture is moistened but no flour is visible. Spread the batter in the pan.

Bake for 45 minutes, or until a wooden toothpick inserted in the center comes out clean. Transfer the pan to a cooling rack. Let cool for 5 minutes. Invert the cake onto a large, flat plate. Let cool for about 30 minutes.

COOK'S TIP ON WHOLE-WHEAT PASTRY FLOUR Whole-wheat pastry flour is lighter than regular whole-wheat flour and thus makes a lighter finished product. Try it in recipes for pancakes, muffins, cakes, and other baked goods. If you don't have the pastry flour, use white flour—regular whole-wheat flour will make the end result too heavy.

PER SERVING

calories 102
total fat 0.0 g
  saturated fat 0.0 g
  trans fat 0.0 g
  polyunsaturated fat 0.0 g
  monounsaturated fat 0.0 g

cholesterol 0 mg
sodium 61 mg
carbohydrates 24 g
  fiber 2 g
  sugars 15 g
  protein 2 g

100   200   300   400

DIETARY EXCHANGES
1½ carbohydrate

orange and almond pudding cake

serves 16; 2 x 2-inch piece per serving

In the mood for a sweet nothing? Then try this cake with its next-to-nothing calories! Enjoy a thin top layer of spongy cake and a second layer with the consistency of pudding or custard for less than 70 calories.

Cooking spray

1 tablespoon sugar and ½ cup sugar, divided use

2 large egg whites, at room temperature

⅛ teaspoon salt

½ cup egg substitute

⅓ cup low-fat buttermilk

1 to 2 tablespoons grated orange zest

½ cup plus 2 tablespoons fresh orange juice, or ½ cup fresh orange juice and 2 tablespoons almond liqueur

1 tablespoon canola or corn oil

¾ to 1 teaspoon almond extract

¼ cup all-purpose flour

1 teaspoon baking soda

3 tablespoons chopped almonds

Preheat the oven to 350°F. Lightly spray an 8-inch square baking pan with cooking spray. Coat the bottom and sides of the pan with 1 tablespoon sugar, shaking out any excess. Set aside.

In a medium mixing bowl, using an electric mixer on medium-high speed, beat the egg whites and salt until stiff peaks form (the peaks stand upright when the beaters are lifted). Set aside.

In a large mixing bowl, using the same beaters (no need to rinse them), beat the egg substitute, buttermilk, orange zest, orange juice, oil, almond extract, and remaining ½ cup sugar at medium speed for 1 minute, or until the mixture is smooth.

Add the flour and baking soda. Beat at low speed for about 30 seconds, just until no flour is visible.

With a rubber scraper, gently fold the egg whites into the batter. Pour into the pan. Sprinkle with the almonds.

Place the filled baking pan in a 13 x 9 x 2-inch baking pan. To avoid spills, put the two pans in the oven, then fill the larger pan with hot water to halfway up the sides of the smaller baking pan. (This is known as a *bain-marie*, or water bath.)

Bake for 30 to 35 minutes, or until the top of the cake is golden brown and slightly spongy to the touch. Remove the cake pan from the water bath and transfer to a cooling rack. Let cool for at least 15 minutes. Serve warm or at room temperature.

COOK'S TIP Substitute an orange liqueur for the almond liqueur; lemon or orange extract for the almond extract; or chopped walnuts with walnut extract or chopped pecans with maple extract for the almonds and almond extract.

COOK'S TIP ON A WATER BATH, OR BAIN-MARIE A water bath, or *bain-marie,* is used for melting ingredients such as butter or chocolate without burning them, or for baking cakes, custards, or cheesecakes when a slow and gentle process is required.

PER SERVING

calories 68
total fat 1.5 g
  saturated fat 0.0 g
  trans fat 0.0 g
  polyunsaturated fat 0.5 g
  monounsaturated fat 1.0 g

cholesterol 0 mg
sodium 125 mg
carbohydrates 11 g
  fiber 0 g
  sugars 9 g
protein 2 g

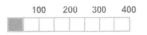

100   200   300   400

DIETARY EXCHANGES
½ carbohydrate, ½ fat

clafouti

serves 8; 1 wedge per serving

You'll find clafouti, usually made with dark cherries, in many French bistros.

Cooking spray
1 pound fresh dark cherries, pitted, or frozen pitted cherries
2 tablespoons firmly packed light brown sugar
½ teaspoon ground cinnamon
¼ teaspoon ground nutmeg
1 cup low-fat buttermilk
¾ cup egg substitute
2 teaspoons grated lemon zest
2 tablespoons almond liqueur or fresh lemon juice
1 tablespoon canola or corn oil
1 teaspoon almond extract
⅓ cup all-purpose flour
⅓ cup sugar
⅛ teaspoon salt

Preheat the oven to 375°F. Lightly spray an 8-inch round cake pan with cooking spray. Place the pan on a rimmed baking sheet.

Place the cherries in the pan. Set aside.

In a small bowl, combine the brown sugar, cinnamon, and nutmeg.

In a food processor, process the buttermilk, egg substitute, lemon zest, liqueur, oil, and almond extract for 30 seconds. Stir in the flour, sugar, and salt. Process for 30 seconds. Pour the batter over the cherries. Top with the brown sugar mixture.

Bake for 55 minutes to 1 hour, or until the clafouti is puffed and golden brown and a wooden toothpick inserted in the center comes out clean. Transfer the pan to a cooling rack. Let cool for about 10 minutes.

PER SERVING

calories 149	cholesterol 1 mg
total fat 2.5 g	sodium 119 mg
saturated fat 0.5 g	carbohydrates 27 g
trans fat 0.0 g	fiber 1 g
polyunsaturated fat 0.5 g	sugars 20 g
monounsaturated fat 1.0 g	protein 4 g

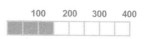

DIETARY EXCHANGES
2 carbohydrate, ½ fat

assorted biscotti

serves 10; 2 cookies per serving

Biscotti are wonderful cookies to dunk in your favorite fat-free milk, coffee, tea, or dessert wine—just remember those calories count, too! Follow the same basic instructions below for whichever of the three delectable flavors you choose.

cinnamon-walnut biscotti

DRY INGREDIENTS

- 2 cups all-purpose flour
- ½ cup sugar
- ½ cup chopped walnuts
- 1½ teaspoons baking powder
- ½ teaspoon ground cinnamon
- ¼ teaspoon salt

WET INGREDIENTS

- 1 large egg
- 2 large egg whites
- ¼ cup fat-free milk

....

- 1 large egg white, lightly beaten

dried fruit and marsala biscotti

DRY INGREDIENTS

- 2 cups all-purpose flour
- ½ cup unsweetened dried cherries, chopped to the size of raisins
- ½ cup dried apricots, chopped to the size of raisins
- ⅓ cup sugar
- 1½ teaspoons baking powder
- ¼ teaspoon salt

WET INGREDIENTS

- 1 large egg
- 2 large egg whites
- ¼ cup dry marsala or unsweetened apple juice

....

- 1 large egg white, lightly beaten

(continued on next page)

chocolate chocolate biscotti

DRY INGREDIENTS

2 cups all-purpose flour

½ cup sugar

½ cup milk chocolate morsels

¼ cup unsweetened cocoa powder (dark preferred)

1½ teaspoons baking powder

¼ teaspoon salt

WET INGREDIENTS

1 large egg

2 large egg whites

¼ cup fat-free milk (plus up to 2 tablespoons as needed)

....

1 large egg white, lightly beaten

Preheat the oven to 375°F. Line a rimmed baking sheet with cooking parchment. Set aside.

In a large bowl, stir together the dry ingredients. For the Dried Fruit and Marsala Biscotti, be sure the pieces of dried fruit are separated.

In a small bowl, whisk together the wet ingredients.

Stir the wet ingredients into the dry ingredients. If the Chocolate Chocolate Biscotti batter doesn't hold together, gradually stir in the extra milk as needed. Divide the dough in half. Form each half into a log 10 to 12 inches long. Place the logs on the baking sheet. Brush with the remaining egg white.

Bake the Cinnamon-Walnut Biscotti and the Dried Fruit and Marsala Biscotti for 15 to 20 minutes, or until the top of the log is golden. Bake the Chocolate Chocolate Biscotti for 20 minutes. Leave the oven on.

Transfer the logs to a cooling rack. Let cool for 5 minutes. Cut each log on the diagonal into 10 slices. Place the slices with one cut side up on the baking sheet.

Bake for 10 to 15 minutes, or until the cut side of the Cinnamon-Walnut Biscotti and the Dried Fruit and Marsala Biscotti is golden and the cut side of the Chocolate Chocolate Biscotti is firm to the touch. Transfer to a cooling rack. Let cool completely. Store the biscotti in an airtight container for up to two weeks at room temperature or freeze them for up to three months.

CINNAMON-WALNUT BISCOTTI
PER SERVING

calories 183	cholesterol 21 mg
total fat 4.5 g	sodium 145 mg
saturated fat 0.5 g	carbohydrates 31 g
trans fat 0.0 g	fiber 1 g
polyunsaturated fat 3.0 g	sugars 11 g
monounsaturated fat 0.5 g	protein 5 g

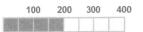

DIETARY EXCHANGES
2 carbohydrate, 1 fat

DRIED FRUIT AND MARSALA BISCOTTI
PER SERVING

calories 177	cholesterol 21 mg
total fat 1.0 g	sodium 143 mg
saturated fat 0.0 g	carbohydrates 36 g
trans fat 0.0 g	fiber 2 g
polyunsaturated fat 0.0 g	sugars 14 g
monounsaturated fat 0.0 g	protein 5 g

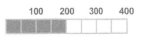

DIETARY EXCHANGES
2½ carbohydrate

CHOCOLATE CHOCOLATE BISCOTTI
PER SERVING

calories 198	cholesterol 23 mg
total fat 3.5 g	sodium 151 mg
saturated fat 2.0 g	carbohydrates 36 g
trans fat 0.0 g	fiber 1 g
polyunsaturated fat 0.5 g	sugars 15 g
monounsaturated fat 1.0 g	protein 6 g

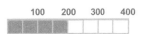

DIETARY EXCHANGES
2½ carbohydrate, ½ fat

pumpkin oatmeal cookies

serves 12; 2 cookies per serving

Pumpkin, rolled oats, and whole-wheat flour make these soft and chewy oatmeal cookies more healthful than most you can buy at the supermarket or bakery. Have two for dessert or for a snack with a glass of fat-free milk.

Cooking spray

2 cups uncooked rolled oats or quick-cooking oatmeal

½ cup all-purpose flour

½ cup whole-wheat flour

1½ teaspoons pumpkin pie spice

½ teaspoon baking powder

½ teaspoon baking soda

⅛ teaspoon salt

¾ cup canned solid-pack pumpkin (not pie filling)

⅓ cup sugar

¼ cup firmly packed light brown sugar

1 large egg white, lightly beaten

1 tablespoon canola or corn oil

1 tablespoon molasses (light or dark)

1 teaspoon vanilla extract

⅓ cup raisins

Preheat the oven to 375°F. Lightly spray two baking sheets with cooking spray. Set aside.

In a medium bowl, stir together the oats, flours, pie spice, baking powder, baking soda, and salt.

In a separate medium bowl, whisk together the remaining ingredients except the raisins.

Add the oat mixture, stirring just until combined but no flour is visible. Stir in the raisins just until blended in. Don't overmix.

Drop the dough by tablespoonfuls, about 1 ½ inches apart, onto the baking sheets. Using your hands or the back of a spoon, lightly flatten the dough until about ¼ inch thick (the dough will be slightly sticky).

Bake for 10 to 12 minutes, or until the cookies begin to lightly brown around the edges. Remove the cookies from the baking sheets and transfer to a cooling rack. For soft, yet slightly crisp (especially around the edges) cookies, let cool for about 10 minutes. For softer cookies that have more the texture of a breakfast bar, let them cool completely, about 1 hour.

······ **PER SERVING** ···

calories 165	cholesterol 0 mg
total fat 2.5 g	sodium 107 mg
saturated fat 0.5 g	carbohydrates 33 g
trans fat 0.0 g	fiber 3 g
polyunsaturated fat 0.5 g	sugars 15 g
monounsaturated fat 1.0 g	protein 4 g

100   200   300   400

DIETARY EXCHANGES
2 carbohydrate, ½ fat

apple and pear strudel

serves 8; 1 slice per serving

Using frozen phyllo dough really reduces the preparation time for this mouthwatering dessert and helps control the calories, saturated fat, and cholesterol, since traditional strudel dough uses lots of butter.

Cooking spray

filling

4 medium baking apples, such as Honey Crisp or Rome, peeled, cored, and thinly sliced

1 medium Anjou or Bartlett pear, thinly sliced

⅓ cup sugar

¼ cup raisins or diced dried apricots

1 tablespoon all-purpose flour

2 teaspoons ground cinnamon

¼ teaspoon ground nutmeg

pastry

1 large egg white

2 tablespoons light olive oil or canola oil

⅛ teaspoon salt

6 sheets frozen phyllo dough (each 18 x 14 inches), thawed

2 tablespoons plain dry bread crumbs (lowest sodium available)

1 teaspoon sugar

Set the oven rack on the upper level of the oven. Preheat the oven to 350°F. Lightly spray a baking sheet with cooking spray. Set aside.

In a large bowl, stir together the filling ingredients. Set aside.

In a small bowl, lightly beat together the egg white, oil, and salt.

Keeping the unused phyllo covered with a damp cloth or damp paper towels to prevent drying, lay a sheet of phyllo with one long side toward you on a flat work surface. Working quickly, use a pastry brush to lightly coat the surface of the phyllo sheet with the egg white mixture. Sprinkle evenly with ½ teaspoon bread crumbs. Repeat with the remaining phyllo and bread crumbs, making a stack of the 6 phyllo sheets.

Spread the filling along the long side of the dough nearest you. Starting at that side, roll up jelly-roll style into a cylinder. Place the roll with the seam side down on the baking sheet. Brush with the remaining egg white mixture. Sprinkle with the remaining 1 teaspoon sugar.

Bake for 25 to 30 minutes, or until golden brown. Transfer the baking sheet to a cooling rack. Let the strudel stand until it has slightly cooled but is still warm. Cut into 8 slices (a bread knife works well for this). Serve warm. If you have leftover strudel, reheat it, uncovered, in a preheated 350°F oven for 10 minutes.

COOK'S TIP ON LIGHT OLIVE OIL Light olive oil has a milder flavor than regular olive oil. The calories and fat are the same, however.

PER SERVING

calories 200	cholesterol 0 mg
total fat 4.0 g	sodium 126 mg
saturated fat 0.5 g	carbohydrates 41 g
trans fat 0.0 g	fiber 3 g
polyunsaturated fat 0.5 g	sugars 23 g
monounsaturated fat 2.5 g	protein 3 g

100 200 300 400

DIETARY EXCHANGES
2½ carbohydrate, 1 fat

lemon-blueberry cream

serves 8 in ramekins; ⅔ cup per serving
serves 10 in pie pan; ½ cup per serving

Serve this light, luscious, lemony dessert immediately in individual ramekins or freeze it in a deep-dish pie pan.

½ cup low-fat graham cracker crumbs

½ teaspoon ground cinnamon

12 ounces fat-free lemon yogurt

8 ounces frozen fat-free whipped topping, thawed in refrigerator

2 teaspoons grated lemon zest

2 tablespoons fresh lemon juice

1 cup fresh or frozen unsweetened blueberries, partially thawed and patted dry if frozen

In a small bowl, stir together the crumbs and cinnamon. Set aside.

In a large bowl, whisk together the yogurt, whipped topping, lemon zest, and lemon juice.

Gently stir the blueberries into the yogurt mixture. Spoon into 8 ramekins or a 9-inch deep-dish pie pan. Sprinkle with the crumb mixture. Serve if using the ramekins; freeze for 2 to 3 hours, or until firm, if using the pie pan. Remove the pie from the freezer 15 to 20 minutes before serving.

RAMEKINS
PER SERVING

calories 177	cholesterol 21 mg
total fat 1.0 g	sodium 143 mg
saturated fat 0.0 g	carbohydrates 36 g
trans fat 0.0 g	fiber 2 g
polyunsaturated fat 0.0 g	sugars 14 g
monounsaturated fat 0.0 g	protein 5 g

100 200 300 400

DIETARY EXCHANGES
2½ carbohydrate

PIE
PER SERVING

calories 99	cholesterol 1 mg
total fat 0.5 g	sodium 58 mg
saturated fat 0.0 g	carbohydrates 20 g
trans fat 0.0 g	fiber 1 g
polyunsaturated fat 0.0 g	sugars 12 g
monounsaturated fat 0.0 g	protein 2 g

100 200 300 400

DIETARY EXCHANGES
1½ carbohydrate

mango-berry sweet cream tarts

serves 5; 3 tarts per serving

These creamy bite-size fruit pastries weigh in just a bit over 100 calories per serving, making them an ideal appetizer, snack, or dessert. If you are having a party, double the recipe. The tarts will brighten your buffet table, and they're so delicious that your guests won't believe they're healthy, too!

- 3 tablespoons fat-free tub cream cheese, at room temperature
- 1 tablespoon sugar
- 1 tablespoon fat-free milk
- ¼ teaspoon vanilla extract
- 1 1.9-ounce package frozen mini phyllo shells (15 mini shells), thawed
- ¼ cup apricot all-fruit spread
- ¼ cup mango chunks, diced
- ½ cup hulled strawberries, diced, or ¼ cup hulled strawberries, diced, and ¼ cup diced pineapple tidbits canned in their own juice, well drained

In a small bowl, stir together the cream cheese, sugar, milk, and vanilla until smooth. Spoon about 1 teaspoon mixture into each shell.

In a small microwaveable bowl, microwave the apricot spread on high for 15 seconds, or until slightly melted. Stir. Spoon over the cream cheese mixture in the shells. Top with the fruit. Serve immediately, or cover and refrigerate for up to 2 hours before serving. (The shells will become soggy if filled too far in advance.)

COOK'S TIP You can make the filling up to 24 hours in advance. Cover and refrigerate until you're ready to assemble the tarts.

PER SERVING

calories 110
total fat 3.0 g
  saturated fat 0.0 g
  trans fat 0.0 g
  polyunsaturated fat 0.0 g
  monounsaturated fat 0.0 g

cholesterol 1 mg
sodium 96 mg
carbohydrates 19 g
  fiber 1 g
  sugars 12 g
  protein 2 g

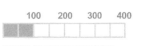

DIETARY EXCHANGES
1½ carbohydrate, ½ fat

pumpkin praline mousse

serves 10; ½ cup per serving

An alternative to traditional pumpkin pie, this mousse is incredibly delicious. If you're in a hurry, leave off the praline topping.

- 1 30-ounce can pumpkin pie filling (not canned solid-pack pumpkin)
- 8 ounces frozen fat-free whipped topping and 4 ounces frozen fat-free whipped topping, thawed in refrigerator, divided use
- ½ teaspoon vanilla extract

Cooking spray

topping

- ¼ cup sugar
- ¼ cup chopped pecans
- ½ teaspoon ground cinnamon

In a large mixing bowl, using an electric mixer on medium-high speed, beat the pie filling, 8 ounces whipped topping, and the vanilla for 2 to 4 minutes, or until light and fluffy. Spoon the mousse into a large serving bowl or 10 ramekins or stemmed glasses. Cover and refrigerate for at least 1 hour before serving.

Meanwhile, line a small baking sheet with aluminum foil. Lightly spray with cooking spray.

In a small, heavy skillet, cook the sugar over medium heat for 6 to 10 minutes, or until it dissolves and liquefies, stirring frequently with a heatproof spoon (a rubber scraper will melt). Stir in the pecans and cinnamon. Reduce the heat to low. Cook for 30 seconds to 1 minute, or until golden. Quickly spread on the baking sheet. Let cool completely, 10 to 15 minutes. Break the praline topping into small pieces.

To serve, spoon the remaining 4 ounces whipped topping over the mousse. Sprinkle with the praline topping.

PER SERVING

calories 186	cholesterol 0 mg
total fat 2.5 g	sodium 134 mg
saturated fat 0.0 g	carbohydrates 37 g
trans fat 0.0 g	fiber 2 g
polyunsaturated fat 0.5 g	sugars 26 g
monounsaturated fat 1.0 g	protein 1 g

100 200 300 400

DIETARY EXCHANGES
2½ carbohydrate, ½ fat

tapioca pudding with blueberries

serves 4; ½ cup pudding and ½ cup blueberries per serving

A creamy layer of tapioca pudding blankets antioxidant-rich blueberries—a full fruit serving per person—in this comforting dessert.

1¼ cups fat-free milk or water

¼ cup egg substitute

3 tablespoons uncooked quick-cooking tapioca

¾ cup fat-free half-and-half

3 tablespoons sugar

1½ teaspoons vanilla extract

2 cups blueberries, patted dry

2 tablespoons all-fruit apricot spread

In a medium saucepan, whisk together the milk, egg substitute, and tapioca. Let stand for 5 minutes. Cook over medium heat for 12 to 15 minutes, or until it comes to a full boil (doesn't stop bubbling when stirred) and begins to thicken, whisking constantly.

Whisk in the half-and-half and sugar. Cook for 2 minutes, whisking constantly. Remove from the heat. Whisk in the vanilla.

Spoon the blueberries into four custard cups, ramekins, or wine glasses, reserving 4 blueberries for a garnish. Spoon the tapioca mixture over the blueberries. Top each serving with the apricot spread. Garnish each with a blueberry. Refrigerate, covered, for at least 2 hours. Serve chilled.

···· **PER SERVING** ····

calories 197

total fat 0.5 g
  saturated fat 0.0 g
  trans fat 0.0 g
  polyunsaturated fat 0.0 g
  monounsaturated fat 0.0 g

cholesterol 2 mg
sodium 109 mg
carbohydrates 43 g
  fiber 2 g
  sugars 28 g
protein 8 g

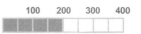

DIETARY EXCHANGES
1 starch, 1 fruit,
1 fat-free milk

mocha meringue shells with raspberries

serves 4; 2 meringues per serving

Vanilla-tinged raspberries nestle in airy, crunchy, chocolaty shells to create a sweet and satisfying dessert for less than 100 calories.

meringues

¼ cup sugar

1 tablespoon unsweetened dark cocoa powder

2 large egg whites, at room temperature

¼ teaspoon cream of tartar

¼ teaspoon vanilla extract

¼ teaspoon almond extract

⅛ teaspoon salt

Cooking spray

filling

1 cup fresh or frozen unsweetened raspberries, thawed and patted dry if frozen

1 tablespoon confectioners' sugar and 1 teaspoon confectioners' sugar, divided use

1 teaspoon vanilla extract

Preheat the oven to 275°F. Line a baking sheet with aluminum foil. Set aside.

In a small bowl, stir together the sugar and cocoa.

In a medium mixing bowl, using an electric mixer on high speed, beat the egg whites until frothy. Add the cream of tartar, extracts, and salt. Beat until soft peaks form. Gradually add the sugar mixture, 1 table-spoon at a time, beating until stiff peaks form (the peaks stand upright when the beaters are lifted). The mixture should remain glossy and not feel grainy when rubbed with your fingers.

Drop the meringue mixture onto the baking sheet to make eight mounds, about 2 inches apart. Lightly coat the back of a tablespoon with cooking spray. Press down gently in the center of each mound to make a well.

Bake for 1 hour. Turn off the oven. Leave the meringues in the oven for 2 hours, or until completely cooled and crisp.

Meanwhile, in a small bowl, gently stir together the raspberries, 1 tablespoon confectioners' sugar, and remaining 1 teaspoon vanilla. Spoon about 2 tablespoons raspberry mixture into each shell. Using a fine-mesh sieve, sprinkle the remaining 1 teaspoon confectioners' sugar over all.

COOK'S TIP ON BEATING EGG WHITES Even a single drop of egg yolk will prevent egg whites from forming peaks when beaten, so separate eggs very carefully.

COOK'S TIP ON MERINGUES Like other meringues, these shells should not be made on a humid day. They will get a little gummy and will lose their crispness.

······ **PER SERVING** ···

calories 93	cholesterol 0 mg	
total fat 0.5 g	sodium 101 mg	
saturated fat 0.0 g	carbohydrates 20 g	
trans fat 0.0 g	fiber 2 g	
polyunsaturated fat 0.0 g	sugars 17 g	
monounsaturated fat 0.0 g	protein 2 g	

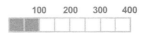

DIETARY EXCHANGES
1½ carbohydrate

chocolate-hazelnut fondue

serves 8; ½ cup fruit and 2 tablespoons fondue per serving

If you're a chocoholic, this recipe is for you. Fresh fruit never had it so good! You can also use the fondue as a sauce to top fat-free frozen vanilla yogurt.

- 1 cup hulled fresh strawberries, halved if large
- 1 cup fresh pineapple chunks
- 1 cup thickly sliced banana
- 1 cup cubed fresh peaches

fondue

- ¾ cup fat-free chocolate syrup
- ¼ cup bottled chocolate-hazelnut spread
- ¼ teaspoon vanilla extract

Put the strawberries, pineapple, banana, and peaches in separate small bowls. Set aside.

In a small, heavy saucepan, stir together the fondue ingredients. Cook over medium heat for 4 to 5 minutes, or until heated through, stirring frequently. Pour into a serving dish or small fondue pot. Serve warm or at room temperature. (As it cools, the sauce will thicken slightly.)

To serve, spear the fruit with fondue forks or wooden skewers and dip into the fondue.

COOK'S TIP ON BANANAS To keep banana slices from turning brown, dip them in a small amount of orange, lemon, or pineapple juice.

PER SERVING

calories 164
total fat 2.5 g
  saturated fat 0.5 g
  trans fat 0.0 g
  polyunsaturated fat 0.5 g
  monounsaturated fat 1.5 g

cholesterol 0 mg
sodium 22 mg
carbohydrates 35 g
  fiber 2 g
  sugars 23 g
protein 1 g

100 200 300 400

DIETARY EXCHANGES
1 fruit, 1½ carbohydrate,
½ fat

fruit sauce

Expand your culinary horizons by experimenting with two classic, fragrant spices—cardamom and nutmeg. This super-easy, velvety sauce is a great place to begin. For rich flavor with few calories, try it on your favorite fruit or stir ½ cup fat-free vanilla yogurt into the finished sauce and serve it chilled.

- 1 medium mango, diced
- ½ cup canned apricot halves in extra-light syrup, drained
- 2 tablespoons fresh orange juice
- 1 tablespoon light brown sugar
- 1 teaspoon grated lemon zest
- ⅛ teaspoon ground cardamom or allspice
- ⅛ teaspoon ground nutmeg

In a food processor or blender, process all the ingredients for 1 to 2 minutes, or until smooth. Serve or cover and refrigerate for up to four days. To serve warm, heat in a small saucepan over medium-low heat for 2 to 3 minutes, or until heated through, stirring occasionally.

COOK'S TIP ON CARDAMOM Cardamom pods hold several small black seeds that are very fragrant. You can grind the seeds with a mortar and pestle or purchase cardamom already ground. Visit a gourmet grocery that sells spices by the ounce so you can experiment with small amounts at a reasonable cost.

PER SERVING

calories 33	cholesterol 0 mg
total fat 0.0 g	sodium 2 mg
saturated fat 0.0 g	carbohydrates 9 g
trans fat 0.0 g	fiber 1 g
polyunsaturated fat 0.0 g	sugars 8 g
monounsaturated fat 0.0 g	protein 0 g

100 200 300 400

DIETARY EXCHANGES
½ fruit

citrus freeze bars

serves 15; 3 x 1¾-inch bar per serving

A nice balance of sweet and tart, this chilled dessert is refreshing and super simple to make. While you take it easy on the prep, the creamy bars take it easy, too—on your waistline.

Cooking spray

25 whole low-fat vanilla wafers and 5 low-fat vanilla wafers, crumbled, divided use

1 14.5-ounce can fat-free sweetened condensed milk

¼ cup egg substitute

1 to 2 teaspoons grated lime or lemon zest

⅔ cup fresh lime or lemon juice

8 ounces frozen fat-free whipped topping, thawed in refrigerator

Lightly spray a 9-inch square baking pan with cooking spray. Arrange 25 cookies in a single layer in the pan. (There will be spaces between the cookies.) Set aside.

Pour the milk and egg substitute into a medium bowl. Add the lime zest and lime juice. Stir for 3 to 4 minutes, or until the mixture begins to thicken.

Fold the whipped topping into the mixture. Pour over the cookies in the baking pan. Sprinkle with the cookie crumbs. Cover and freeze for about 4 hours, or until frozen. Before serving, let the mixture thaw for 4 to 5 minutes, or just until you can easily cut it into bars.

PER SERVING

calories 137
total fat 0.5 g
  saturated fat 0.0 g
  trans fat 0.0 g
  polyunsaturated fat 0.0 g
  monounsaturated fat 0.0 g

cholesterol 1 mg
sodium 71 mg
carbohydrates 29 g
  fiber 0 g
  sugars 22 g
protein 3 g

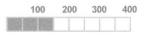

DIETARY EXCHANGES
2 carbohydrate

part III
No-Fad Toolkit

my personal weight-loss plan

Date: _____ My current weight is _____.

My long-term weight-loss goal is

to lose _____ pounds by _____.

My short-term weight-loss goals are to lose

1. _____ pounds by_____.

2. _____ pounds by_____.

3. _____ pounds by_____.

I will achieve my goals through these specific actions.
(Be sure to include what, when, and how.)

1. _____

2. _____

3. _____

I will evaluate my progress at these two-week intervals.

1. _____

2. _____

3. _____

The rewards for reaching my goals are

1. _____

2. _____

3. _____

my daily food diary

TIME/PLACE	FOOD OR BEVERAGE (TYPE AND AMOUNT)	CALORIES	WHAT PROMPTED YOU TO EAT? WHY THIS FOOD CHOICE?
Date: ❏ Mon ❏ Tues ❏ Wed ❏ Thurs ❏ Fri ❏ Sat ❏ Sun			
BREAKFAST			
SNACK			
LUNCH			
SNACK			
DINNER			
SNACK			
TOTAL DAILY CALORIES:			

switch and swap food substitutions

FOR BREAKFAST, INSTEAD OF . . .	CALORIES	TRY . . .	CALORIES	CALORIE SAVINGS!
1 large bakery blueberry muffin	490	1 slice whole-grain toast with 2 teaspoons all-fruit blueberry spread	97	393
1 large plain bagel with 2 tablespoons cream cheese	459	2 plain mini bagels with 1 tablespoon light tub cream cheese	164	295
1 fast-food egg biscuit	350	1 *Cheesy Florentine Egg Cup* (page 386)	73	277
1 bakery cinnamon roll	410	1 whole-grain cinnamon raisin English muffin with 2 teaspoons light tub margarine	161	249
1 bakery apple Danish pastry	300	1 slice *Apple and Dried Cherry Quick Bread* (page 379) with 1 teaspoon cherry all-fruit spread	95	205
8 ounces low-fat vanilla yogurt	220	8 ounces fat-free, sugar-free vanilla yogurt	125	100

FOR A BEVERAGE, INSTEAD OF . . .	CALORIES	TRY . . .	CALORIES	CALORIE SAVINGS!
16 ounces cola	205	16 ounces diet cola	2	203
8 ounces fast-food strawberry milk shake	280	8 ounces *Cran-Raspberry Smoothies* (page 138)	127	153
8 ounces store-bought café mocha	165	6 ounces coffee with 2 ounces fat-free milk and 1 tablespoon light chocolate syrup	48	177
8 ounces whole milk	146	8 ounces fat-free milk	83	63

FOR AN ENTRÉE, INSTEAD OF . . .	CALORIES	TRY . . .	CALORIES	CALORIE SAVINGS!
1 frozen chicken pot pie	667	1 wedge *Chicken Pot Pie* (page 270)	219	448
1 large fast-food hamburger patty (without the bun) with lettuce, tomato, and condiments	430	1 patty and ½ cup vegetables from *Italian Veggie Burgers* (page 320)	177	253
1 fast-food 6-inch meatball sub	580	1 fast-food 6-inch turkey breast sub	280	300
1 fast-food fish sandwich with tartar sauce and cheese	470	1 serving *Cornmeal-Crusted Catfish with Lemon-Ginger Tartar Sauce* (page 190)	235	235
1 fast-food fried chicken sandwich	530	1 fast-food grilled chicken sandwich	420	110
3 cups tossed salad with 2 tablespoons creamy Caesar salad dressing	157	3 cups tossed salad with 2 tablespoons light Italian salad dressing	75	82
1 cup takeout Chinese Orange Beef	283	1 serving *Orange Beef Stir-Fry* (page 280)	235	48

FOR A SNACK, INSTEAD OF . . .	CALORIES	TRY . . .	CALORIES	CALORIE SAVINGS!
½ cup store-bought trail mix	427	½ cup *Lemon-Ginger Trail Mix* (page 136)	160	267
20 potato chips	310	20 baked potato chips	200	110
¼ cup dry-roasted macadamia nuts with salt	237	¼ cup dry-roasted edamame, lightly salted	130	107
½ cup chocolate ice cream	130	1 sugar-free frozen fudge bar	50	80

FOR A SIDE DISH, INSTEAD OF . . .	CALORIES	TRY . . .	CALORIES	CALORIE SAVINGS!
¾ cup restaurant creamed spinach	260	¾ cup spinach cooked with 1 teaspoon olive oil and minced garlic	70	190
½ cup restaurant baked cinnamon apples	250	1 medium apple, sliced, warmed, sprinkled with cinnamon	95	155
1 medium baked potato with skin, topped with 1 tablespoon each sour cream, butter, shredded Cheddar cheese, and chopped chives	321	1 medium baked potato with skin, topped with 2 tablespoons each light sour cream and salsa	211	110
½ cup store-bought coleslaw	180	½ cup *Multicolored Marinated Slaw* (page 171)	82	98
¾ cup store-bought broccoli-cheese soup	148	¾ cup *Creamy Broccoli Soup with Sour Cream and Cheddar* (page 147)	88	60

FOR DESSERT, INSTEAD OF . . .	CALORIES	TRY . . .	CALORIES	CALORIE SAVINGS!
1 serving bakery pineapple upside-down cake	367	1 piece *Peach and Pineapple Upside-Down Cake* (page 392)	102	265
1 slice traditional pumpkin pie with 2 tablespoons whipped cream	368	½ cup *Pumpkin Praline Mousse* (page 406)	186	182
1 fast-food hot fudge sundae	330	½ cup fat-free frozen vanilla yogurt with 2 tablespoons fat-free chocolate syrup	190	140
½ cup instant vanilla pudding prepared with whole milk	162	½ cup fat-free, sugar-free instant vanilla pudding prepared with fat-free milk	64	98

my menu planner

DATE:	CALORIES	FOOD GROUP*
BREAKFAST		
SNACK		
LUNCH		
SNACK		
DINNER		
DAILY TOTALS:		

*The food groups can be abbreviated as follows:

PRO = Protein from seafood, lean meat or poultry, or vegetarian source

GR = Grain

VG = Vegetable / legume

FR = Fruit

DA = Dairy

FAT = Healthy fats and oils

menu planner chart by food group

1,200 Daily Calories: Aim to include at least 3 vegetable, 3 fruit, 3 grain, 1 to 2 dairy, and 2 protein servings most days.*

	Sample Food Group Combinations	Calories
Breakfast	1 grain, 1 dairy, 1 fruit	about 300
Snack	1 fruit	about 100
Lunch	1 protein, 1 grain, 1 vegetable	about 300
Snack	1 dairy [+1 grain if possible]	about 100
Dinner	1 protein, 1 grain, 2 vegetable	about 400

1,600 Daily Calories: Aim to include at least 3 to 4 vegetable, 3 to 4 fruit, 5 to 6 grain, 2 to 3 dairy, and 2 protein servings most days.*

	Sample Food Group Combinations	Calories
Breakfast	2 grain, 1 dairy, 1 fruit	about 400
Snack	1 fruit	about 100
Lunch	1 protein, 2 grain, 2 vegetable	about 400
Snack	1 dairy, 1 grain	about 200
Dinner	1 protein, 1 grain, 2 vegetable, 1 fruit	about 500

2,000 Daily Calories: Aim to include 4 to 5 vegetable, 4 to 5 fruit, 6 to 8 grain, 2 to 3 dairy, and 2 protein servings most days.*

	Sample Food Group Combinations	Calories
Breakfast	1 grain, 1 dairy, 1 fruit	about 450
Snack	1 dairy, 1 fruit	about 200
Lunch	1 protein, 2 grain, 2 vegetable	about 500
Snack	1 dairy, 1 grain, 1 fruit	about 250
Dinner	1 protein, 2 grain, 2 vegetable, 1 fruit	about 600

*Include at least two servings of fish, preferably oily fish, such as salmon, trout, and tuna, each week. Add up to 2 daily servings of healthy fat if your calorie count allows.

entrée recipes by calorie count and food group*

SOUPS	PER SERVING	
	CALORIES	FOOD GROUP
Egg Drop Soup with Crabmeat and Vegetables (page 152)	122	1 PRO, 1 VG
Wild Rice and Chicken Chowder (page 153)	243	1 PRO, 1 GR, 1 VG
Market-Fresh Fish and Vegetable Soup (page 154)	239	1 PRO, 1 GR, 1 VG
Chicken Minestrone (page 156)	228	1 PRO, 1 GR, 1 VG
Bayou Andouille and Chicken Chowder (page 158)	196	1 PRO, 1 GR, 1 VG
Vegetable Beef Soup (page 160)	240	1 PRO, 1 GR, 1 VG
Slow-Cooker Lentil Soup (page 161)	229	1 PRO, 2 VG

SALADS	PER SERVING	
	CALORIES	FOOD GROUP
Spinach and Salmon Salad with Spicy Orange Dressing (page 179)	212	1 PRO, 1 GR, 2 VG
Tuna Pasta Provençal (page 180)	329	1 PRO, 1 GR, 2 VG
Chicken and Toasted Walnut Salad (page 181)	246	1 PRO, 1 FR
Grilled Chicken and Raspberry Salad (page 182)	305	1 PRO, 2 FR
Flank Steak Salad with Sesame-Lime Dressing (page 184)	231	1 PRO, 2 VG
Cannellini and Black Bean Salad (page 185)	212	1 PRO, 3 VG, ½ FR
Taco Salad with Avocado Dressing (page 186)	328	1 PRO, 1 GR, 1 VG

*PRO indicates protein from seafood, lean meat or poultry, or vegetarian source; GR, grain; VG, vegetable or legume; FR, fruit; DA, dairy; and FAT, healthy fats and oils.

	PER SERVING	
SEAFOOD	**CALORIES**	**FOOD GROUP**
Cornmeal-Crusted Catfish with Lemon-Ginger Tartar Sauce (page 190)	235	1 PRO, 1 GR, 1 FAT
Baked Almond-Crunch Halibut (page 192)	319	1 PRO, 2 VG
Grilled Fish with Cucumber Salsa (page 194)	183	1 PRO, 1 VG
Pasta with Salmon, Roasted Mushrooms, and Asparagus (page 196)	301	1 PRO, 1 GR, 2 VG
Salmon-and-Veggie Patties with Mustard Cream (page 198)	205	1 PRO, 1 GR
Salmon Florentine (page 200)	189	1 PRO, 1 VG
Salmon with Creamy Caper Sauce (page 201)	148	1 PRO
Skillet-Poached Salmon with Wasabi and Soy Sauce (page 202)	205	1 PRO, 1 VG
Tilapia Champignon (page 203)	170	1 PRO, 1 VG
Tilapia en Papillote (page 204)	128	1 PRO
Tilapia and Spinach Roll-Ups with Shallot and White Wine Sauce (page 206)	234	1 PRO, 1 VG
Fish Tacos with Tomato and Avocado Salsa (page 208)	340	1 PRO, 2 GR, 1 VG
Lime-Cilantro Swordfish with Mixed Bean and Pineapple Salsa (page 210)	296	1 PRO, 1 VG, ½ FR
Hazelnut-Crusted Trout with Balsamic Glaze (page 212)	267	1 PRO, 1 GR
Grilled Trout with Horseradish Sour Cream (page 214)	209	1 PRO, 1 FAT
Sweet-Heat Broiled Trout (page 216)	163	1 PRO
Gourmet Tuna-Noodle Casserole (page 217)	323	1 PRO, 2 GR, 1 VG
Tuna Lettuce Wraps with Asian Sauce (page 218)	196	1 PRO
Tuna and Broccoli with Lemon-Caper Brown Rice (page 219)	266	1 PRO, 1 GR, 1 VG
Orange-Ginger Tuna Steaks (page 220)	119	1 PRO
Tuna Steaks with Tarragon Sour Cream (page 221)	175	1 PRO
Scallop and Spinach Sauté (page 222)	188	1 PRO, 2 VG
Tomato-Caper Shrimp with Herbed Feta (page 223)	300	1 PRO, 2 GR, 1 VG
Cumin Shrimp and Rice Toss (page 224)	245	1 PRO, 1 GR, 2 VG

POULTRY	PER SERVING	
	CALORIES	FOOD GROUP
Turkey Cutlets with Chutney Sauce (page 228)	242	1 PRO, 1 FR
Turkey Burgers with Mediterranean Tomato Relish (page 230)	192	1 PRO, 1 VG
Turkish Meatballs (page 232)	220	1 PRO, 1 VG
Turkey Sausage and Lentils with Brown Rice (page 234)	253	1 PRO, 1 GR, 1 VG
Artichoke and Bell Pepper Lasagna (page 236)	212	1 PRO, 1 GR, 2 VG
Slow-Roasted Sage Turkey Breast (page 238)	125	1 PRO
Black-Pepper Chicken (page 239)	155	1 PRO
Southwest Lime Chicken (page 240)	173	1 PRO
Chicken with Zesty Apricot Sauce (page 241)	230	1 PRO, 1 FR
Bistro Chicken with Fresh Asparagus (page 242)	268	1 PRO, 1 GR, 1 VG
Grilled Honey Mustard Chicken with Pineapple Salsa (page 244)	168	1 PRO
Salsa Chicken (page 246)	227	1 PRO, 1 GR, ½ VG
Slow-Cooker White Chili (page 248)	322	1 PRO, 1 GR, 1 VG
Chicken with Herbed Mustard and Green Onion Sauce (page 250)	211	1 PRO
Chicken Breasts with Spinach, Apricots, and Pine Nuts (page 252)	315	1 PRO, 1 GR, 1 VG, ½ FR
Chicken Breasts Stuffed with Goat Cheese, Dates, and Spinach (page 254)	193	1 PRO
Chicken Breasts Stuffed with Fresh Basil and Red Bell Pepper (page 255)	146	1 PRO
Stuffed Chicken Breasts in Lemon-Oregano Tomato Sauce (page 256)	177	1 PRO, 1 VG
Chicken and Snow Pea Stir-Fry (page 258)	222	1 PRO, 1 VG
Chicken and Bow-Ties with Green Beans (page 259)	301	1 PRO, 1 GR, 1 VG
Cheesy Chicken and Quinoa Stir-Fry (page 260)	303	1 PRO, 1 GR, 2 VG
Chicken Fajitas (page 262)	315	1 PRO, 2 GR, 1 VG
Risotto with Porcini Mushrooms and Chicken (page 264)	413	1 PRO, 2 GR, 1 VG
Chicken and Veggies with Noodles (page 266)	311	1 PRO, 1 GR, 1 VG
Chicken Enchiladas (page 268)	312	1 PRO, 2 GR, 2 VG
Chicken Pot Pie (page 270)	219	1 PRO, 2 VG

	PER SERVING	
MEATS	**CALORIES**	**FOOD GROUP**
Beef Tenderloin with Horseradish Cream (page 274)	174	1 PRO
Filet Mignon with Balsamic Berry Sauce (page 276)	215	1 PRO
Honey-Lime Flank Steak (page 278)	188	1 PRO
Broiled Flank Steak in Barbecue-Style Marinade (page 279)	161	1 PRO
Orange Beef Stir-Fry (page 280)	235	1 PRO
Grilled Sirloin Kebabs with Creamy Herb Dipping Sauce (page 282)	222	1 PRO, 1 VG
Satay-Style Sirloin with Peanut Dipping Sauce (page 284)	206	1 PRO
Greek-Style Sirloin Cubes and Olive-Feta Rice (page 286)	356	1 PRO, 1 GR, 1 VG
Beef Stroganoff with Baby Bella Mushrooms (page 288)	340	1 PRO, 1 GR, 1 VG
Slow-Cooker Steak-and-Bean Chili (page 290)	313	1 PRO, 3 VG
Slow-Cooker Barbecue Beef in Pitas (page 292)	255	1 PRO, 1 GR
Meat Loaf with a Twist (page 294)	175	1 PRO
Ground Beef Goulash with Red Wine (page 296)	364	1 PRO, 1 GR, 1 VG
Moussaka-Style Eggplant Casserole (page 298)	287	1 PRO, 1 GR, 2 VG
Chicken-Fried Steak with Creamy Gravy (page 300)	285	1 PRO
Saucy Cube Steaks (page 302)	172	1 PRO
Cube Steaks with Avocado Salsa (page 304)	199	1 PRO, 1 VG
Chopped Beef Hash (page 305)	256	1 PRO, 2 VG
Pork Tenderloin with Cranberry Salsa (page 306)	206	1 PRO, 1 FR
Pork Tenderloin with Orange-Ginger Sweet Potatoes (page 308)	159	1 PRO, 1 VG, ½ FR
Thai Coconut Curry with Pork and Vegetables (page 310)	320	1 PRO, 1 GR, 1 VG
Pork Chops Parmesan (page 312)	237	1 PRO
Ham and Broccoli with Rotini (page 314)	270	1 PRO, 2 GR, 1 VG
Sausage and White Beans with Spinach (page 315)	286	1 PRO, 1 GR

	PER SERVING	
VEGETARIAN ENTRÉES	CALORIES	FOOD GROUP
Fresh Veggie Marinara with Feta (page 318)	373	1 PRO, 1 GR, 3 VG
Italian Veggie Burgers (page 320)	177	1 PRO, 1 VG
Pesto Florentine Pasta (page 321)	250	½ PRO, 1 GR
Pasta e Fagioli Stew (page 322)	312	1 PRO, 1 GR, 2 VG
Stuffed Shells with Arugula and Four Cheeses (page 324)	280	1 PRO, 1 GR, 1 DA
Make-Ahead Manicotti (page 326)	284	1 PRO, 1 GR, 2 VG
Soba Noodles in Peanut Sauce (page 328)	373	1 PRO, 1 GR, 1 VG
Lentils with Basil and Feta (page 329)	251	1 PRO, 1 GR, 1 VG
Spinach and Bean Quesadillas with Homemade Salsa (without sour cream) (page 330)	287	1 PRO, 1 GR, 1 VG
Slow-Cooker Black Bean Chili (page 332)	356	1 PRO, 2 GR, 1 VG
Braised Edamame with Bok Choy (page 334)	288	1 PRO, 1 GR, 2 VG
Mediterranean Wraps (page 335)	311	1 PRO, 1 GR, 3 VG
Miami Pita Sandwiches (page 336)	326	1 PRO, 2 GR, 1 VG
Mediterranean Vegetable Stew (page 337)	184	1 PRO, 3 VG
Broccoli Bake with Three Cheeses (page 338)	206	1 PRO, 2 VG
Spinach and Ricotta Frittata (page 340)	91	1 PRO, ½ DA, 1 VG
One-Pot Vegetable and Grain Medley (page 341)	226	1 PRO, 1½ GR, 2 VG
Cajun Red Beans and Brown Rice (page 342)	277	1 PRO, 1 GR, 3 VG
Fried Rice with Snow Peas, Bell Pepper, and Water Chestnuts (page 344)	199	½ PRO, ½ GR, 2 VG
Almond-Topped Bok Choy, Sugar Snap Pea, and Tofu Stir-Fry (page 346)	229	1 PRO, 1 GR, 1 VG
Speed-Dial Stuffed Peppers (page 348)	258	½ PRO, 1 GR, 2 VG
Creole Ratatouille (page 350)	196	1 PRO, 1 GR, 2 VG
Vegetable and Bulgur Curry (page 352)	375	½ PRO, 2 GR, 1 VG, ½ FR

snack ideas: 50 calories and under

1 cup sugar-free gelatin, any flavor	20
1 medium tomato	20
12 grape tomatoes	24
1 slice fresh pineapple	25
½ cup raw baby carrots	25
½ cup cubed cantaloupe	27
¼ cup green grapes (try these frozen, too!)	28
½ cup sliced peaches	30
½ cup blackberries	31
1 large green bell pepper	33
2 medium apricots	34
1 medium plum	35
¾ cup *Quick Mexican-Style Soup* (page 143)	35
½ cup fruit cocktail, packed in water	38
8 medium strawberries with 1 tablespoon fat-free frozen whipped topping	39
½ cup low-sodium mixed vegetable juice	40
1 whole-wheat breadstick	40
½ cup blueberries	40
1 medium rib of celery with 1 teaspoon low-sodium peanut butter	43
½ cup broccoli florets with 2 tablespoons *Cucumber and Avocado Dip* (page 127)	44
1 ounce fat-free Cheddar cheese	45
1 medium kiwifruit	46
1 cup cubed watermelon	46
1 ounce fat-free Colby cheese	49
3 to 4 ounces fat-free plain yogurt or fat-free, sugar-free yogurt, any flavor	48

snack ideas: 51 to 100 calories

1 rye crispbread with 1 teaspoon all-fruit spread, any flavor	51
1 Asian pear	51
10 sweet cherries	52
½ medium cucumber with 2 tablespoons *Creamy Cannellini Dip* (page 129)	53
½ medium banana	55
½ medium grapefruit	60
2 graham crackers	60
½ cup *Zingy Carrot Salad* (page 169)	60
2 tablespoons raisins	60
½ cup *Cran-Raspberry Smoothies* (page 138)	63
4 ounces fat-free plain yogurt or fat-free, sugar-free yogurt, any flavor	65
2 cups leafy greens with 2 tablespoons light Italian salad dressing	65
2 clementines	70
4 *Crunchy Cinnamon Chips* (page 131)	73
1 large yellow bell pepper with 2 tablespoons *Artichoke and Spinach Dip* (page 128)	74
½ cup raw baby carrots and 2 tablespoons hummus	75
1 *Fruit Kebab with Yucatán Dipping Sauce* (page 132)	75
1 *Fruit Kebab with Poppy Seed Dipping Sauce* (page 133)	79
½ ounce dry-roasted unsalted pistachios (20 kernels)	80
¾ cup *Smoky Roasted Tomato Soup* (page 148)	81
½ medium apple with 1 teaspoon low-sodium peanut butter	81
1 slice *Apple and Dried Cherry Quick Bread* (page 379)	82
¼ cup *Lemon-Ginger Trail Mix* (page 136)	82
2 pieces unsalted whole-grain melba toast with 1 ounce fat-free Swiss cheese	85
½ ounce unsalted almonds	88
1 1-ounce 2% milk mozzarella cheese stick with 1 Roma tomato and fresh basil	90
½ ounce unsalted hazelnuts	92
¼ cup fat-free ranch dressing mixed with 1 cup chopped mixed fresh veggies	92
½ cup *Asian Citrus Salad* (page 173)	93
½ ounce unsalted walnuts	95
1 medium apple	95
2 *Crunchy Cinnamon Chips* (page 131) with ¼ cup *Kiwi-Banana Dip* (page 130)	97
¼ cup dried sweetened cranberries	99
½ cup cooked edamame sprinkled with fresh herbs	100

common foods by calorie count

BEVERAGES	CALORIES
1 cup fat-free milk	85
1 cup frozen lemonade, prepared with water	100
1 cup hot cocoa, made with fat-free milk and 1 tablespoon light chocolate syrup	103
12 ounces light beer	110
1 cup orange juice	112
1 cup unsweetened apple juice	116
5 ounces red wine	120
1 cup pineapple juice	140
BREADS AND BREAKFAST DISHES	
1 piece melba toast, any flavor	20
¼ cup liquid egg substitute	30
1 slice whole-grain bread, light	40
1 medium breadstick (hard)	41
½ cup cooked oat bran	44
1 6-inch corn tortilla	56
1-ounce slice whole-grain bread, regular	69
2 meatless soy protein breakfast link sausages	70
1 small (1 ounce) whole-wheat pita	76
1-ounce slice raisin bread	78
1 medium multigrain hamburger bun (1½ ounces)	113
2 frozen fat-free waffles	120
¾ cup regular or quick-cooking oatmeal, prepared with water	125
1 whole-wheat English muffin	134
2-ounce whole-wheat baguette	140
¾ cup bran nuggets (without milk)	170
1¼ cups high-fiber cereal (without milk)	175
1 3½-inch plain bagel	195

DAIRY PRODUCTS	CALORIES
1 ounce fat-free Cheddar or Colby cheese	45
1 ounce part-skim mozzarella cheese	72
½ cup 1% cottage cheese	82
½ cup fat-free ice cream	100
1 ounce grated Parmesan cheese	129
FRUITS	
½ cup cubed watermelon	23
½ cup sliced strawberries	23
½ cup cubed cantaloupe	27
½ cup blackberries	31
10 grapes	34
1 plum	36
½ medium grapefruit	38
½ cup blueberries	41
1 medium kiwifruit	46
10 sweet cherries	48
½ cup unsweetened applesauce	53
½ cup mango slices	54
1 medium peach	58
½ cup pineapple tidbits canned in their own juice	60
1 medium orange	70
1 medium apple	80
¼ medium avocado	81
10 dried apricot halves	83
1 Bartlett pear	100
1 medium banana	105
MEATS	
2 ounces lean Canadian bacon	62
3 ounces roasted lean pork tenderloin	122
3 ounces broiled 95% lean hamburger patty	132
3 ounces broiled flank steak without fat	158

NUTS	CALORIES
1 ounce unsalted pistachios	162
1 ounce unsalted cashews	163
1 ounce unsalted almonds	169
1 ounce unsalted peanuts	170
1 ounce unsalted English walnut halves	185
1 ounce unsalted pecan halves	196
PASTA AND GRAINS	
½ cup cooked whole-wheat pasta	87
½ cup cooked barley	97
½ cup cooked brown rice	108
POULTRY	
1 turkey hot dog without bun (1.5 ounces)	109
3 ounces roasted turkey breast, without skin	115
3 ounces roasted chicken breast, without skin	142
SALADS AND SALAD DRESSINGS	
2 cups mixed salad greens	20
1 tablespoon light mayonnaise	34
2 tablespoons light Italian dressing	40
SEAFOOD	
3 ounces cooked orange roughy	81
3 ounces cooked flounder or sole	99
3 ounces low-sodium albacore tuna canned in water	109
3 ounces cooked halibut	125
3 ounces drained canned Sockeye salmon with bones	148
3 ounces cooked Atlantic or coho salmon	156

SNACKS	CALORIES
½ cup fat-free, sugar-free flavored gelatin	10
10 pretzel sticks	20
1 cup 94% fat-free microwave popcorn	21
6 ounces fat-free yogurt, plain or sugar-free	95
1 ounce baked potato chips	110

VEGETABLES	
1 raw baby carrot	3
1 celery rib	6
½ cup shredded raw green cabbage	9
½ cup canned sliced bamboo shoots	13
½ cup raw fresh cauliflower	13
½ cup cooked zucchini	14
1 cup sliced raw button mushrooms	15
½ cup cooked yellow summer squash	18
½ cup cooked spinach	21
½ cup cooked green beans	22
½ cup cooked broccoli	22
½ cup cooked asparagus	25
1 medium tomato	27
1 medium cucumber (11 ounces)	38
½ cup cooked artichoke hearts	40
1 large bell pepper	44
½ cup cooked frozen green peas	52
1 medium ear cooked yellow corn	77
½ cup cooked lima beans	97
½ cup cooked black-eyed peas	99
10 frozen french fries, baked	111
½ cup cooked dried beans	114
½ cup cooked green soybeans (edamame)	127
1 medium baked sweet potato with skin (5 ounces)	130
1 medium baked potato with skin (5 ounces)	132

my personal physical activity plan

Date: _____ My current activity level is _____.

My average number of daily steps is _____.

My long-term activity goals are to

1. _____ by _____.

2. _____ by _____.

3. _____ by _____.

I will achieve my goals by

Doing this: _____

This often: _____

At this level: _____

For this long: _____

I will evaluate my progress at these two-week intervals.

1. _____

2. _____

3. _____

The rewards for reaching my goals are

1. _____

2. _____

3. _____

my activity tracker

Date:	❑ Mon ❑ Tues ❑ Wed ❑ Thurs ❑ Fri ❑ Sat ❑ Sun			
Time of Day	Activity	Duration	Level of Perceived Effort	Level of Enjoyment

TOTAL DAILY ACTIVITY IN MINUTES:

TOTAL DAILY NUMBER OF STEPS:

Notes

If You Did Not Exercise Today, Why?

❑ Not enough time

❑ Didn't want to

❑ Other:

Level of Perceived Effort	Level of Enjoyment
0 = Nothing at all	1 = Did not enjoy
1 = Very, very light	2 = Neutral
2 = Very light	3 = Did enjoy
3 = Light	
4 = Moderate/brisk	
5 = Somewhat hard	
6 = Hard	
7 = Very hard	
8 = Very, very hard	
9 = Extremely hard	
10 = Absolute maximal effort	

calories burned in 30 minutes of continuous activity*

ACTIVITY	150 LB	175 LB	200 LB	225 LB
Walking (strolling at 1 mph)	70	80	90	100
Yoga/Hatha (introductory)	85	100	115	130
Stretching	85	100	115	130
Washing a car	100	120	140	155
Dancing, ballroom (slow)	100	120	140	155
Weight lifting (light to moderate)	100	120	140	155
Housecleaning (general)	100	120	140	155
Mopping	120	140	160	180
Vacuuming	120	140	160	180
Walking (at 3½ mph)	130	150	170	190
Cleaning windows	135	160	180	200
Water aerobics	140	160	180	205
Gardening	140	160	180	205
Raking leaves	150	170	195	220
Baseball and softball	170	200	230	260
Skiing (light downhill)	170	200	230	260
Golfing (carrying the clubs)	190	220	250	280
Bicycling (10 to 12 mph)	205	240	270	310
Hiking and backpacking	205	240	270	310
Shoveling snow	205	240	270	310
Swimming	240	280	320	360
Aerobics (high impact)	240	280	320	360
Jogging (at 5 mph)	270	320	360	410
Tennis (singles)	270	320	360	410
Basketball	270	320	360	410
Treadmill (stair)	310	360	410	460
Running (at 6 mph)	340	400	455	510
Jumping rope	340	400	455	510

* Calorie numbers are rounded to the nearest multiple of 5 and are intended as estimates. The actual number of calories burned will differ for each individual.

Dunn Public Library

index

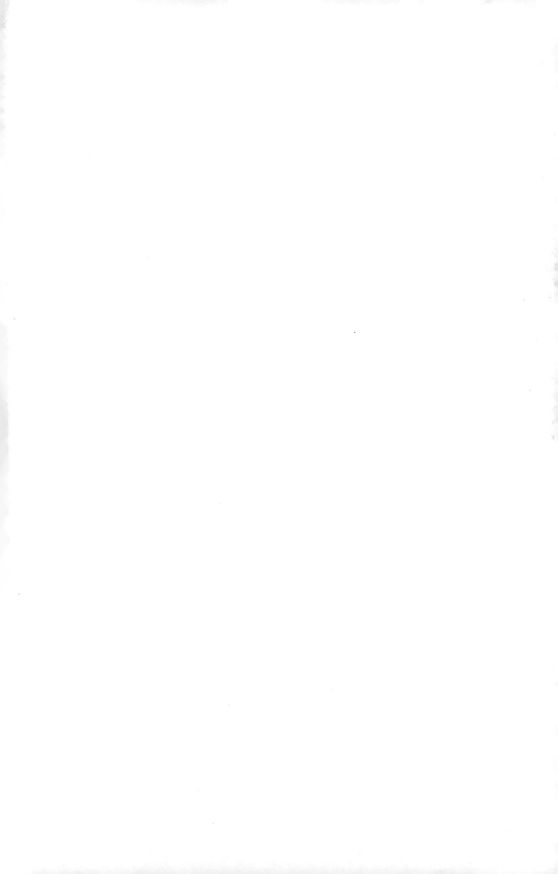

Dunn Public Library
110 E. Divine St.
Dunn, NC 28334
892-2899